W0081256

Extreme and Rare Sports
Performance Demands, Drivers, Functional Foods, and Nutrition

Extreme and Rare Sports
Performance Demands, Drivers, Functional Foods, and Nutrition

Edited by
Sourya Datta, BE, MBA
Debasis Bagchi, PhD, MACN, CNS, MAIChE

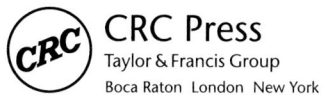

CRC Press
Taylor & Francis Group
Boca Raton London New York

CRC Press is an imprint of the
Taylor & Francis Group, an **informa** business

CRC Press
Taylor & Francis Group
6000 Broken Sound Parkway NW, Suite 300
Boca Raton, FL 33487-2742

First issued in paperback 2021

© 2019 by Taylor & Francis Group, LLC
CRC Press is an imprint of Taylor & Francis Group, an Informa business

No claim to original U.S. Government works

ISBN-13: 978-1-03-209256-0 (pbk)
ISBN-13: 978-1-138-09144-3 (hbk)

This book contains information obtained from authentic and highly regarded sources. Reasonable efforts have been made to publish reliable data and information, but the author and publisher cannot assume responsibility for the validity of all materials or the consequences of their use. The authors and publishers have attempted to trace the copyright holders of all material reproduced in this publication and apologize to copyright holders if permission to publish in this form has not been obtained. If any copyright material has not been acknowledged please write and let us know so we may rectify in any future reprint.

Except as permitted under U.S. Copyright Law, no part of this book may be reprinted, reproduced, transmitted, or utilized in any form by any electronic, mechanical, or other means, now known or hereafter invented, including photocopying, microfilming, and recording, or in any information storage or retrieval system, without written permission from the publishers.

For permission to photocopy or use material electronically from this work, please access www.copyright.com (http://www.copyright.com/) or contact the Copyright Clearance Center, Inc. (CCC), 222 Rosewood Drive, Danvers, MA 01923, 978-750-8400. CCC is a not-for-profit organization that provides licenses and registration for a variety of users. For organizations that have been granted a photocopy license by the CCC, a separate system of payment has been arranged.

Trademark Notice: Product or corporate names may be trademarks or registered trademarks, and are used only for identification and explanation without intent to infringe.

Publisher's Note
The publisher has gone to great lengths to ensure the quality of this reprint but points out that some imperfections in the original copies may be apparent.

Library of Congress Cataloging-in-Publication Data

Names: Datta, Sourya, editor. | Bagchi, Debasis, 1954- editor.
Title: Extreme and rare sports : performance demands, drivers, functional foods, and nutrition / [edited by] Sourya Datta and Debasis Bagchi.
Description: First edition. | Boca Raton : Taylor & Francis, [2019] | Includes bibliographical references.
Identifiers: LCCN 2018056848 | ISBN 9781138091443 (hardback)
Subjects: | MESH: Sports Nutritional Physiological Phenomena | Athletic Performance | Sports | Risk-Taking
Classification: LCC RA784 | NLM QT 263 | DDC 613.2--dc23
LC record available at https://lccn.loc.gov/2018056848

Visit the Taylor & Francis Web site at
http://www.taylorandfrancis.com

and the CRC Press Web site at
http://www.crcpress.com

Dedicated to Respected Mr. Santosh Kumar Biswas (ex-Berger)

Debasis Bagchi

Contents

Preface...xi
Editors..xv
Contributors xvii

SECTION I   Introduction to Extreme Sports

Chapter 1   Extreme Endurance Sports – Why Not Just Sports?...........................3

   David Townes

SECTION II   Extreme Sports: Swimming, Contact, and Combat Sports and Factors Affecting Extreme Sports

Chapter 2   Open-Water Swimming...11

   *Paola Zamparo, Roberto Baldassarre, Marco Bonifazi, and
   Maria Francesca Piacentini*

Chapter 3   Contact and Combat Sports: Sports Nutrition Benefits.....................35

   Jonathan Mike

Chapter 4   An Overview on the Nutritional Requirements for Athletes
   Engaged in Extreme Endurance Events 49

   Chad Kerksick

SECTION III   Overview of Food and Nutritional Requirements for Diverse Extreme Sports

Chapter 5   Functional Foods: Role in Endurance Sports.....................................73

   Kamesh Venkatakrishnan and Chin-Kun Wang

Chapter 6   Prosthetics and Limb Health in Extreme Sports.............................. 115

   Sashwati Roy, Shomita S. Mathew-Steiner, and Chandan K. Sen

Chapter 7   Nutritional Requirements in Extreme Sports 127

Matthew Butawan, Jade L. Caldwell, and Richard J. Bloomer

Chapter 8   Dietary Supplements for Use in Extreme Sports 143

Nicholas J.G. Smith, Matthew Butawan, and Richard J. Bloomer

Chapter 9   Intake of Selected Nutrients and Some Morphological and
Biochemical Blood Parameters of Professional Athletes 177

*Estera Nowacka-Polaczyk, Teresa Leszczyńska, Aneta Kopeć,
and Jerzy Zawistowski*

Chapter 10 Testosterone in Sport: The Androgen Response to Extreme
Endurance Exercise 193

*Jake Shelley, Christopher Howe, Hannah Jayne Moir, and
Andrea Petróczi*

Chapter 11 Physical Performance and Antioxidants 205

Wataru Aoi and Yuji Naito

SECTION IV   Olympic Sports and Evolution of Current Extreme Sports

Chapter 12 Greek Olympic Sports: The Beginning of Modern
Extreme Sports 219

Sourya Datta and Debasis Bagchi

Chapter 13 An Overview of Extreme Sports 237

Sourya Datta and Debasis Bagchi

Chapter 14 An Overview of Challenging Mountain and High Altitude Sports 259

Sourya Datta and Debasis Bagchi

Chapter 15 Structurally Diverse Water Sports in Extreme Conditions 277

Sourya Datta and Debasis Bagchi

SECTION V Importance of Hydration and Use of Gelatin

Chapter 16 An Overview on the Beneficial Effects of Hydration 297

Douglas S. Kalman

Chapter 17 Versatile Use of Gelatin in Functional Food and Nutraceuticals..... 311

Douglas S. Kalman

SECTION VI Impact of Eccentric Exercise on Muscle and Adaption of Body and Muscles

Chapter 18 Skeletal Muscle Damage and Recovery from Eccentric Contractions 321

Eisuke Ochi and Yosuke Tsuchiya

SECTION VII Growth, Marketing Techniques, and Future of Extreme Sports

Chapter 19 Extreme Sports: Growth Prospect, Marketing Potential, and Opportunities: A Commentary 341

Sourya Datta and Debasis Bagchi

Index 353

Preface

"If you want to experience all of the success and pleasure in life, you have to be willing to accept the pain and failure that comes with it."

– Mat Hoffman

Extreme and Rare Sports: Performance Demands, Drivers, Functional Foods, and Nutrition covers a wide variety of definitions, philosophies, thoughts, and practices involved with structurally diverse extreme sports. For some, extreme sports could be a 26.2-mile marathon, while for others a sport is extreme only if there is a threat or danger to life. Extreme sports are two words which signify sport or activities that are done which involve a high degree of risk.

An extreme sport needs to be exciting, thrilling, daring and challenging. In an extreme sport, a participant must demonstrate both mental and physical skills. This type of activity gives an adrenaline rush to individuals who are part of the community of extreme sportsmen.

The two most important factors of a healthy life are (1) appropriate nutrition and (2) physical exercise and skill development. If these two can be managed properly, there will be great positive influence in the current and future generations. Sports and physical activities will keep everyone healthy, lively, and happy.

Extreme sports are a unique way to keep one active and fit; it also provides the enjoyment of doing something fun that might have an added advantage of providing an extra level of thrill and passion. Extreme sports also help to boost immunity and resistance to common infections, and studies have shown sports help in managing an effective work–life balance as well. This book merges the importance of sports with the food and nutrition that are important to make healthy individuals.

This book covers both the sports as well as nutrition. It talks about some traditional sports and then goes in-depth about some types of sports that are non-traditional and unusual in everyday life. This book covers different types of extreme sports and food and nutrition requirements for athletes who take part in these types of sports.

The target audience for this book will be sports enthusiasts and sports nutritionists, nutrition and functional food researchers, sport practitioners, food experts, health professionals, endocrinologists, nurses, general practitioners, public health officials, and sports organizers.

This book is useful to understand the types of extreme sports along with food and nutritional requirements for different types of athletes. Not only does this book demonstrate requirements for different athletes but it also goes into detail about the food and nutritional requirements for particular types of sports, such as for extreme water sports, land sports and high altitude sports.

The book can be broadly divided into seven major sections:

- Section 1 provides an introduction of extreme sports.
- Section 2 demonstrates swimming, contact and combat sports along with factors that affect athletes in extreme sports.

- Section 3 provides an overview on food and nutritional requirements for diverse sports activities especially extreme sports. Section 3 also captures the importance of dietary supplements and antioxidants as well as androgen response to endurance training.
- Section 4 captures the start of Olympic sports and outlines the evolution of current extreme sports in different conditions (land, water and high altitude).
- Section 5 discusses the importance of hydration in diverse sports activities and the use of gelatin in functional foods and nutraceuticals.
- Section 6 exhibits the impact of eccentric exercise on muscle and adaptation of body and muscles to extreme and eccentric exercises.
- Section 7 is the concluding section that captures the growth, marketing techniques and future of extreme sports.

The book starts with the definition of extreme sports followed by their evolution over the years and then describes the current forms and features of extreme sports. It covers diverse extreme sports and the nutrition and food requirements for athletes involved. The demographic of extreme sports is generally younger than other sports, and the book provides in detail the differences between regular and extreme sports. Diet, food, and nutrition are extremely important for success in this type of sport, and are important for vitality, vigor, endurance, focus, and strength. A section of the book details the activities for high-intensity, life-threatening occupations and the importance of nutrition for such occupations. The book concludes with the marketing techniques for increasing the interests of extreme sports and finally with the future of extreme sports.

Section 1 of the book introduces 'extreme sports' to the readers. The introductory chapter in this book introduces the concept of extreme sports, which is authored by Dr. David A. Townes, a veteran in the field of sports medicine, currently at University of Washington School of Medicine. Dr. Townes has worked in Antarctica, Costa Rica, Ethiopia, Ghana, Guatemala, Haiti, Indonesia, Jordan, Kenya, Malawi, Mozambique, Russia, Senegal, Tanzania, Turkey, the West Indies, and Zambia; he extensively discusses and highlights his past research and experience in introducing extreme sports, as well as what exactly it stands for and the evolution of extreme sports.

The second chapter is by Dr. Paola Zamparo, Dr. Roberto Baldassarre, Dr. Marco Bonifazi, and Dr. Maria Francesca Piacentini and gives extensive detail on open-water swimming. Dr. Zamparo works in the Department of Neuroscience at Università degli Studi di Verona while Dr. Bonifazi is based in the Department of Medical, Surgical, and Neuro Sciences. Dr. Baldassarre and Dr. Piacentini are associated with University of Rome Foro Italico, Rome. Chapter 3 delivers intricate aspects of sports and introduces fundamental concepts of extreme sports, like contact and combat sports. Authored by Dr. Jonathan Mike of Grand Canyon University, this chapter goes in detail about both contact and combat sports as well as nutritional aspects of both types of sports. Chapter 4 is written by Dr. Chad Kerksick, a well-renowned researcher and professor in the School of Sport, Recreation, and Exercises, Lindenwood University, St. Charles, Missouri. This chapter covers the various factors that affect athletes. Dr. Kerksick has been instrumental in depicting the intricate features of extreme sports athletes.

Chapter 5 talks about the food and nutritional requirements of extreme sportspersons. Authored by distinguished professors Dr. Chin-Kun Wang and Dr. Kamesh Venkatakrishnan of Chung Shan Medical University, this chapter describes functional foods and role of functional foods in endurance sports. Chapter 6 is written by Dr. Chandan Sen, Dr. Sashwati Roy, and Dr. Shomita Steiner and reveals details on prosthetics. Dr. Sen has been associated with sports medicine, especially in the field of wound healing, for a considerable period, and Dr. Sen, Dr. Roy, and Dr. Steiner have contributed a very intriguing chapter on prosthetics. Chapter 7 is written by Dr. Richard Bloomer, Dr. Matthew Butawan, and Dr. Jade Caldwell, and Chapter 8 is written by Dr. Bloomer, Dr. Butawan, and Dr. Nicholas Smith. These chapters cover the nutritional and dietary aspects of extreme sports and give us a complete flavor of functional food and nutritional requirements for extreme sports athletes. Dr. Bloomer is a distinguished professor and dean in the Department of Health and Sport Sciences in The University of Memphis. Dr. Butwana, Dr. Caldwell, and Dr. Smith are associated with the very renowned School of Health studies at The University of Memphis. Chapter 9 takes a very interesting approach and talks about impact of selected nutrients and is authored by Dr. Jerzy Zawistowski, academic director of Food, Nutrition, and Health, University of British Columbia, along with Dr. Estera Nowacka-Polaczyk, Dr. Teresa Leszczyńska, and Dr. Aneta Kopeć. This chapter provides in-depth research about selected nutrients and biochemical parameters for professional athletes.

Chapters 10 and 11 explore other parts of sports apart from the food and nutritional aspects. Chapter 10 demonstrates another very important aspect, testosterone, and its role in response to extreme sports and exercise, written by Dr. Jake Shelley, Dr. Christopher Howe, Dr. Hannah Jayne Moir, and Dr. Andrea Petróczi from Kingston University, London. Section 3 ends with a chapter from Dr. Yuji Naito and Dr. Watari Aoi on the role of antioxidants in extreme sports.

Section 4 covers extreme sports in different scenarios and conditions. Chapter 12 gives us the history of the evolution of sports and goes into the Greek sports which evolved into the early Olympics and finally the current Olympic games. Chapters 13, 14, and 15 talk about extreme sports in different conditions and capture the food and nutritional aspects of such sports in different situations. Extreme sports are differentiated based on weather conditions, and these chapters go deeper into (a) water sports, (b) high-altitude sports, and (c) land-based extreme sports. These chapters are authored by Sourya Datta, supply chain manager at eBay and avid follower and participant in extreme sports activities, and Dr. Debasis Bagchi, director of scientific affairs for VNI, Inc., as well as a faculty member of the Department of Pharmacological and Pharmaceutical Sciences at the University of Houston College of Pharmacy in Houston, Texas.

Section 5 consists of Chapters 16 and 17, which emphasize the benefits of hydration in different extreme sports activities, and the versatile use of gelatin in diverse foods and nutraceuticals. Dr. Douglas Kalman, a distinguished faculty member in the Robert Stempel School of Public Health, Florida International University, Miami, Florida, has authored both these chapters.

Section 6 consists of Chapter 18, written by Dr. Eisuke Ochi and Dr. Yosuke Tsuchiya, Faculty of Bioscience, Hosei University in Tokyo, Japan. This chapter discusses the intricate aspects of skeletal muscle injury and recovery from eccentric contractions.

Finally, Section 7 is authored by the editors, which looks at the essence of extreme sports, marketing aspects, and growth and future prospects.

Sourya Datta, BE, MBA
eBay, Inc.,
Supply Chain Management, San Jose, CA

Debasis Bagchi, PhD, MACN, CNS, MAIChE
Department of Pharmacological and Pharmaceutical Sciences, University of Houston College of Pharmacy, Houston, TX, and Victory Nutrition International, Inc., Lederach, PA

Editors

Sourya Datta is part of the Strategic Deals team at Apple where he is responsible for managing the procurement of a number of components for Apple. Prior to joining Apple, he managed the finances for eBay's North American division. This included managing P&L, budgeting, forecasting, and closing the month and quarters for eBay. He was also responsible for leading the analytics for Latam and Canada for eBay. Prior to that, Sourya was the supply chain manager in the Business Operations and Strategy Group at eBay. He received his Masters in Business Administration from the University of Pittsburgh, Pennsylvania, in Operations and his Bachelors of Engineering from Anna University, India, and worked in various consulting firms before doing his MBA. Sourya was featured in Poets and Quants as one of the best MBAs in 2015 and has won a number of awards in his tenure at eBay.

He is an avid sports fan and has completed a number of marathons and Spartan races since 2007. He has been swimming since he was seven years old and has participated in and won numerous state level competitions. He has also taken active part in mountaineering and trekking since he was in elementary school. He has participated in various marathons in California and has been intricately associated with nutrition and functional food requirements for sports performance. He is also the author of two chapters in *Developing New Functional Food and Nutraceutical Products* that was published by Elsevier/Academic Press in October 2016.

He is also the author of a chapter in the second edition of *Nutrition and Enhanced Sports Performance* published by Elsevier/Academic Press in September 2018.

Debasis Bagchi, PhD, MACN, CNS, MAIChE, received his PhD in Medicinal Chemistry in 1982. He is the director of scientific affairs at Victory Nutrition International, Inc., Lederach, Pennsylvania; a professor in the Department of Pharmacological and Pharmaceutical Sciences at the University of Houston College of Pharmacy, Houston, Texas, and, an adjunct faculty member in Texas Southern University, Houston, Texas. He served as the senior vice president of Research & Development of InterHealth Nutraceuticals Inc, Benicia, California, from 1998 until February 2011, and then as director of innovation and clinical affairs of Iovate Health Sciences, Oakville, Ontario, until June 2013, and then chief scientific officer at Cepham, Inc., Somerset, New Jersey from June 2013 until December 2018. Dr. Bagchi received the Master of American College of Nutrition Award in October 2010. He is the past chairman of the International Society of Nutraceuticals and Functional Foods (ISNFF), past president of the American College of Nutrition, Clearwater, Florida, and past chair of the Nutraceuticals and Functional Foods Division of Institute of Food Technologists (IFT), Chicago, Illionois. He is currently serving as a distinguished advisor on the Japanese Institute for Health Food Standards (JIHFS), Tokyo, Japan. Dr. Bagchi is a member of the Study Section and Peer Review Committee of the National Institutes of Health (NIH), Bethesda, Maryland. He has 352 papers in peer reviewed journals, 37 books, and 20 patents. Dr. Bagchi is also a member of the Society of Toxicology, member of the New York Academy of Sciences, fellow of the Nutrition Research Academy, and member of the TCE stakeholder committee of the Wright Patterson Air Force Base, Ohio. Dr. Bagchi is an associate editor of the *Journal of Functional Foods, Journal of the American College of Nutrition,* and *Archives of Medical and Biomedical Research,* and an editorial board member of numerous peer reviewed journals, including *Antioxidants & Redox Signaling, Cancer Letters, Food & Nutrition Research, Toxicology Mechanisms and Methods, The Original Internist*, and other peer reviewed journals.

Contributors

Wataru Aoi
Laboratory of Nutritional Science,
    Graduate School of Life and
    Environmental Sciences
Kyoto Prefectural University
Kyoto, Japan

Debasis Bagchi
College of Pharmacy
University of Houston
Houston, Texas

Roberto Baldassarre
University of Rome Foro Italico
Rome, Italy

Richard J. Bloomer
School of Health Studies
University of Memphis
Memphis, Tennessee

Marco Bonifazi
Department of Medical, Surgical and
    Neuro Sciences
University of Siena
Siena, Italy

Matthew Butawan
School of Health Studies
University of Memphis
Memphis, Tennessee

Jade L. Caldwell
School of Health Studies
University of Memphis
Memphis, Tennessee

Sourya Datta
eBay
San Jose, California

Christopher Howe
Kingston University London
Kingston upon Thames, UK

Douglas Kalman
Dr. Pallavi Patel College of Health
    Care Sciences, Health and Human
    Performance
Nova Southeastern University
Davie, Florida

Chad M. Kerksick
School of Health Sciences
Lindenwood University
St. Charles, Missouri

Aneta Kopeć
Department of Human Nutrition
University of Agriculture in Krakow
Krakow, Poland

Teresa Leszczyńska
Department of Human Nutrition
University of Agriculture in Krakow
Krakow, Poland

Jonathan Mike
Department of Exercise Science and
    Sports Performance
Grand Canyon University
Phoenix, Arizona

Hannah Jayne Moir
Kingston University London
Kingston upon Thames, UK

Yuji Naito
Department of Molecular
    Gastroenterology and Hepatology,
    Graduate School of Medical Science
Kyoto Prefectural University of Medicine
Kyoto, Japan

Eisuke Ochi
Faculty of Bioscience and Applied
   Chemistry
Hosei University
Tokyo, Japan

Estera Nowacka-Polaczyk
Department of Human Nutrition
University of Agriculture in Krakow
Krakow, Poland

Andrea Petróczi
Kingston University London
Kingston upon Thames, UK

Maria Francesca Piacentini
University of Rome Foro Italico
Rome, Italy

Sashwati Roy
Department of Surgery
Indiana University School of Medicine
Indianapolis, Indiana

Chandan Sen
Department of Surgery
Indiana University School of Medicine
Indianapolis, Indiana

Jake Shelley
Kingston University London
Kingston upon Thames, UK

Nicolas J.G. Smith
School of Health Studies
University of Memphis
Memphis, Tennessee

Shomita S. Mathew-Steiner
Department of Surgery
Indiana University School of Medicine
Indianapolis, Indiana

David Townes
Department of Emergency Medicine
University of Washington School of
   Medicine
Seattle, Washington

Yosuke Tsuchiya
Faculty of Modern Life, Trainer and
   Sports Management
Teikyo Heisei University
Tokyo, Japan

Kamesh Venkatakrishnan
School of Nutrition
Chung Shan Medical University
Taichung City, Taiwan

Chin-Kun Wang
School of Nutrition
Chung Shan Medical University
Taichung City, Taiwan

Paola Zamparo
Department of Neuroscience,
   Biomedicine and Movement Sciences
Università degli Studi di Verona
Verona, Italy

Jerzy Zawistowski
Faculty of Land and Food Systems,
   Food, Nutrition and Health
University of British Columbia
Vancouver, British Columbia, Canada

Section I

Introduction to Extreme Sports

1 Extreme Endurance Sports – Why Not Just Sports?

David Townes

CONTENTS

1.1   Introduction 3
1.2   Running 4
1.3   Cycling 5
1.4   Swimming 5
1.5   Triathlon 5
1.6   Adventure Races/Multi-Sport 6
1.7   Health and Medical Support 7
1.8   Training and Nutrition 7
1.9   Conclusion 8
References 8

1.1 INTRODUCTION

While there is no universally accepted definition of 'extreme sports', many are considered extreme due to their unusual and dangerous nature, such as parkour and zorbing, while others, 'extreme endurance sports', are considered extreme as they push the limits of human endurance.

Successful participation in extreme sports requires specialized skills acquired through a combination of natural ability, education and training, trial and error, dedication, and perseverance. For extreme endurance sports, this also requires a comprehensive training program including nutrition. This text explores the origins and history of extreme endurance sports and describes some of the training and nutrition theories and practices that result in successful participation.

Extreme endurance sports have grown significantly in popularity worldwide in the past several decades and today there are events held throughout the world, on every continent, covering a wide variety of athletic disciplines. There are several potential explanations for this trend. First, economic prosperity, for at least some populations, particularly in Western countries, has resulted in disposable income and time to participate in these activities.[1] Second, this prosperity, in combination with relatively inexpensive and readily available air travel, has made even the most remote areas of the world accessible to amateur adventurers and athletes. Third, the gear and equipment necessary for participation in these extreme sports are more readily available, more sophisticated and user-friendly, and relatively affordable. Finally, some of the growth is undoubtedly driven by the adventure tourism industry, valued at greater than $400 million in 2016, which plays a role in marketing and promoting extreme sports events.[2]

Perhaps the oldest endurance event is the marathon, which traces its roots back to ancient Greece in 490 B.C. when, as legend has it, a soldier named Pheidippides ran from the battlefield near the town of Marathon to Athens to announce the defeat of the Persians. After covering the approximately 25 miles on foot, he delivered the message 'Niki' or 'victory' before dying of exhaustion. The modern marathon as we know it today is based on this legend.

The first organized marathon was held in Athens at the 1896 Olympic Games. For the 1908 London Olympic Games, the distance was increased from 25 miles to 26 miles 385 yards so the race would finish in front of the Royal Box inside the Olympic Stadium, thus establishing the marathon as we know it today as a race of 26.2 miles.

From these beginnings have grown extreme endurance events that test the limits of human endurance.

1.2 RUNNING

Marathons have grown in popularity to the point that there are currently 4,192 such races worldwide.[3] These include well-known traditional marathons such as the Boston Marathon, the New York City Marathon, and the London Marathon, as well as more extreme but perhaps lesser-known marathons such as the Everest Marathon, the North Pole Marathon, the Great Wall of China Marathon, and the Big Five Marathon in South Africa. Today, marathons are held on every continent in almost every environment imaginable from mountains to valleys, from the cold tundra to the hot desert.

In addition, longer races, or ultramarathons, have become increasingly popular. Many of these races are 50–100 kilometers or 50–100 miles and are run without a break. While some of these resemble traditional marathons run on paved surfaces, runs through desert, jungle or mountains have become increasingly popular. Examples include the Badwater Ultramarathon, first run in 1987, which covers 135 miles through Death Valley; the Leadville Trail 100, run in the heart of the Rocky Mountains; and the Western States Endurance Run, which starts in Squaw Valley, California, and covers 100 miles with 18,090 feet of elevation gain and 22,970 feet of descent. The latter race has been completed in less than 24 hours.

Some extreme endurance running events combine running with adventure tourism and more closely resemble adventure races, described below, rather than traditional marathons or ultramarathons. Examples include the Marathon des Sables, a six-day, 155-mile run through the Moroccan Sahara; the Jungle Ultra, a five-day, 143-mile trek through Peru from the Andes to the Amazon; the 6633 Arctic Ultra, during which runners must support themselves, pulling all of their food, clothing and other supplies on a sled over the 120- or 350-mile course, both of which cross the Arctic Circle at 66 degrees, 33 minutes. In the 350-mile race, participants are allowed two drop bags to resupply at miles 120 and 230.[4]

1.3 CYCLING

Similar to running, endurance cycling events, or 'ultra-distance cycling', has grown in popularity. This term is generally reserved for races longer than 100 miles, the distance commonly referred to as a century among cyclists. Some of these events are held without a break while others are stage events with intervening rest periods for participants. Events may take place on paved roads, gravel roads or trails. Some are races while many are non-competitive rides. Examples of non-competitive events include the RAGBRAI, covering over 400 miles in six days across Iowa, perhaps the oldest and longest recreational cycling event in the world; the Seattle to Portland (STP), which takes one or two days, with the majority of the 9,000 participants taking two days to cover the 200 miles. Examples of competitive events include the Race Across America, a competitive event covering over 3,000 miles; the Transcontinental Race in Europe, a competitive event covering between 3,200 and 4,200 kilometers; the Leadville Trail 100 MTB, a competitive mountain-bike event covering 100 miles of unpaved trails in the Rocky Mountains, similar to The Leadville Trail 100 run.

1.4 SWIMMING

Long-distance swimming involves distances longer than those typically swum in pool competitions. Ultradistance swimming events, also referred to as marathon swimming events, generally begin at distances greater than 10 kilometers. In some of these events, called solo-swims, there is one swimmer who starts at a given date and time, while others involve a group swimming at the same time or as part of a relay team. Well-known solo-swims include swimming across the English Channel, swimming from Cuba to Florida, and swimming the length of the Amazon River. Swimmers have crossed the Atlantic Ocean and attempts at crossing the Pacific Ocean are ongoing.

1.5 TRIATHLON

Triathlons are perhaps a natural progression from endurance running, cycling and swimming. Triathlons include a combination of three different, sequential, continuous endurance events, most commonly swimming, cycling, and running. Triathlons thus have transition areas where the participant transitions from one discipline to another. This normally involves a change in clothing and equipment and the time taken for changing is included in the participant's overall time.

Triathlons take place over different distances, but standard races include the Sprint (750 meter [0.465 mi] swim; 20 kilometer [12.5 mi] bike; 5 km [3.1 mi] run), Standard or Olympic (1.5 kilometer [0.93 mi] swim; 40 km [25 mi] bike; 10 km [6.2 mi] run), Half-Ironman (1.9 kilometer [1.2 mi] swim; 90 km [56 mi] bike; 21.1 km [13.1 mi] run), and Ironman (3.8 kilometer [2.4 mi] swim; 180.2 km [112 mi] bike; 42.2 km [26.2 mi] run).

Well-known triathlons include the Ironman Triathlon in Hawaii; the Escape from Alcatraz Triathlon and the Wildflower Triathlon, both in California; and the Norseman Triathlon in Norway. The triathlon has been an Olympic event since 2000.

1.6   ADVENTURE RACES/MULTI-SPORT

Adventure races or multi-sport competitions combine aspects of triathlons, outdoor activities, extreme endurance sports, and adventure travel. Adventure races are competitive events in which teams compete over a course including multiple disciplines, commonly trekking, mountain biking, flat- and white-water paddling, orienteering/navigation, and ropes travel. Additional, less common disciplines may also be included, such as horseback riding, river boarding, in-line skating, paragliding, mountaineering, and caving.

Common race lengths include sprint (2–6 hours), 12-hour, 24-hour, multi-day (36–48 hour), and expedition length (3–10 days). Races are continuous, with no built-in rest periods, and in many cases, especially for expedition length races, there is no set course – instead a team must pass through a series of ordered check points and transition areas where they change disciplines, as in triathlons, and the team to complete the course successfully in the least amount of time is the winner. Teams are left to strategize if and when to rest and how to get from one check point to another. For example, a team with strong climbers may opt to go over a ridge while another team may decide to go around it. Some teams may opt to rest on a set schedule while others may rest more spontaneously.

Examples of adventure races include the Coast to Coast and the Raid Gauloises, started in New Zealand in 1980 and 1989 respectively; the Eco-Challenge and the Primal Quest, started in the United States in 1995 and 2002 respectively; and, more recently, urban series races such as the Tough Mudder.

Teams are governed by the 'rules of travel' that dictate what type of travel is allowed, and outline penalties for breach of these rules. For example, the rules of travel may dictate that travel on paved roads is not allowed on a section of the course. Similarly, the rules of travel may dictate that personal floatation devices (PFD) must be worn during a paddling section of the course and helmets worn while biking. Breaching these rules results in penalties. Minor infractions such as travel on a section of paved road may result in a time penalty where time is added on to the team's overall time. More serious infractions, such as not wearing required safety equipment such as helmets or PFDs, may result in expulsion from the race.

In addition, the rules of travel outline penalties for acceptance of medical care during the event. If too strict, the rules of travel may discourage participants from seeking necessary medical care. If too lenient, however, teams might request medical care that is not medically indicated but instead to enhance performance. A common example is the use of intravenous fluids (IVF) to maximize hydration and electrolyte balance to optimize performance.

An example rule of travel used in many expedition-length adventure races is the IVF fluid rule: If a participant requires 1–2 liters of IVF they must wait 4 hours after completion of the infusion and then be cleared by a member of the medical staff before continuing to race. Participants requiring more than 2 liters of IVF at one time or IVF at more than one point during the race are eliminated from the event. The purpose of this rule is to deter the use of IVF unless medically indicated but to avoid penalizing teams so much that they might forgo necessary medical treatment.

1.7 HEALTH AND MEDICAL SUPPORT

With the development and growth of extreme endurance sports have come challenges in providing medical support for these events. Previously, the field of event medicine, dedicated to the provision of medical support for mass gatherings and events, divided events into three categories: Category 1 events are those in which participants remain seated or stationary during the duration of the event (common examples include concerts and stadium sporting events); Category 2 events are those in which participants are mobile, such as spectators at a golf tournament or carnival celebration; and Category 3 events, such as marathons, are those in which participants are mobile, on a set course, and are often outnumbered by spectators.

Expedition-length adventure races, with no set course and no built-in rest periods, are particularly challenging in terms of provision of medical support. Locating and communicating with ill or injured participants is inherently difficult, and search and rescue may be necessary to access participants in need of medical assistance. These Category 4 events require sophisticated and compressive medical support plans including advanced communication with participants often with duplicative systems consisting of mobile phones, radios with repeaters, and satellite phones. In addition, medical and other support personnel must be familiar with search-and-rescue techniques and have supplies and equipment to perform at least basic search and rescue to access ill and injured participants and provide definitive care for simple medical problems and initial stabilization and evacuation for medical problems requiring a higher level of care.

From the standpoint of the participants themselves, they should be prepared to be self-sufficient for many hours to several days while awaiting assistance. This includes sufficient nutritional resources to maximize physical and mental functioning until assistance arrives.

1.8 TRAINING AND NUTRITION

Extreme endurance sports require proper nutrition both in the setting of training and competition. While variable from athlete to athlete and dependent on environmental conditions, the caloric requirements for extreme endurance sports is significant. It has been estimated that the average runner burns about 100 calories per mile for a marathon, resulting in 2,600 calories burned for the duration of the race.[5] For an Ironman Triathlon, this is estimated at 7,000–10,000 calories.[6] For expedition-length adventure races, this can climb to more than 12,000 calories per day.[7] It can be challenging for athletes to maintain enough caloric intake to meet this demand, especially during multi-day events with no built-in rest periods to eat or sleep, such as expedition-length adventure races.

There is no single, widely agreed-upon diet for maximizing performance in extreme endurance events.[8] Athletes have experimented with different diets both during training and competition. Most of these have varied the balance and timing of intake of the three major macronutrients, fat, protein and carbohydrates.[9] These include extremes in carbohydrate intake from a very low, essentially a ketogenic diet, to the more traditional approach of 'carbohydrate loading' prior to hard training or competition.[10,11]

1.9 CONCLUSION

There are general consensus and evidence that a diet balanced in macronutrients is preferred over dietary extremes in intake of macronutrients to optimize endurance performance.[12–14] In addition to macronutrients, athletes have used nutritional supplements to optimize performance.[15] This text will examine some approaches to nutritional practices for extreme endurance athletes.

REFERENCES

1. Outside. Why do rich people love endurance sports? 2018. https://www.outsideonline.com/2229791/why-are-most-endurance-athletes-rich (accessed August 23, 2018).
2. Ciston PR Newswire. Global adventure tourism market expected to reach $1,335,738 million by 2023 – Allied Market Research. 2018. https://www.prnewswire.com/news-releases/global-adventure-tourism-market-expected-to-reach-1335738-million-by-2023-allied-market-research-672335923.html (accessed August 23, 2018).
3. World's Marathons. Find your next race. 2018. https://worldsmarathons.com (accessed August 23, 2018).
4. Sports Management Degree Hub. The 10 longest races in the world. 2018. https://www.sportsmanagementdegreehub.com/10-longest-races-world/ (accessed August 23, 2018).
5. Runner's World. Calories burned running calculator. 2018. https://www.runnersworld.com/training/a20801301/calories-burned-running-calculator/ (accessed August 23, 2018).
6. Life. Ironman 101: Building your race-day fueling plan. 2018. http://www.ironman.com/triathlon/news/articles/2014/07/bonk-breaker-race-day-fueling.aspx#axzz5OvSdYakc (accessed August 23, 2018).
7. Red Bull. Plan your fuel. 2018. https://www.redbull.com/gb-en/15-things-to-know-before-your-first-adventure-race (accessed August 23, 2018).
8. The Endurance Edge. Macronutrient needs for athletes. 2018. http://www.theenduranceedge.com/2017/08/macronutrient-needs-athletes/ (accessed August 23, 2018).
9. Ormsbee, M. J., Back, C. W. and Baur, D. A. 2014. Pre-exercise nutrition: The role of macronutrients, modified starches, and supplements on metabolism and endurance performance. *Nutrients* 6.5, 1782–1808.
10. Stellingwerff, T. 2015. Competition nutrition practices of elite ultramarathon runners. *International Journal of Sports Nutrition and Exercise Metabolism* 26.1, 93–99.
11. Horvath, P. J., Eagen, C. K., Fisher, N. M., Leddy, J. J. and Pendergast, D. R. 2000. The effects of varying dietary fat on performance and metabolism in trained male and female runners. *Journal of the American College of Nutrition* 19.1, 52–60.
12. Pendergast, D. R., Leddy, J. J. and Venkatraman, J. T. 2000. A perspective on fat intake in athletes. *Journal of the American College of Nutrition* 19.3, 345–350.
13. Kanter, M. 2018. High-quality carbohydrates and physical performance. *Nutrition and Physical Activity* 53.1, 35–39.
14. Lambert, E. V. and Goedecke, J. H. 2003. The role of dietary macronutrients in optimizing endurance performance. *Current Sports Medicine Reports* 2.4, 194–201.
15. Casazza, G. A., Tovar, A. P., Richardson, C. E., Cortez, A. N. and Davis, B. A. 2018. Energy availability, macronutrient intake, and nutritional supplementation for improving exercise performance in endurance athletes. *Current Sports Medicine Reports* 17.6, 215–223.

Section II

Extreme Sports

Swimming, Contact, and Combat Sports and Factors Affecting Extreme Sports

2 Open-Water Swimming

Paola Zamparo, Roberto Baldassarre, Marco Bonifazi, and Maria Francesca Piacentini

CONTENTS

2.1 General Introduction 11
2.2 Energetics and Biomechanics of (Endurance) Swimming 12
2.3 Anthropometric Characteristics of OW Swimmers and Gender
    Differences 15
2.4 Open-Water Swimming: Performance Analysis and Pacing Strategies
    during Official Competitions 16
2.5 Ultra-Endurance OWS Races 20
    2.5.1 The English Channel Swim 20
    2.5.2 The Catalina Channel Swim 21
    2.5.3 The Manhattan Island Marathon Swim 21
    2.5.4 The Lake Zurich Marathon Swim 21
2.6 Psychological Aspects 21
2.7 Risk Factors, Water Temperature and Hypothermia 22
    2.7.1 Risk Factors 22
    2.7.2 Water Temperature and Hypothermia 22
2.8 Roles of Appropriate Nutrition 24
    2.8.1 Energy Intake Requirements 24
    2.8.2 Carbohydrate Requirements 25
    2.8.3 Estimation of Energy Requirement in the 10 km Race 25
2.9 Appropriate Nutrition during Competitions 26
    2.9.1 Pre-Race Nutrition 26
    2.9.2 Nutrition During the Race 27
        2.9.2.1 Short Races (5 km or Less) 28
        2.9.2.2 Olympic Races (10 km) 28
        2.9.2.3 Longer Races (up to 25 km or More) 28
2.10 Nutrition for Recovery 29
References 29

2.1 GENERAL INTRODUCTION

On August 23, 1875, Captain Matthew Webb entered the waters of Dover for what was to be a history-making swim of immense courage. He arrived in Calais 21 hours and 4 minutes after leaving the English mainland. His effort, without special training, sport nutrition or modern navigational technology, is still the standard by which many contemporary open-water marathon swimmers set their goal (Gerrard 1999). His legacy inspired people to discover the unknown of the ocean and set in place the general principles and rules of modern open-water swimming competitions (Munatones 2011).

Nowadays, open-water swimming (OWS) is an outdoor endurance discipline that takes place in oceans, seas, rivers and lakes. Conventional races take place over distances of 5, 10 and 25 km and are present in the World and European championships, while only the 10-km race is an Olympic event (since 2008). In recent years, the popularity of ultra-endurance events has significantly increased and the three most challenging open-water swims worldwide are the 21 mile (34 km) English Channel swim, the 20.1 mile (32.2 km) Catalina Channel swim and the 28.5 mile (45.9 km) Manhattan Island Marathon Swim, known collectively as the "Triple Crown of Open Water Swimming".

OWS involves physiological issues (thermoregulatory challenges, significant fluid losses, muscle fuel depletion) and environmental challenges (unpredictable waves, tides and currents) not typically seen in other events within aquatic sports. However, performance in OWS is determined/affected by the specific challenges of aquatic locomotion; this chapter will thus be introduced by general principles regarding the bioenergetics and biomechanics of swimming with a specific focus on the physiological and biomechanical determinants of endurance speed.

2.2 ENERGETICS AND BIOMECHANICS OF (ENDURANCE) SWIMMING

In swimming, as in other cyclic forms of locomotion in water or on land (e.g. running, cycling and kayaking), endurance speed (V_{end}) depends essentially on two factors, as formally described by di Prampero (1986):

$$V_{end} = F \cdot V'O_{2\,max}/C \tag{2.1}$$

where F is the fraction of $V'O_{2\,max}$ (maximal oxygen uptake) that can be sustained during the race and C is the energy cost (i.e. the energy expended to cover one unit distance, or the economy of locomotion) at a given speed (i.e. V_{end}). This equation indicates that larger values of V_{end} would be attained by swimmers with larger values of $F \cdot V'O_{2\,max}$ and/or lower values of C.

As reviewed by Baldassarre et al. (2017) the $V'O_{2\,max}$ values of elite middle-distance and open-water swimmers are comparable to those reported for athletes specialized in endurance events on land (e.g. marathon runners): about 60 and 70 ml·min^{-1}·kg^{-1} for female and male swimmers, respectively. However, is the ability to sustain an elevated percentage of $V'O_{2\,max}$, rather than a high $V'O_{2\,max}$ per se, the factor associated with a good performance in endurance events (Dwyer 1983; di Prampero 1986), as recently pointed out for marathon runners (Tam et al. 2012).

Since $F \cdot V'O_{2\,max}$ corresponds to the ratio of the speed attained at the lactate threshold (LT) to V_{end} (e.g. Tam et al. 2012), Eq. 2.1 indicates that larger values of V_{end} would be attained by swimmers with larger values of $F \cdot V'O_{2\,max}$ and/or with higher speeds at LT. In elite open-water swimmers, VanHeest et al. (2004) reported that lactate threshold occurred at a pace equal to 88.75% of peak pace for males and 93.75% for females; as these authors suggest, training programs for these athletes should be designed to increase LT velocity as a percentage of peak swimming velocity.

As indicated by Eq. 2.1, larger values of V_{end} are associated with lower values of C; in water locomotion C depends essentially on three factors, as formally described by Zamparo et al. (2011):

$$C = W_D / (\eta_P \cdot \eta_O) \qquad (2.2)$$

where W_D is hydrodynamic resistance (drag), η_P is propelling efficiency and η_O is overall efficiency.

At a given speed, women have a lower hydrodynamic resistance (W_D) than men due to their smaller size, higher fat percentage (lower body density) and more buoyant/horizontal position in water (Pendergast et al. 1977; Zamparo et al. 2000, 2011). According to Eq. 2.1 and 2.2, this explains why, in endurance and ultra endurance swimming events, women could swim faster than men or, in more general terms, explains why gender differences in endurance swimming are trivial compared to other endurance events on land (e.g. Rüst et al. 2014; Knechtle et al. 2014).

Gender differences in the anthropometric and physiological characteristics are not observed before puberty; therefore in the pre-pubertal age there is a substantial equality in swimming performance between males and females. The earlier changes in sexual maturation (earlier increase in $V'O_{2\,max}$ with no major changes in hydrodynamic resistance) constitute an advantage for females so that in the 11–13 age range female swimmers can out-swim males, particularly so in long-distance races. This advantage is quickly lost due to the steeper growth in $V'O_{2\,max}$ (as well as in muscle size and power) compared to females after puberty, particularly so in short distance races (Fox et al. 1989), even if their growth is accompanied by a substantial increase in hydrodynamic resistance compared to females.

To put it another way, in short-distance swimming races it is important to maximize the nominator of Eq. 2.1 (high metabolic – and mechanical – power is required for a short time and C plays a less important role) whereas in long-distance swimming races C (i.e. the denominator of Eq. 2.1) is of paramount importance (less metabolic – and mechanical – power is required but it should be maintained for a long time; in this case economy is a big issue). Accordingly, the differences in V_{end} between genders are expected to decrease in long-distance races, covered at progressively lower speed (see Figures 2.1 and 2.2); this state of affairs is specific for swimming since the differences in C between genders are far larger in water than on land (e.g. in running or cycling).

It goes without saying that, regardless of the gender and the age of the swimmers, those with better "anthropometric characteristics", as well as those more able to maintain a buoyant/horizontal position in water, will encounter lower hydrodynamic resistance and hence will be characterized by a lower C at a given swimming speed.

Besides hydrodynamic resistance, the energy cost of swimming also depends on propelling and overall efficiency (Eq. 2.2). These two parameters are quite difficult to measure and a detailed description on how they can be calculated/estimated is beyond the aims of this chapter; the reader is referred to Zamparo et al. (2011) for a detailed discussion about this point.

It suffices here to say that propelling efficiency defines the capability of a swimmer to transform the mechanical power produced by his/her muscles into useful

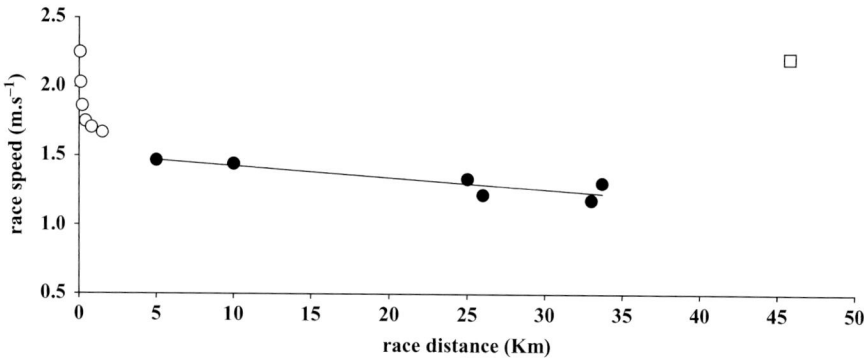

FIGURE 2.1 Race speed (m·s⁻¹, average of male and female swimmers) as a function of race distance (km): the longer the race the lower the speed, except for the Manhattan Island race (empty square) where the current of the Hudson River and the tides favor the swimmers. Full circles and empty square: OWS races (data are taken from Tables 2.1 and 2.2). Open circles: 50-m pool world records in freestyle (data are taken from http://www.fina.org/sites/default/files/wr_50m_oct_11_2017).

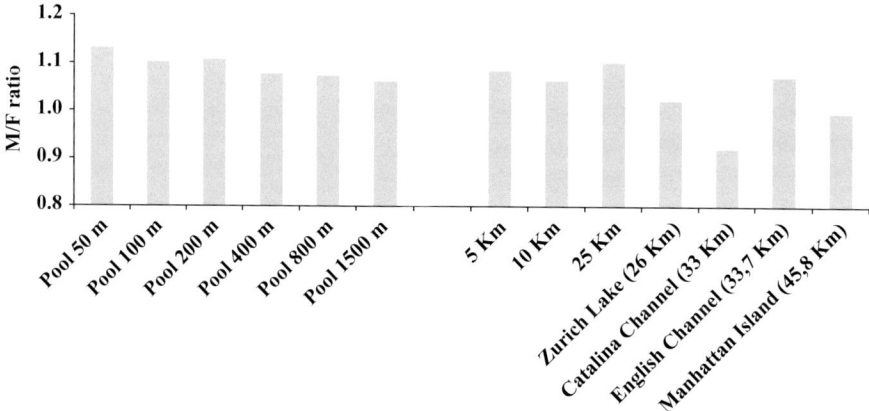

FIGURE 2.2 M/F ratio (in swimming speed) in pool events (50-m pool world records in freestyle, http://www.fina.org/sites/default/files/wr_50m_oct_11_2017), in conventional OWS races (5, 10 and 25 km) and in endurance OWS events (data are taken from Tables 2.1 and 2.2).

power to move in water (e.g. to overcome drag) and that, according to Eq. 2.2, the greater this capability (e.g. the larger the η_P) the lower the energy cost of swimming (and hence the larger V_{end}, according to Eq. 2.1).

Since propelling efficiency decreases with fatigue, C is bound to increase in fatigued swimmers and V_{end} is thus expected to decrease. The distance covered per stroke (the stroke length [SL]) is an index of propelling efficiency (e.g. Toussaint and Beek 1992; Zamparo et al. 2005, 2011) and thus the deterioration of stroke mechanics in fatigued subjects could be expected to lead to a progressive increase in C, and to a decrease in V_{end}; this was indeed observed in different studies (e.g. Zamparo et al. 2005; Barbosa et al. 2008; Figueiredo et al. 2011).

As an example, Zamparo et al. (2005) evaluated changes in C, stroke rate (SR) and SL during three 400-m swims performed at increasing speed, with or without a pre-fatiguing 2 km trial performed at 10 km race pace. The authors noted an increase in C and SR due to development of fatigue and a consequent decrease in SL. Similar results were reported by De Ioannon et al. (2015), who monitored SR, SL and speed of a master athlete while solo crossing the Adriatic Sea (78 km). After the first three hours, SL and velocity started to decrease while SR increased. Although the swimmer self-selected the velocity to complete the event in the established time, several environmental conditions (water temperature, tides, currents and waves) other than fatigue may have affected swimming technique. In any case these data show that SL was critical in influencing ultra-endurance swimming performance, similar to what was already seen in pool events (e.g. by Zamparo et al. 2005). Thus, by learning to manipulate their SL and SR, and eventually the arm coordination, swimmers can achieve a larger velocity with a lower C (e.g. Barbosa et al. 2008; Figueiredo et al. 2011)

2.3 ANTHROPOMETRIC CHARACTERISTICS OF OW SWIMMERS AND GENDER DIFFERENCES

Data regarding these athletes are scarce, compared to those competing in other disciplines of the same time duration (marathon, triathlon). Early data, collected during the English Channel race in 1954, showed that subcutaneous fat was thicker in open-water swimmers and that their anthropometric profile was characterized by a large body weight in relation to stature, causing a better tolerance to cold water (Pugh and Edholm 1955). More recent studies reported OW swimmers as smaller and leaner than pool swimmers (VanHeest et al. 2004) and indicate that OW swimmers possess a wide range of adiposity that did not seem to impact swimming success (Shaw and Mujika 2018). It could be hypothesized that the higher body fat and lower muscle mass compared to pool swimmers might be dictated by the necessity of these athletes to adapt to wide ranges of water temperatures.

However, since the introduction of OWS in the Olympic Games, several athletes perform both in the pool and in open water events. (Shaw and Mujika 2018). Oussama Mellouli, Ferry Weertman, Jordan Wilimovsky, Sharon Van Rouwendaal and Samantha Arevalo are some examples of male and female swimmers that have raced in the pool and OW swimming events in the same edition of World Championships and Olympic Games. Oussama Mellouli is the first swimmer to win a gold medal in both pool and OW swimming events in the Olympic Games (https://www.olympic.org). In ultra-endurance events the increase in the number of participants over the years is associated with an increase in the average age of the participants, meaning a massive participation of non-professional OW swimmers (e.g. of master athletes).

Although women generally do not outperform men in endurance events, open-water ultra-endurance swimming offers an exception (see Figure 2.2): in the Catalina Channel Swim and the Manhattan Island Marathon Swim, the fastest women ever were faster than the best-performing men (Sandbakk et al. 2018). The fastest person ever to complete the Triple Crown was a woman who finished the three races within 36 days in 2008, in a total time of 70 hours and 50 minutes (Knechtle et al. 2015).

As indicated above, the smaller body size and greater body fat percentage in females results in less drag and lower energy cost than males. The higher body fat may also improve women's swimming performance in cold water by acting as insulation against the cold (Knechtle et al. 2014).

2.4 OPEN-WATER SWIMMING: PERFORMANCE ANALYSIS AND PACING STRATEGIES DURING OFFICIAL COMPETITIONS

Conventional races take place over 5, 10 and 25 km, and are present in the World and European championships. OW swimming became an official event at the Beijing Olympic Games (2008), with the distance of 10 km. For these races a multi-lap 2500-m course is used, and depending on the length of the race a certain number of laps need to be completed. The environmental challenges (unpredictable waves, tides and currents) explain why geographical distance and real distance might differ in these events (this is even more the case in ultra-endurance races). Most of the ultra-endurance OW races have similar regulations: athletes have to be accompanied by a support boat to guarantee their safety and provide for their nutrition, and wetsuits are prohibited.

In individual sports, record marks as finishing times are of great interest but in OWS the Fédération Internationale de Natation (FINA) does not hold official world records since weather, water conditions, temperature and tides can considerably affect race time (Zingg et al. 2014b). Therefore, comparison among different races is more difficult than in other disciplines. Nevertheless, different studies analysed performance (Vogt et al. 2013; Zingg et al. 2014a, 2014b; Baldassarre et al. 2017) or pacing profiles (Baldassarre et al. 2017, 2018; Rodriguez and Veiga 2017) of the 5, 10 and 25 km races (official competitions).

As an example, Vogt et al. (2013) analysed swimming performance and corresponding sex differences of elite OW swimmers competing in all FINA 10 km competitions between 2008 and 2012 (World Cup, European Championship, World Championship and Olympic Games.) The main finding was that performance remained stable over the years (1.35 ± 0.09 m·s^{-1} for the fastest women and 1.45 ± 0.10 m·s^{-1} for the fastest men), and that sex difference in performance was about 7%. Regarding the Olympic Games, the swimming speed improved for both sexes from Beijing to London (Vogt et al. 2013); in Rio the swimming speed of female athletes remained stable while it decreased in males (Baldassarre et al. 2017) (Table 2.1).

As indicated above, a comparison of swimming speed (V_{end}) in different races can be misleading due to environmental factors such as water temperature and tides (see Figure 2.1) but sex differences in performance, performance density and pacing strategies can indeed be compared and are of interest.

When compared to other endurance disciplines, in conventional OWS races sex differences in performance are rather low (about 7%, as indicated above). For example, at the Ironman Hawaii the speed difference between the sexes is smaller in swimming (10–12%) than in cycling (13–15%) or in running (13–18%) (Lepers 2008;

TABLE 2.1

Swimming Speed and Performance Density of the 10 Fastest 10 km Swimmers in the Three Olympic Races (modified from (Baldassarre et al. 2017))

Competition	Velocity (m·s⁻¹)		Performance Density (%)		References
	Women	Men	Women	Men	
Beijing (2008)	1.39 ± 0.00	1.49 ± 0.00	0.18	0.33	Vogt et al. (2013)
London (2012)	1.41 ± 0.01	1.51 ± 0.01	1.06	0.81	Vogt et al. (2013)
Rio (2016)	1.41 ± 0.02	1.47 ± 0.02	0.81	0.07	https://www.olympic.org/rio-2016

TABLE 2.2

Ultra-swim Races: Distances, Best Times and Sex Differences (M, Men; W, Women)

Race	Distance (km)	Water Temperature (°C)	Best Performance (h:min:s)	Sex difference (%)	References
English Channel swim	34	14–18	M 06:55:00 W 07:25:15	7	https://www.dover.uk.com/channel-swimming/records
Catalina Channel swim	32.2	15–21	M 08:05:44 W 07:27:25	9	https://swimcatalina.org/individuals-records/
Manhattan Island Swim	45.9	16–20	M 05:44:02 W 05:44:47	0.2	https://www.nyopenwater.org/20-bridgesmanhattan-island-swim-solo-swim-results/
Marathon-Swim Lake Zurich	26	16–26	M 05:51:41 W 05:59:43	2	https://ch.srichinmoyraces.org/veranstaltungen/zhlake

Lepers and Maffiuletti 2011; Lepers et al. 2013). As shown in Figure 2.2 and Table 2.2 sex differences are further reduced in ultra-endurance OW races. Possible reasons for this are reported above.

Performance density is defined as the difference between the competitors finishing in first and tenth places (or first and last): a high performance density indicates a small difference in speed between the winner and the competitor finishing in tenth (or last) place. A higher performance density is observed in OWS compared to other disciplines (e.g. running). As an example, in the 10 km OWS Olympic event in Rio, performance density was 0.07% and 0.81% (for men and women, respectively) between the first- and tenth-placed finishers, and 5.27% and 7% (for men and women, respectively) between the first and the last finishers (see Table 2.1, adapted from (Baldassarre et al. 2017)). As a comparison, during the Olympic marathon in Rio, performance density was 2.91% and 3.15% between the first- and tenth-placed finishers, and 29.18% and 36.18% between the first and the last finishers, for men and women respectively (https://www.olympic.org/rio-2016).

The high density observed during OWS races indicates that OWS is a tactical event; split data from the Rio Olympic race (https://www.rio2016.com) indeed show that the medallists adopted a "conservative tactic" increasing the speed in the last lap; the swimmers in the lead group swam together until the last buoy (350m before the finish) to benefit from drafting (see section 2.4).

Pacing strategy has a significant impact on performance and can differentiate successful and less successful athletes in a variety of sporting events. Pacing strategies can be categorised as positive pacing (the athlete's speed decreases during the competition), negative pacing (the athlete speeds up), even pacing (a stable speed is maintained), variable pacing (speed is varied throughout) and parabolic-shaped pacing (Hanley 2016).

Rodriguez and Veiga (2017) analysed pacing strategy in the 10 km race at the World Championship in Kazan, an important race that decided which athletes qualified for the Olympic Games in Rio. They reported that the most successful males adopted a negative pacing and the females an even pacing, with the less successful athletes dropping off throughout the race. The most successful OW swimmers increased their speed in the last split.

In Figure 2.3 the pacing strategy OW swimmers (males and females) during the World Championships in Budapest (2017) are reported, as a further example. Data were obtained from the official website of Omega (http://www.omegatiming.com/) and thereafter analysed.

Split times were obtained for each 2.5 km (1st = 2.5 km, 2nd = 5 km, 3rd = 7.5 km …) and the mean speed (m·s⁻¹) for each split was calculated. Swimmers were divided into four groups based on finishing time, and each swimmer assigned to one group only. Group 1 (the swimmers whose finishing times were within 0.50% of the winner's time); Group 2 (between 0.51% and 1% slower than winner's time); Group 3 (between 1.1% and 2% slower than winner's time); Group 4 (more than 2% slower than winner's time). These percentages were selected according to the performance density of OWS competitions observed in previous studies (Zingg et al. 2014a, 2014b).

Figure 2.3 indicates that in the 5 km race, both genders, independently of performance level, adopted a negative pacing, increasing their speed in the second part of the race. Over the 10 km distance the best swimmers (Groups 1, 2 and 3) adopted a negative pacing, increasing their speed in the last part of the race. Over the 25 km distance all groups adopted the same pacing strategy up to approximately the halfway point in the race; thereafter Groups 1 and 2 were able to increase and maintain their speed whereas Groups 3 and 4 decreased their speed. Thus, in OWS, exercise duration appears to be an important factor influencing both optimal and self-selected pacing.

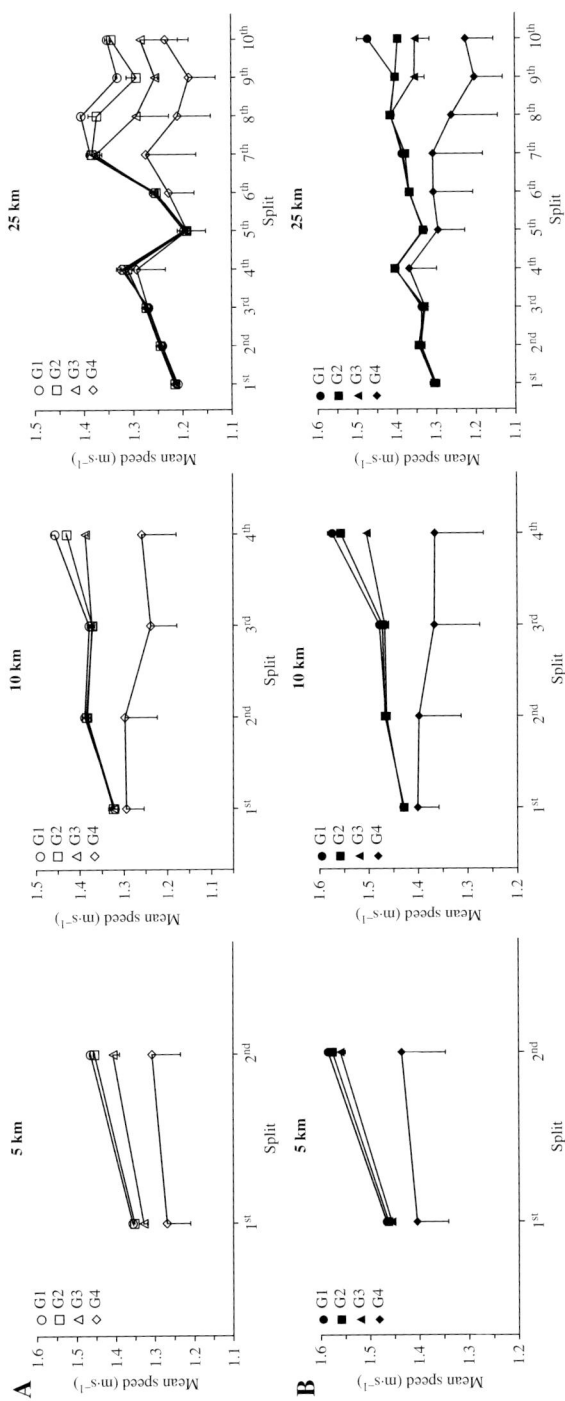

FIGURE 2.3 Pacing strategy of open-water swimmers (5, 10 and 25 km races) during the World Championships of Budapest (2017). A, women; B, men. Group 1 (the swimmers whose finishing times were within 0.50% of the winner's time); Group 2 (between 0.51% and 1% slower than winner's time); Group 3 (between 1.1% and 2% slower than winner's time); Group 4 (more than 2% slower than the winner's time). (See text for details).

As a comparison, studies that analysed the pacing strategies of runners or triathletes showed that athletes adopt an even or positive pacing. As an example, Hanley (2016) showed that marathon runners of both sexes maintained an even pace in Olympic and World Championship races; whereas Angehrn et al. (2016) reported that elite Ironman athletes adopt a positive pacing, decreasing their speed in cycling and running in most races in 2014.

Pacing strategies in OWS depend, among other factors, on the benefits of drafting. Swimming behind another swimmer at a distance of up to 50 cm reduces by 11% the metabolic response of the draftee (Chatard and Wilson 2003). A sheltered position allows the swimmer to control the race and to save energy for the "final sprint" (Chatard and Wilson 2003); this tactic is very similar to what was previously reported for sprinters in road cycling, where the last 10 minutes of the race are the most crucial part of the competition (Menaspà et al. 2015).

OWS is in fact a head-to-head competition where finishing position rather than finishing time is important and where the differences between the winner and the other competitors may be only marginal (Rodriguez and Veiga 2017). Although official split times are every 2.5 km, it is evident that the final end spurt occurs over a much shorter distance. During the men's 10 km Olympic race in Rio (2016, https://www.olympic.org/rio-2016), the swimmers in the head group swam together until the last buoy at 350 m from the finish and only five seconds separated the winner from the tenth-placed athlete (Baldassarre et al. 2017). Similarly, at the 2012 Olympic Games, Mellouli Oussama from Tunisia won the 10 km in just under two hours, with less than a 1% time difference from the following 12 athletes. Therefore, solo swims and wins are unheard of in official OWS races (Zingg et al. 2014b).

2.5 ULTRA-ENDURANCE OWS RACES

Nowadays, the three most challenging open-water swims worldwide are the English Channel Swim, the Catalina Channel Swim and the Manhattan Island Marathon Swim, collectively termed the "Triple Crown of Open Water Swimming". In 2008 the female American swimmer Rendy Lynn Opdycke completed all three events within 36 days in a total time of 70 h 50 min, which was faster than any man's attempt so far (Knechtle et al. 2015).

2.5.1 THE ENGLISH CHANNEL SWIM

In the English Channel Swim, one of the oldest open-water races in the world, competitors swim between England and France, a distance of 34 km. The number of participants has increased over the years and, in recent decades, more than 50 men and 20 women have successfully completed the event each year. About 30% of the participants have been women (Eichenberger et al. 2012a, 2012b), a lower percentage than in other ultra-endurance races (e.g. Ironman or 160 km run). Swim speed has increased over the years for both men and women, which is also due to greater support from sports science regarding pre-race preparation, training, and nutrition. Speed differences between sexes in the Channel Swim have remained stable over the years: around 7% for the best performers and around 12% for the top three males and females; however, the best annual performances did not differ between the sexes (men 0.89 m·s⁻¹ and women 0.84 m·s⁻¹) (Eichenberger et al. 2012a; Fischer et al. 2013).

2.5.2 THE CATALINA CHANNEL SWIM

This is a 32.2 km swim between Avalon on Santa Catalina Island to Point Vicente, a landmark on the Californian coast. From the first edition in 1927, won by George Young in 15:44:30 h:min:s, until the end of 2014, a total of 370 swimmers successfully crossed the Catalina Channel (Knechtle et al. 2015). For this event, independently of the direction of the swim, the fastest woman ever was faster than the fastest man. This result is interesting considering that both the English Channel and the Catalina Channel are solo swims, meaning athletes are not able to draft. Only one study measured heart rate (HR), speed and perceptual responses during the event in one female participant. The athlete completed the event in 9 h and 2 min with an average HR ranging between 81–86% of HR_{max} and an average speed of 1 m·s⁻¹, indicating the ability to maintain elevated exercise intensities for long durations (Judelson et al. 2015).

2.5.3 THE MANHATTAN ISLAND MARATHON SWIM

This is a 46-km swim that covers a full counter-clockwise circumnavigation of the island of Manhattan, normally held in June. Water temperature in this event is normally below 20°C. Women represent approximately 30% of participants and, on average, 18 men and 8 women finish the race each year (Knechtle et al. 2014). The race record for women was set in 1995 (345 minutes) a time that is 14% faster than the men's record set in 1985. Also, when considering the first 10 performances, women are faster than men (Knechtle et al. 2014). Compared to the other two races of the Triple Crown, the Manhattan Island Swim is a draft legal swim, therefore it can be hypothesized that women benefit from the drafting of the male leaders, thus further reducing their energy cost of swimming.

2.5.4 THE LAKE ZURICH MARATHON SWIM

This 26 km swim is another participant event that takes place at the beginning of August with a cut-off time of 12 hours. In an analysis performed between 1987 and 2011, it appears that the number of participants increased over the years (women representing 33% of the total), but that performance by males and females did not change (Eichenberger et al. 2012b). The mean sex difference in swimming performance during this time period was around 11% (Eichenberger et al. 2012b).

2.6 PSYCHOLOGICAL ASPECTS

Psychological and emotional experiences before and during a competition may have a significant effect on performance (Allen et al. 2013). Anxiety has been the most investigated emotion in sport, because it is an important element in the attention system and in decision- making processes (Allen et al. 2013).

The effects of long-distance swimming on psychological state were studied through rating of perceived exertion (RPE) and profile of mood states (POMS) (Invernizzi et al. 2014; De Ioannon et al. 2015). In the first study, eight short- and mid-distance male swimmers swam 25 km in a swimming pool while in the second study, one subject swam in solo 78.1 km; in both studies participants had no previous experience in completing such distances. In both studies, the POMS profile post-race showed an increase in fatigue and a decrease in other parameters (tension, depression, anger, vigour and confusion). These authors showed that satisfaction at having completed the trial could have a significant impact on the emotional aspects, especially when the knowledge of the endpoint is vague or missing. Training and knowledge about the specific distance in a competition could thus have direct effects on psychological and emotional aspects of performance. However, there is a lack of studies that focus specifically on OWS.

2.7 RISK FACTORS, WATER TEMPERATURE AND HYPOTHERMIA

2.7.1 RISK FACTORS

With an increasing number of participants in OWS events, the rate of adverse medical events has also increased. This has already been shown in triathlon, where most deaths between 2003 and 2011 occurred during swimming, with unexplained sudden cardiac death (USAT 2012; Tipton 2014). Interestingly, these adverse events are unrelated to swimming ability, anxiety or medical problems such as stroke, seizure or syncope (USAT 2012; Tipton 2014). It has therefore been hypothesized that circumstances such as anger, competition and extended breath-holding may increase the likelihood of an autonomic conflict (Tipton 2014) in competitions (but not in training), but more research is necessary to underpin the causes of sudden cardiac deaths that occur in some OW swimmers.

2.7.2 WATER TEMPERATURE AND HYPOTHERMIA

According to FINA rules, during official events the water temperature should not be lower than 16°C or higher than 31°C and should be checked before the start of the race, as well as periodically during the race, in the middle of the course, at a depth of 40 cm (FINA 2005). If the water temperature is not within these limits the race should be stopped for the swimmers' safety. In ultra-endurance races there is no water temperature limit.

A common risk in OWS is hypothermia; according to the American Heart Association (Desk and Williams 2005) hypothermia is defined as a core body temperature below 35°C. Specifically, mild hypothermia refers to a core body temperature between 32 and 35°C, and moderate hypothermia to a core body temperature between 28 and 32°C (Gerrard 1999). Other factors apart from water temperature may increase the risk of hypothermia, such as wind chill, the ability of the swimmer to conserve body heat, the duration of exposure and the occurrence of fatigue (Gerrard 1999). Tachycardia and shivering are the most common signs of mild hypothermia but are difficult for medical staff to recognize immediately. Moderate hypothermia is more recognizable considering that athletes at this stage often swim off course and present signs of altered cognition (Gerrard 1999).

Analysing the core body temperature of 12 nationally ranked OW swimmers after a 10 km race (with water temperature of 21°C), Castro et al. (2009) reported that three athletes finished the race with mild hypothermia (34–35°C) and seven with moderate hypothermia (30–34°C). Branningan et al. (2009) also reported signs of hypothermia when analysing the oral temperature of solo participants in the Rottnest Channel Swim (a 19.2 km race with water temperature of 19–22°C) in Western Australia; they found that hypothermia was more frequent with increasing race time and in swimmers with a low body mass index. Therefore, even if the water temperature in both studies was relatively warm and well within the limits imposed by FINA, medical staff must be aware of the risk of hypothermia in elite swimmers both during 10 km open-water competitions and during ultra-endurance races.

Expert cold-water swimmers are able to swim in water temperatures of less than 11°C for a relatively long time, without suffering from hypothermia (Keatinge et al. 2001). However, immersion in cold water could provoke a shock response that includes hyperventilation, gasp response, tachycardia and an increase in stress hormone response (Tipton and Bradford 2014), factors that can be a precursor to drowning. Moreover, the energy expenditure of swimming increases in cold water. Holmér and Bergh (1974) reported an increase of 0.5 L·min^{-1} in V'O_2 during sub-maximal swimming at the same intensity in cold water (18°C) compared to swimming in warm water (34°C). The increase of V'O_2 has been attributed to thermogenesis and to the superimposition of shivering on swimming metabolism (Tipton and Bradford 2014). Moreover, the viscosity of water increases with decreasing water temperature (leading to an increase in W_D), and this could partly be responsible for the increased energy cost measured while swimming at lower water temperatures (Tipton and Bradford 2014).

For medical staff it is important to continue to monitor swimmers that have raced in very cold water after the race because deep body temperature continues to fall (Golden et al. 1991). Therefore, acclimatization to cold water is an important element for these athletes.

The individual ability to develop an adaptation against environmental stress may be the basis of natural selection in marathon swimmers (Dwyer 1983), and the bias toward high levels of adipose tissue in early studies (Pugh and Edholm 1955). According to Judelson et al. (2015), OW swimmers have a unique combination of fatness and fitness that allows them to maintain a high level of heat production and retain it below significant levels of insulation (Tipton and Bradford 2014). More research is needed to explain the effect of extreme conditions on endurance and ultra-endurance performances.

There are not many studies that investigated the physiological responses while swimming at high intensities (e.g. race pace) in warm water; many studies in fact investigated lower intensities or shorter durations (Tipton and Bradford 2014). However, many competitions take place in water of about 32°C, so it is necessary to have a more precise idea of the increase in core temperature during these events.

Hue et al. (2015) recently investigated the effects of cold-water ingestion during a 5 km swim in warm water (28.8°C) at 10 km race pace, on core temperature and thermal sensation. Increasing fluid ingestions, and specifically increasing the amount of cold fluids, significantly decreased core temperature and prevented hyperthermia.

2.8 ROLES OF APPROPRIATE NUTRITION

2.8.1 ENERGY INTAKE REQUIREMENTS

Daily energy intake in elite swimmers can show great variability, especially between men and women, despite a similar training volume. For example, Van Handel et al. (1984) reported that elite swimmers training more than three hours per day had a self-reported daily energy intake ranging from 3000 to 6800 kcal·day^{-1} for males and from 1500 to 3300 kcal·day^{-1} for females. More recently, (self-reported) energy intakes of elite male and female swimmers have been reported to be 15–20 MJ·day^{-1} (3600–4800 kcal·day^{-1}) and 8–11 MJ·day^{-1} (1900–2600 kcal·day^{-1}), respectively (see Shaw et al. 2014a).

The fact that female swimmers usually report energy intakes less than expected with stable body composition or less than males undertaking similar training has often been considered (see Shaw et al. 2014a). These differences could be explained by the large individual variability of C values among swimmers and by the lower C values usually observed in women compared to men (e.g. (Zamparo et al. 2011)). Another possible explanation for this remark could be related to underestimating dietary intake: female athletes in other weight-conscious sports have been often described as underreporting their dietary intakes on self-reported food diaries (see Shaw et al. 2014a).

Differences between men and women were also reported in the ability to match changes in energy requirements during periods of different training volumes. In this respect, male swimmers seem to be able to appropriately increase energy intake during periods of increased training (by increasing the intake of carbohydrates), while female swimmers appear less able to spontaneously make such adjustments (see Shaw et al. 2014a).

Hence, especially in female swimmers, the risks of an inadequate calorie intake should be taken into account. In this respect, it should be taken into account that if the energy intake is too low to support the optimal functioning of the body (once the energy cost of exercise is subtracted), negative health consequences such as reductions in metabolic rate, hormonal disturbances, menstrual dysfunction and an increased risk of illness and injury can occur (see Shaw et al. 2014a).

In addition, it is not enough that the body mass remains stable over time for considering that the energy intake is sufficient for the needs of the body under a hard training regimen. For instance, VanHeest et al. (2004) recently reported that a low energy availability in junior elite female swimmers, in which ovarian suppression occurred, was associated with poor performance despite body mass remaining stable during the 12 weeks of the study. According to the same authors, the observed reduction in circulating thyroid hormones leads to a reduction in metabolic rate, which can counteract the expected positive effects of training on performance.

2.8.2 Carbohydrate Requirements

Muscle glycogen stores can be depleted by repeated swimming training sessions at high volume and intensity. Costill et al. (1988) showed that swimmers who were not able to increase carbohydrate intake following a sharp increase in training volume reported muscle fatigue and soreness and difficulty in performing scheduled training workouts. This indicates that swimmers should be able to adapt carbohydrate intake to the change in training workload to ensure adequate muscle glycogen restoration. Therefore, swimmers must be encouraged to ingest carbohydrate according to sports nutrition guidelines (6–10 g·kg^{-1} of body mass per day), particularly during hard training periods (see Shaw et al. 2014b). It must also be considered that reduced carbohydrate availability, associated with high training volume and intensity, can impair immune system responses (Pyne et al. 2014).

Consequently, training sessions should always start with adequate stores of muscle glycogen, and fluid-containing carbohydrates should be consumed during each session. Some sessions might be deliberately performed with low muscle glycogen stores or in fasting conditions to stimulate a greater metabolic adaptation of fats utilization. However, such interventions should be carefully programmed and, according Mujika et al. (2014), should follow a careful consideration of a cost-benefit analysis and appropriate periodization to avoid compromising training adaptations and/or immune functions.

2.8.3 Estimation of Energy Requirement in the 10 km Race

Based on data in the literature, an attempt to estimate the amount of energy needed to cover the requirements for a swimming competition in open water can be proposed. As an example, at the 2016 Olympic Games in Rio de Janeiro, the male winner of the OWS race covered the 10 km distance in about 113 minutes, corresponding to an average speed of 1.475 m·s^{-1}. According to the C vs. V relationship reported by Capelli et al. (1998) in elite crawl male swimmers, this speed corresponds to a value of C of 1.20 KJ·m^{-1} and consequently to an overall energy expenditure of about 12000 KJ (2868 kcal). Assuming that ATP is fully resynthesized via oxidative metabolism and that an average respiratory exchange ratio (RER) of 0.85 can be maintained during the 10 km race, the contributions of carbohydrates (FG) and fats (FL) used as fuel are of about 49% (5880 KJ) and 51% (6120 KJ), respectively. According to this estimation, the absolute amounts of carbohydrates and fats used are hence of about 340 g and 160 g, respectively (considering 38.9 KJ·g^{-1} for fat and 17.2 KJ·g^{-1} for carbohydrates).

Nevertheless, as previously reported, it should be considered that C could show, even among elite swimmers, considerable individual variability. For instance, the 2016 Olympic champion at 1500 meters, at the same speed of 1.475 m·s^{-1}, showed a C value of 0.84 KJ·m^{-1} (calculated directly by measuring V'O$_2$ in a swimming flume, personal data). According to the previous calculations, this swimmer, in a 10 km race, should have an overall energy expenditure of about 8400 KJ (2008 kcal) supplied from about 240 g of carbohydrates and 110 g of fats.

In addition, as previously specified, OW swimmers are able to take advantage of swimming directly behind another swimmer. Drafting allows C to be reduced and hence glycogen stores to be saved at equal speed. It has been calculated that C is reduced by about 11% when the drafting distance is 50 cm or less (measured from the toes of the lead swimmer to the fingertips of the drafting swimmer) and about 8% when the drafting distance is between 50 and 150 cm (Chatard and Wilson 2003).

Furthermore, as previously pointed out, during standardized exercise V'O$_2$ increases by about 16% in cold water (18°C, a temperature which is not uncommon during OW competitions) compared to in water at 25°C (McArdle et al. 1976).

Even if these calculations are based on a simplified approach and on different methods of V'O$_2$ determination, they can indicate a quantitative range of values to be considered for feeding strategies during competitions for elite OW swimmers.

2.9 APPROPRIATE NUTRITION DURING COMPETITIONS

According to their duration, OW events are usually able to induce consistent, if not complete, muscle glycogen depletion. It has long been reported that glycogen depletion in active muscles, consequent to prolonged swimming at high intensity, reduces the distance per stroke (Costill et al. 1988). Since swimming efficiency is correlated to distance per stroke and it is considered a key factor limiting C in OW swimming (Zamparo et al. 2005), the amount of muscle glycogen stores is crucial. It can be protected through nutritional strategies: pre-race (to optimize glycogen stores), during race (to save stores) and for recovery (to restore stores when the swimmer is engaged in more events in the same championship).

2.9.1 PRE-RACE NUTRITION

In endurance exercise lasting more than 90 minutes, it is well known that elevated muscle glycogen contents at the beginning of the event will delay the onset of fatigue; in fact, during exercise of this duration, exhaustion usually occurs when muscle glycogen content becomes critically low (see Hawley et al. 1997). This outcome could occur during races of 10 km or more, challenging the swimmer to maintain adequate speeds. For this reason, several carbohydrate-loading regimens have been developed since the late 1960s to increase muscle glycogen stores (super-compensation). More recently, Bussau et al. (2002) have shown that only one day of physical inactivity combined with a high intake of carbohydrate (10 g per kg of body mass) enables trained athletes to attain maximal muscle glycogen contents. To summarize this aspect, it has been reported that a carbohydrate intake of 10–12 g per kg of body mass per day in the 36–48 hours before the event, combined with a normal training schedule (tapering), should be enough to achieve a super-compensation in muscle glycogen content (see Shaw et al. 2014b).

As Hawley et al. (1997) reported in their review, several studies have shown that exhaustion time decreases during intense exercise of short duration (less than 15 minutes) after a low intake of carbohydrates and this suggests that nutrition strategies to achieve maximum individual glycogen content are probably also useful for the shorter distances of OWS competitions.

It has been reported that the last meal, 1–4 hours before a race, can represent a final opportunity to start the race with optimal carbohydrate availability: general recommendations for a prerace meal involve well-tolerated foods providing 1–4 g per kg of body mass of carbohydrates (Burke et al. 2011). However, several studies have shown reduced rates of fat oxidation during exercise following ingestion of carbohydrates (see Wu et al. 2003). This is mainly due to hyperglycaemia and hyperinsulinaemia during the postprandial period, which exert inhibition of lipolysis and lipid oxidation within the muscles (Coyle et al. 1997; Horowitz et al. 1997).

Wu et al. (2003) have shown that a carbohydrate meal three hours before exercise resulted in lower rates of fat oxidation during subsequent exercise than when exercise is performed in the fasting state. Interestingly, higher fat oxidation was observed after a carbohydrate meal composed of low-glycaemic index food than a high-glycaemic index one. From a practical point of view, Hargreaves et al. (2004) claimed that there is no convincing evidence that insulin-mediated inhibition of lipolysis is always associated with impaired performance in prolonged exercise. However, individual experience should address individual practice.

Men and women seem to respond differently to carbohydrate loading: it has been reported that women do not increase their muscle glycogen content in response of elevation from 55–60% to 75% in dietary carbohydrates for a period of four days, while men submitted to the same regimen, increased muscle glycogen concentration by 41% (Tarnopolsky et al. 1995).

High-intensity prolonged swimming can determine high rates of fluid loss (up to 1.2 L·h^{-1}) depending on water temperature. For instance, moderate levels (2% of body mass) of dehydration can occur when swimming 5 km in 32°C water. Hence, swimmers should begin a race with an optimal hydration status especially if water temperature is high (see Shaw et al. 2014b).

The swimmers who compete in water above 30°C can benefit from strategies that help them to tolerate the hot environmental conditions. It has been suggested that the ingestion of cold beverages (less than 4°C) and/or ice slurries in the 30 minutes before exercise can be useful to improve endurance capacity in terrestrial exercise (see Shaw et al. 2014b). On the other hand, hot drinks can be expected to be useful in cold environmental conditions even if, at present, there are no studies that demonstrate that these interventions influence performance in cold conditions.

2.9.2 Nutrition During the Race

To ensure appropriate nutrition during the race, feeding platforms are usually placed at regular intervals on the swimming course, every 1.25 km or at least every 2.5 km, as is the case in FINA competitions. According to the rules, a swimmer's approved representative stays on the platform and the swimmer shall receive feeding directly from his/her representative by a feeding pole, not exceeding 5 m in length when extended, with a cup or vessel attached to one end. However, in other races, an individual support boat could handle feeding.

2.9.2.1 Short Races (5 km or Less)

An event lasting less than one hour could still have (little) benefit from carbohydrate ingestion during the effort, despite the value of exogenous carbohydrate being questionable during exercise of this duration if glycogen levels are optimal before the start. A possible explanation of this paradox comes from several studies (see Chambers et al. 2009) showing that performance during exercise lasting 45–75 min is improved by rinsing the mouth with a carbohydrate solution during the effort. According to Chambers et al. (2009), the improvement observed may be due to the activation of brain regions involved in reward and motor control. However, swimmers participating in events lasting less than one hour should be encouraged to focus on prerace nutrition to optimize glycogen stores, and to consider using the feeding stations only if it could be tactically advantageous (Shaw et al. 2014b). In fact, elite OW swimmers usually do not supply during official 5 km races; evidently, the time lost when taking food or fluids is not considered to be compensated by any benefit related to feeding.

2.9.2.2 Olympic Races (10 km)

Since the duration and intensity of the 10 km Olympic race is limited by muscle glycogen content, carbohydrate intake during the race should be theoretically useful to save glycogen stores by providing an additional source of muscle fuel. Carbohydrate sources can be sports drinks, gels, confectionary or other kinds of food according to the swimmer's preference. It should be considered that the absorption of carbohydrate products is improved when such products contain mixtures of different kinds of sugars (the so-called "multiple transportable carbohydrates"). However, it is very important that foodstuffs are tested in training, before competition, to check their tolerability and to personalize their content (see Shaw et al. 2014b). Actually, many elite swimmers rely less on feeding platforms to take nutritional support, carrying gel containers tucked into their swimwear; this arrangement gives them the opportunity to choose the most tactically advantageous moment for feeding. However, this practice raises the problem of disposing of the containers, hence the increased risk of environmental aquatic pollution, and it should require specific rules.

General guidelines for endurance exercise of two hours' duration suggest carbohydrate intake of 30–60 g per hour (Burke et al. 2011). Usually, during international competitions, the swimmers feed 2–3 times during the race (on average every 30 minutes).

2.9.2.3 Longer Races (up to 25 km or More)

For events lasting 3–5 hours or more, swimmers should be encouraged to increase their reliance on feeding platforms to take nutritional support at least every 30–35 minutes, reducing the stress related to environmental exposure. Intakes of carbohydrates (up to 90 g·h^{-1} from multiple carbohydrate sources), proteins, electrolytes and water therefore assume a more significant role for longer races (Shaw et al. 2014b).

Studies examining nutrition in ultra-endurance swimming are very scarce. Recently, Kumstát et al. (2016) described the feeding strategies of an elite female swimmer participating in seven events (ranging from 15 to 88 km and lasting 3–12 hours) during the 2014 FINA Open Water Grand Prix. The study reported a mean in-race energy intake of 394 ± 26 kcal per hour provided by carbohydrate (gels, fluids, bananas) and protein (protein drinks, branched chain amminoacids) mean intake of 83 ± 5 and 12 ± 8 g·h^{-1}, respectively. Fluid ingestion reached a mean value of 662 ± 27 ml·h^{-1} with a mean sodium intake of 423 ± 16 mg·h^{-1}. Fat intake was neglected (~1 g·h^{-1}) and timing of feeding was not predetermined.

2.10 NUTRITION FOR RECOVERY

Swimmers competing in different events in one meeting (for example during World Championships) should pay particular attention to nutritional strategies for recovery, aiming to restore glycogen stores as fast as possible.

It is well known that in the first few hours immediately following exercise, high rates of muscle glycogen synthesis occur as a result of the activation of glycogen synthase enzyme and increases in muscle membrane permeability to glucose, while, after this time, refuelling rates decrease (see Burke and Mujika 2014). However, according to the same authors, it should be considered that carbohydrate intake after exercise provides an immediate source of substrates to start effective recovery within muscles rather than simply to determine a few hours of moderately enhanced glycogen synthesis. For appropriate recovery, an intake of carbohydrates of about 1 g per kg of body mass per hour has been recommended to maximize glycogen replenishment in the first two hours following exercise, together with high-quality proteins in an amount of about 0.2–0.3 g per kg of body mass (Burke and Mujika 2014).

REFERENCES

Allen, M. S., M. Jones, P. J. McCarthy, S. Sheehan-Mansfield, and D. Sheffield. 2013. Emotions correlate with perceived mental effort and concentration disruption in adult sport performers. *European Journal of Sport Science* 13 (6): 697–706.

Angehrn, N., C. A. Rüst, P. T. Nikolaidis, T. Rosemann, and B. Knechtle. 2016. Positive pacing in elite ironman triathletes. *The Chinese Journal of Physiology* 59 (6): 305–314.

Baldassarre, R., M. Bonifazi, M. F. Piacentini. 2018. Pacing profile in the main international open-water swimming competitions. *European Journal of Sports Science* 19 (4): 422–431.

Baldassarre, R., M. Bonifazi, P. Zamparo, and M. F. Piacentini. 2017. Characteristics and challenges of open-water swimming performance: A review. *International Journal of Sports Physiology and Performance* 12 (10): 1275–1284.

Barbosa, T. M., R. J. Fernandes, K. L. Keskinen, and J. P. Vilas-Boas. 2008. The influence of stroke mechanics into energy cost of elite swimmers. *European Journal of Applied Physiology* 103 (2): 139–149.

Branningan, D., I. R. Rogers, I. Jacobs, A. Montgomery, A. Williams, and N. Khangure. 2009. Hypothermia is a significant medical risk of mass participation long-distance open water swimming. *Wilderness and Environmental Medicine* 20 (1): 14–18.

Burke, L. M., J. A. Hawley, S. H. S. Wong, and A. E. Jeukendrup. 2011. Carbohydrates for training and competition. *Journal of Sports Sciences* 29 (suppl 1): S17–27.

Burke, L. M., and I. Mujika. 2014. Nutrition for recovery in aquatic sports. *International Journal of Sport Nutrition and Exercise Metabolism* 24 (4): 425–436. doi:10.1123/ijsnem.2014-0022.

Bussau, V., T. Fairchild, A. Rao, P. Steele, and P. Fournier. 2002. Carbohydrate loading in human muscle: An improved 1 day protocol. *European Journal of Applied Physiology* 87 (3): 290–295.

Capelli, C., D. R. Pendergast, and B. Termin. 1998. Energetics of swimming at maximal speeds in humans. *European Journal of Applied Physiology and Occupational Physiology* 78 (5): 385–393.

Castro, R. R. T., F. S. Mendes, and A. C. L. Nobrega. 2009. Risk of hypothermia in a new Olympic event: The 10-km marathon swim. *Clinics (Sao Paulo, Brazil)* 64 (4): 351–356.

Chambers, E. S., M. W. Bridge, and D. A. Jones. 2009. Carbohydrate sensing in the human mouth: Effects on exercise performance and brain activity. *The Journal of Physiology* 587 (8): 1779–1794.

Chatard, J. C., and B. Wilson. 2003. Drafting distance in swimming. *Medicine and Science in Sports and Exercise* 35 (7): 1176–1181.

Costill, D. L., M. G. Flynn, J. P. Kirwan, et al. 1988. Effects of repeated days of intensified training on muscle glycogen and swimming performance. *Medicine and Science in Sports and Exercise* 20 (3): 249–254.

Coyle, E. F., A. E. Jeukendrup, A. J. Wagenmakers, and W. H. Saris. 1997. Fatty acid oxidation is directly regulated by carbohydrate metabolism during exercise. *The American Journal of Physiology* 273 (2 Pt 1): E268–275.

De Ioannon, G., G. Cibelli, S. Mignardi, A. Antonelli, L. Capranica, and M. F. Piacentini. 2015. Pacing and mood changes while crossing the Adriatic Sea from Italy to Albania: A case study. *International Journal of Sports Physiology and Performance* 10 (4): 520–523.

Desk, R., and L. Williams. 2005. 2005 American Heart Association guidelines for cardiopulmonary resuscitation and emergency cardiovascular care. *Circulation* 112 (24 suppl) 203: IV1.

di Prampero, P. E. 1986. The energy cost of human locomotion on land and in water. *International Journal of Sports Medicine* 7 (2): 55–72.

Dwyer, J. 1983. Marathon swimmers: Physiologic characteristics. *The Journal of Sports Medicine and Physical Fitness* 23 (3): 263–272.

Eichenberger, E., B. Knechtle, P. Knechtle, C. A. Rüst, T. Rosemann, and R. Lepers. 2012a. Best performances by men and women open water swimmers during the 'English Channel Swim' from 1900 to 2010. *Journal of Sports Sciences* 30 (12): 1295–1301.

Eichenberger, E., B. Knechtle, C. A. Rüst, P. Knechtle, R. Lepers, and T. Rosemann. 2012b. No gender difference in peak performance in ultra-endurance swimming performance - Analysis of the 'Zurich 12-H Swim' from 1996 to 2010. *The Chinese Journal of Physiology* 55 (5): 346–351.

Figueiredo, P., P. Zamparo, A. Sousa, J. P. Vilas-Boas, and R. J. Fernandes. 2011. An energy balance of the 200 m front crawl race. *European Journal of Applied Physiology* 111 (5): 767–777.

FINA. 2005. Open-water swimming rules 2005–2009 FINA Handbook. In *Constitution and Rules*, edited by Fédération Internationale de Natation, 146–553. Lausanne.

Fischer, G. B., C. A. Knechtle, C. A. Rüst, and T. Rosemann. 2013. Male swimmers cross the english channel faster than female swimmers. *Scandinavian Journal of Medicine and Science in Sports* 23 (1): e48–e55.

Fox, E. L., R. W. Bowers, and M. L. Foss. 1989. *The Physiological Basis of Physical Education and Athletics*. Dubuque, IA: W.B. Saunders Company.

Gerrard, D. F. 1999. Open water swimming: Particular medical problems. *Clinics in Sports Medicine* 18 (2): 337–347.

Golden, F. S., G. R. Hervey, and M. J. Tipton. 1991. Circum rescue-collapse: Collapse, sometimes fatal, associated with rescue of immersion victims. *Journal of the Royal Naval Medical Service* 77 (3): 139–149.

Hanley, B. 2016. Pacing, packing and sex-based differences in Olympic and IAAF world championship marathons". *Journal of Sports Sciences* 34 (17): 1675–1681.

Hargreaves, M., J. A. Hawley, and A. Jeukendrup. 2004. Pre-exercise carbohydrate and fat ingestion: Effects on metabolism and performance. *Journal of Sports Sciences* 22 (1): 31–38.

Hawley, J., E. J. Schabort, T. D. Noakes, and S. C. Dennis. 1997. Carbohydrate-loading and exercise performance. *Sports Medicine* 24 (2): 73–81.

Holmér, I., and U. Bergh. 1974. Metabolic and thermal response to swimming in water at varying temperatures. *Journal of Applied Physiology* 37 (5): 702–705.

Horowitz, J. F., R. Mora-Rodriguez, L. O. Byerley, and E. F. Coyle. 1997. Lipolytic suppression following carbohydrate ingestion limits fat oxidation during exercise. *The American Journal of Physiology* 273 (4 Pt 1): E768–775.

Hue, O., R. Monjo, and F. Riera. 2015. Imposed cold-water ingestion during open water swimming in internationally ranked swimmers. *International Journal of Sports Medicine* 36 (11): 941–946.

Invernizzi, P. L., E. Limonta, A. Bosio, R. Scurati, A. Veicsteinas, and F. Esposito. 2014. Effects of a 25-km trial on psychological, physiological and stroke characteristics of short- and mid-distance swimmers. *The Journal of Sports Medicine and Physical Fitness* 54 (1): 53–62.

Judelson, D. A., J. R. Bagley, J. M. Schumacher, and L. D. Wiersma. 2015. Cardiovascular and perceptual responses to an ultraendurance channel swim: A case study. *Wilderness and Environmental Medicine* 26 (3): 359–365.

Keatinge, W. R., M. Khartchenko, N. Lando, and V. Lioutov. 2001. Hypothermia during sports swimming in water below 11 degrees C. *British Journal of Sports Medicine* 35 (5): 352–353.

Knechtle, B., T. Rosemann, R. Lepers, and C. A. Rüst. 2014. Women outperform men in ultradistance swimming: The Manhattan Island marathon swim from 1983 to 2013. *International Journal of Sports Physiology and Performance* 9 (6): 913–924.

Knechtle, B., T. Rosemann, and C. A. Rüst. 2015. Women cross the 'Catalina Channel' faster than men. *SpringerPlus* 4 (1): 332. eCollection 2015.

Kumstát, M., S. Rybářová, A. Thomas, and J. Novotný. 2016. Case study: Competition nutrition intakes during the open water swimming grand prix races in elite female swimmer. *International Journal of Sport Nutrition and Exercise Metabolism* 26 (4): 370–376.

Lepers, R. 2008. Analysis of Hawaii Ironman performances in elite triathletes from 1981 to 2007. *Medicine and Science in Sports and Exercise* 40 (10): 1828–1834.

Lepers, R., B. Knechtle, and P. J. Stapley. 2013. Trends in triathlon performance: Effects of sex and age. *Sports Medicine* 43 (9): 851–863.

Lepers, R., and N. Maffiuletti. 2011. Age and gender interactions in ultraendurance performance: Insight from the triathlon. *Medicine and Science in Sports and Exercise* 43 (1): 134–139.

McArdle, W. D., J. R. Magel, G. R. Lesmes, and G. S. Pechar. 1976. Metabolic and cardiovascular adjustment to work in air and water at 18, 25, and 33 degrees C *Journal of Applied Physiology* 40 (1): 85–90.

Menaspà, P., M. Quod, D. T. Martin, J. J. Peiffer, and C. R. Abbiss. 2015. Physical demands of sprinting in professional road cycling. *International Journal of Sports Medicine* 36 (13): 1058–1062.

Mujika, I., T. Stellingwerff, and K. Tipton. 2014. Nutrition and training adaptations in aquatic sports. *International Journal of Sport Nutrition and Exercise Metabolism* 24 (4): 414–424.

Munatones, S. 2011. *Open Water Swimming: Improve Your Time, Improve Your Performance.* Champaign, IL: Human Kinetics.

Pendergast, D. R., P. E. di Prampero, A. B. Craig, D. R. Wilson, and D. W. Rennie. 1977. Quantitative analysis of the front crawl in men and women. *Journal of Applied Physiology: Respiratory, Environmental and Exercise Physiology* 43 (3): 475–479.

Pugh, L. G., and O. G. Edholm. 1955. Summary for policymakers. In *Climate Change 2013 – The Physical Science Basis,* edited by Intergovernmental Panel on Climate Change. Cambridge: Cambridge University Press.

Pyne, D. B., E. A. Verhagen, and M. Mountjoy. 2014. Nutrition, illness, and injury in aquatic sports. *International Journal of Sport Nutrition and Exercise Metabolism* 24 (4): 460–469.

Rodriguez, L., and S. Veiga. 2017. Effect of the pacing strategies on the open water 10-km World swimming championships performances. *International Journal of Sports Physiology and Performance* 16: 1–19.

Rüst, C. A., B. Knechtle, P. Knechtle, R. Lepers, T. Rosemann, and V. Onywera. 2014. European athletes dominate performances in Double Iron ultra-triathlons – A retrospective data analysis from 1985 to 2010. *European Journal of Sport Science* 14 (suppl 1): s39–50.

Sandbakk, Ø., G. S. Solli, and H. C. Holmberg. 2018. Sex differences in world record performance: The influence of sport discipline and competition duration. *International Journal of Sports Physiology and Performance* 13: 2–8.

Shaw, G., K. T. Boyd, L. M. Burke, and A. Koivisto. 2014a. Nutrition for swimming. *International Journal of Sport Nutrition and Exercise Metabolism* 24 (4): 360–372.

Shaw, G., A. Koivisto, D. Gerrard, and L. M. Burke. 2014b. Nutrition considerations for open-water swimming. *International Journal of Sport Nutrition and Exercise Metabolism* 24 (4): 373–381.

Shaw, G., and I. Mujika. 2018. Anthropometric profiles of elite open water swimmers. *International Journal of Sports Physiology and Performance* 11: 1–4.

Tam, E., H. Rossi, C. Moia, et al. 2012. Energetics of running in top-level marathon runners from Kenya. *European Journal of Applied Physiology* 112 (11): 3797–3806.

Tarnopolsky, M. A., S. A. Atkinson, S. M. Phillips, and J. D. MacDougall. 1995. Carbohydrate loading and metabolism during exercise in men and women. *Journal of Applied Physiology* 78 (4): 1360–1368.

Tipton, M. 2014. Sudden cardiac death during open water swimming. *British Journal of Sports Medicine* 48 (15): 1134–1135.

Tipton, M., and C. Bradford. 2014. Moving in extreme environments: Open water swimming in cold and warm water. *Extreme Physiology and Medicine Jun* 11 (3: 12).

Toussaint, H. M., and P. J. Beek. 1992. Biomechanics of competitive front crawl swimming. *Sports Medicine* 13 (1):8–24.

USAT, USA Triathlon. 2012. USA triathlon fatality incidents study. *USA Triathlon.* https:// www.teamusa.org/USA-Triathlon/News/Articles-and-Releases/2012/October/25/1025 12-Medical-Panel-Report.

Van Handel, P. J., K. A. Cells, P. W. Bradley, and J. P. Troup. 1984. Nutritional status of elite swimmers. *Journal of Swimming Research* 1 (1): 27–31.

VanHeest, J. L., C. E. Mahoney, and L. Herr. 2004. Characteristics of elite open-water swimmers. *The Journal of Strength and Conditioning Research* 18 (2): 302.

Vogt, P., C. A. Rüst, T. Rosemann, R. Lepers, and B. Knechtle. 2013. Analysis of 10 km swimming performance of elite male and female open-water swimmers. *SpringerPlus* 2 (1): 603.

Wu, C. L., C. Nicholas, C. Williams, A. Took, and L. Hardy. 2003. The influence of high-carbohydrate meals with different glycaemic indices on substrate utilisation during subsequent exercise. *British Journal of Nutrition* 90 (6): 1049–1056.

Zamparo, P., M. Bonifazi, M. Faina et al. 2005. Energy cost of swimming of elite long-distance swimmers. *European Journal of Applied Physiology* 94 (5–6): 697–704.

Zamparo, P., C. Capelli, M. Cautero, and A. Di Nino. 2000. Energy cost of front-crawl swimming at supra-maximal speeds and underwater torque in young swimmers. *European Journal of Applied Physiology* 83 (6): 487–491.

Zamparo, P., C. Capelli, and D. Pendergast. 2011. Energetics of swimming: A historical perspective. *European Journal of Applied Physiology* 111 (3): 367–378.

Zingg, M. A., C. A. Rüst, T. Rosemann, R. Lepers, and B. Knechtle. 2014a. Analysis of swimming performance in FINA World Cup long-distance open water races. *Extreme Physiology and Medicine* 3 (1): 2.

Zingg, M. A., C. A. Rüst, T. Rosemann, R. Lepers, and B. Knechtle. 2014b. Analysis of sex differences in open-water ultra-distance swimming performances in the fina world cup races in 5 km, 10 km and 25 km from 2000 to 2012. *BMC Sports Science, Medicine and Rehabilitation* 6 (1): 7.

3 Contact and Combat Sports
Sports Nutrition Benefits

Jonathan Mike

CONTENTS

3.1 Combat Sports 35
    3.1.1 Boxing...35
        3.1.1.1 Training and Nutrition for Boxing....................................36
3.2 Hydration 39
    3.2.1 Kickboxing 39
3.3 Sport Supplements Strategies for Boxing and Kickboxing 40
    3.3.1 Creatine..40
    3.3.2 Caffeine 41
    3.3.3 Beta-Alanine..42
    3.3.4 Mixed Martial Arts (MMA)...43
3.4 The Fighter Diet Plan 44
    3.4.1 Wake Up 44
    3.4.2 Breakfast (Pre-Workout)...44
    3.4.3 Post-Workout...45
    3.4.4 Lunch 45
    3.4.5 Snack 45
    3.4.6 Dinner..45
    3.4.7 Evening Snack (Only If Hungry) 45
References..45

3.1 COMBAT SPORTS

3.1.1 BOXING

Boxing is a striking combat sport characterized by high-paced, high-intensity muscular actions demanding both aerobic and anaerobic capacity as well as considerable skill. In fact, this energy system contributes to the boxers' ability to repeat attacks with the highest strength and speed over the total duration of the combat (1). Recent studies indicated that the aerobic pathway also ensures the recovery process during the brief periods of rest, particularly the recovery of the high-energy phosphate system, and also an effective recovery between rounds (1, 2). Thus, the anaerobic metabolic pathway provides energy for short and intense attacks of maximal power.

Boxing is contested in both amateur and professional competitions, with the Olympic Games the pinnacle of amateur boxing. Bouts consist of three 3-min rounds for men and four 2-min rounds for women with a 1-min rest between rounds. Successive bouts in a tournament are fought over a number of days with one bout per day. The format in professional boxing varies widely and may include up to 10 or more rounds in a bout. Boxing is also considered a contact sport in which the athletes compete in weight categories. The athletes use different strategies to achieve their desired weight, some of which may affect their sports performance.

A key feature of boxing competition is the grouping of athletes into weight divisions in an attempt to create a match-level playing field in which one competitor does not have a significant size or strength advantage (Table 3.1). To ensure athletes have "made weight", official weigh-ins are held prior to competition. Generally, the weigh-in occurs on the morning of the competition in amateur boxing, or the day before the competition in professional boxing. It is common for boxers to attempt to lose weight in order to compete in a lighter weight division against smaller opponents.

In addition to long-term weight loss or body-fat reduction, some athletes engage in extremely rapid weight-loss practices in the hours and days prior to the weigh-in that can negatively alter performance and affect both health and the outcome of the competition. Extreme dehydration, vomiting, starvation, and laxative and diuretic use all significantly decrease performance and can be dangerous to health, so they are strongly discouraged.

3.1.1.1 Training and Nutrition for Boxing

In order to benefit the most from training sessions, boxers need to ensure they are properly fueled and hydrated. Guaranteeing adequate intake of a wide variety of fruits and vegetables will provide many of the vitamins and minerals required to prevent illness and promote good health and recovery. Consuming adequate carbohydrate-containing foods, particularly before and after training sessions, will help fuel and promote recovery. Protein intake that contains a high biological value (BV) and various protein stores

TABLE 3.1
Boxing Weight Divisions

Male Weight Divisions	Female Weight Divisions
46–49 kg	45–48 kg*
49–52 kg	48–51 kg*
52–56 kg	51–54 kg*
56–60 kg	54–57 kg*
60–64 kg	57–60 kg*
64–69 kg	60–64 kg*
69–75 kg	64–69 kg*
75–81 kg	69–75 kg*
81–91 kg	75–81 kg*
>91 kg	>81 kg*

*Weight divisions not contested at Olympic Games.

that possess a high Protein Digestibility Corrected Amino Acid Score (PDCAA) are recommended to best facilitate recovery and growth (Table 3.2). Care needs to be taken to prevent excessive body-fat gain between competitions, while fueling training sessions, achieving recovery post-training and promoting a healthy body image and attitude towards food intake and weight management are all important. It is common for athletes to feel nervous or find it hard to eat before a bout. Choosing light, easy-to-digest, low-fat, low-fiber foods or liquid foods (e.g. meal-replacement drinks, sports bars, simple sandwiches, dry biscuits, etc.) close to competition can be a suitable strategy to provide energy while minimizing gut discomfort. Following their bout, if a boxer needs to make weight again the following day, they should check their weight and if further weight loss is required then they should adjust total volume/weight of food and fluid consumed over the rest of the day. Preference should be given to low-fiber/low-weight foods that provide carbohydrate and protein for energy and recovery while avoiding excessively large/heavy meals and large fluid intakes in order to make weight again.

The protein requirements for these types of combat and contact sports have been the subject of much debate. According to the International Society of Sports Nutrition (ISSN), their Position Stand on Protein (3), specifically states that "protein intakes of 1.4–2.0 g/kg/day for physically active individuals is not only safe, but may improve the training adaptations to exercise training". Other investigators have suggested a 1.2–1.4 g/kg/day and 1.6–1.7 g/kg/day for endurance and strength-trained athletes, respectively (4). Thus, a ceiling of 2.0 g/kg/day is the consensus in relation to the protein needs of athletic individuals. Data on high-protein diets are somewhat misleading in that investigators operationally define "high" incorrectly. The definitions of a high protein diet include intakes greater than 15–16% of total energy, as high as 35% of total calories or intakes that merely exceed the RDA (5). Basing a diet solely on percentages can be quite misleading. Instead, one should operationally define what a "high" protein diet is via the amount consumed daily per kilogram of body weight. Further, as 2.0 g/kg/d seems to be the upper limit of what active

TABLE 3.2

A Comparison of Protein Quality of Selected Foods and Protein Sources

Protein	BV	PER	PDCAAS
Hydrolyzed whey	100	>3.0	1.00
Whey concentrate	100	>3.0	1.00
Whole egg	100	2.8	1.00
Milk	91	2.8	1.00
Beef/poultry, fish	79–83	2.0–2.9	0.80–0.92
Soy	74	1.8–2.3	0.91–1.00
Casein	71	2.9	1.00

*BV= Biological Value.
*PER= Protein Efficiency Ratio.
*PDCAA = Protein Digestibility Corrected Amino Acid Score.

individuals purportedly need, it is our contention that for a diet to truly be considered high in protein, daily consumption should necessarily exceed 2.0 g/kg/d.

Carbohydrates play a critical role in fueling exercise, either by being the primary energy source to fuel anaerobic exercise via glycolysis or as a gateway to oxidative phosphorylation. This is particularly important for boxing and other, similar sports. Thus, during high-intensity training (similar to what is typically performed by combat sport athletes), carbohydrates can provide energy for only a relatively short duration of time. This places a large emphasis on maximizing carbohydrate storage before training and competition and replenishing them after exercise and competition (3). There are several types of carbohydrates available, all of which are metabolized differently by the body. According to the recent ISSN Position Stand on Nutrient Timing, the following abbreviated strategies should be used for both combat and contact sports in efforts to both optimally adapt and optimize performance:

- Meeting the total daily intake of protein, preferably with evenly spaced protein feedings (approximately every 3 h during the day), should be viewed as a primary area of emphasis for exercising individuals.
- If rapid restoration of glycogen is required (<4 h of recovery time) then the following strategies should be considered:
  a. aggressive carbohydrate refeeding (1.2 g/kg/h) with a preference for carbohydrate sources that have a high (>70) glycemic index
  b. the addition of caffeine (3–8 mg/kg)
  c. combining carbohydrates (0.8 g/kg/h) with protein (0.2–0.4 g/kg/h)
- Extended (>60 min) bouts of high intensity (>70% $VO_{2\ max}$) carbohydrate should be consumed at a rate of ~30–60 g of carbohydrate/h in a 6–8% carbohydrate–electrolyte solution (6–12 fluid ounces) every 10–15 minutes throughout the entire exercise bout, particularly in those exercise bouts that extend beyond 70 mins.
- When carbohydrate delivery is inadequate, adding protein may help increase performance, ameliorate muscle damage, promote euglycemia and facilitate glycogen re-synthesis.
- Pre- and/or post-exercise nutritional interventions (carbohydrate + protein or protein alone) may operate as an effective strategy to support increases in strength and improvements in body composition. However, the size and timing of a pre-exercise meal may impact the extent to which post-exercise protein feeding is required.
- Ingesting a 20–40 g protein dose (0.25–0.40 g/kg body mass/dose) of a high-quality source every three to four hours appears to have the most favorable effect on MPS rates when compared to other dietary patterns and is associated with improved body composition and performance outcomes.
- Consuming casein protein (~30–40 g) prior to sleep can acutely increase MPS and metabolic rate throughout the night without influencing lipolysis.
- Protein consumption during the peri-workout period is a pragmatic and sensible strategy for athletes, particularly those who perform high volumes of exercise. Not consuming protein post-workout (e.g. waiting for several hours post-exercise) offers no benefits.

3.2   HYDRATION

Replacement of this fluid mostly depends on drinking behavior, but research has shown for decades that a person's desire to drink does not normally occur until water loss reaches 1–2% of body mass (6). Even this mild degree of dehydration will impair both exercise (7) and cognitive performance (8, 9) while increasing the physiological strain (i.e., heart rate and core body temperature) associated with a given intensity of exercise. According to an ACSM roundtable discussion, hypohydration also impairs and delays the thermoregulatory benefits that characterize heat acclimatization and physical fitness (10). Therefore, it is common for combat athletes to withhold fluid as part of a strategy to further reduce body weight for competition in lower weight classes. This practice inflicts greater levels of dehydration and thermal strain that may lead to non-favorable outcomes. To combat these potentially dangerous situations with respect to hydration, the following strategies should be considered for optimal hydration before exercise:

- Before exercise, the athlete should be well hydrated, with replenished muscle glycogen stores.
- Chronic dehydration may occur in athletes who perform repeated bouts of intense training or competition on the same day or on consecutive days
- The athlete should drink 500–600 mL of fluid 2–3 hours before exercise, providing ample time to urinate excess fluid. Then, 10–20 minutes before exercise, an additional 200–300 mL of fluids should be consumed (11).
- Changes in body weight, urine color (12), and urine specific gravity are each valid indicators of hydration status, and athletes, coaches, and trainers should routinely use these methods to assess pre-exercise hydration status.

3.2.1   KICKBOXING

Similar to other striking and combat sports, kickboxing simulates most of the technical and tactical aspects of competition, facilitating discrimination of winners and defeated athletes, and can be used for specific cardiovascular conditioning in combat sports (13, 14). The distance between opponents plays an important role that might affect technical and tactical actions. For this reason, during combat sports' technical and tactically focused sparring sessions, coaches must adjust the size of the sparring ring to suit the desired training outcomes. Moreover, to increase the rhythm of the sparring and attain higher intensities to obtain specific cardiovascular conditioning, coaches sometimes use multiple partners during sparring bouts (15), but no scientific evidence is available concerning these strategies.

Kickboxing includes basic techniques, technical combinations, sparring (skill) drills, and free sparring (15). In kickboxing, sparring drills are mainly incorporated by coaches for technical and tactical skill development to mimic their behaviors during actual combat (16). To date, no studies have investigated the physiological effects of specific kickboxing activities (sparring games) that can target both the physical and technical and tactical development. Furthermore, no studies have quantified the effect of ring size variation and the use of different numbers of sparring partners during sparring drills. Therefore, it is imperative to find alternative methods for kickboxing-specific exercises and conditioning protocols to further advance the technique of these types of athletes. A recent study by Ouergui (17) showed that small combat games can be a good form of exercise to provide optimal cardiovascular conditioning specific to kickboxing. Nonetheless, nutritional strategies should be used in similar fashion to the boxing strategies outlined above, as these sports are nearly identical in terms of their prospective sports nutrition needs for pre-, peri-, and post-exercise strategies.

3.3 SPORT SUPPLEMENTS STRATEGIES FOR BOXING AND KICKBOXING

The consumption of certain dietary supplements, taken in conjunction with a properly designed strength and conditioning program, may further optimize these attributes. Combat sports such as boxing, kickboxing wrestling, judo, Brazilian jujitsu, Muay Thai kickboxing, and mixed martial arts (MMA) are dynamic sports that can challenge and potentially tax various physiological systems of the body. Therefore, this section will address various sports supplements and their effects on recovery with respect to these various sports. Note, many of these supplements elicit their effects on many types of sports. Although not exclusive to combat and contact sport, the following supplements have been shown to enhance performance and can benefit these types of athletes (Table 3.3).

3.3.1 CREATINE

Creatine is synthesized from the amino acids arginine, glycine, and methionine in the human liver and pancreas. In an average adult (weighing 154 pounds), the total amount of existing creatine is 120 grams, most of which (95%) is comprised in skeletal muscle. It is estimated that 65% of intracellular creatine is phosphorylated (i.e., phosphocreatine), and the remainder exists as free creatine. According to

---

TABLE 3.3
Dietary Supplements Marketed to Combat Sport Athletes, and Their Benefits

Dietary Supplement	Potential Benefit to Combat Sport Athletes
Creatine monohydrate (Combined with Resistance Training)	Increases strength, high-intensity exercise capacity, and upper-body and lower-body power production
B-Alanine	Increases high-intensity exercise capacity.
Protein (Combined with Resistance Training)	Increases strength.
Caffeine	May improve reaction time and power production in trained athletes
Sodium bicarbonate	Improves short-duration, high-intensity exercise performance

the ISSN position stand (3), creatine monohydrate is the most effective ergogenic nutritional supplement currently available to athletes for increasing high-intensity exercise performance and lean body mass during training. Today, several hundred peer-reviewed research studies exist that have examined the effectiveness of creatine supplementation. According to Kreider, (17), of those studies, nearly 70% have reported a significant improvement in exercise performance. While it is safe to say that the remaining 30% of those studies did not show any benefit, research reports that this is likely due to the lack of an increase in skeletal muscle creatine content (18).

3.3.2 Caffeine

Consumed in coffee, tea, soda, and energy drinks, caffeine (1,3,7-trimethylxanthine) is a powerful stimulant, and is the most widely consumed drug in the world. Its ability to increase muscular work has been evident since the early 1900s. It has also been used since the Stone Age (19), and its ability to enhance muscular work was first recognized over 100 years ago (20). Upon ingestion, caffeine is rapidly absorbed and increases in plasma concentrations, generally observed between 30 to 60 minutes following ingestion (3). Early work reported that the variability in absorption time is dependent on the physicochemical formulation properties of the product dose (21). Caffeine exhibits a strong cardiovascular effect that stimulates an increase in epinephrine (adrenaline) output to a greater extent when ingested via its anhydrous formulation when compared to an equal amount of brewed or instant caffeinated coffee (McLellan 2004). The ISSN (2017) summarized many of the effects of caffeine on exercise performance as follows:

1. Caffeine is effective for enhancing sports performance in trained athletes when consumed in low-to-moderate dosages (~3–6 mg/kg/BM) and overall does not result in further enhancement in performance when consumed in higher dosages (≥9 mg/kg/BM).
2. Caffeine exerts a greater ergogenic effect when consumed in an anhydrous state as compared to coffee.
3. Caffeine supplementation is beneficial for high-intensity exercise, including team sports such as soccer and rugby, both of which are categorized by intermittent activity within a period of prolonged duration.
4. Caffeine is ergogenic for sustained maximal endurance exercise and has been shown to be highly effective for time-trial performance.
5. The literature is equivocal when considering the effects of caffeine supplementation on strength-power performance, and additional research in this area is warranted.
6. The overall scientific literature does not support caffeine-induced diuresis during exercise, or any harmful change in fluid balance that would negatively impact performance.
7. It has been shown that caffeine can enhance vigilance during bouts of extended exhaustive exercise, as well as periods of sustained sleep deprivation.

A significant increase in maximal bench-press strength has been observed in resistance-trained women after caffeine ingestion (22). Astorino (23) reported increases in training volume after acute caffeine consumption in the first two sets of performing the leg press to exhaustion, and knee extension/flexion (24), while Duncan (25) reported an increase in bench press to exhaustion at 60% of 1RM. However, Hendrix (26) found no changes in 1RM in the bench press and leg extension exercises in untrained males after consumption of 400 mg of caffeine.

3.3.3   BETA-ALANINE

Beta-alanine, or 3-aminopropionic acid, is a naturally occurring beta-amino acid and a component of the histidine dipeptides carnosine and anserine, as well as vitamin B5 or pantothenic acid. Structurally, beta-alanine is a hybrid between the potent neurotransmitters L-glycine and GABA, which may explain why consumers often claim to experience a caffeine-like response from it. Beta-alanine is even gaining support within the scientific community for being secondarily classified as a neurotransmitter.

Your body can produce beta-alanine in at least three ways. It can be released during the breakdown of histidine dipeptides, such as carnosine or anserine, or it can be formed as a secondary byproduct of a reaction that converts L-alanine to pyruvate. Additionally, beta-alanine can be formed during digestion, when intestinal microbes remove a carbon atom from L-aspartate, releasing both beta-alanine and CO_2.

However, the most notable method of increasing beta-alanine is through supplementation. Carnosine increases muscle function and performance mainly through its ability to reduce acidity in muscles during prolonged high-intensity exercise. Carnosine is highly prevalent in skeletal muscle, primarily fast-twitch muscle fibers. During high-intensity exercise, certain metabolites accumulate that cause fatigue (e.g. hydrogen ions). As the concentration of hydrogen ions increases, pH drops and reduces muscle function and power output. Muscle carnosine concentration is also linked with having a high percentage of Type II fast-twitch muscle fibers. For this reason, you will find higher levels of muscle carnosine among sprinters, MMA fighters, boxers, and many combat and contact sport athletes.

Carnosine serves as a buffer to hydrogen ions, reducing their accumulation and delaying fatigue. Compared to creatine, however, beta-alanine does not seem to improve maximal strength (27–29). Although aerobic power is not improved, there is some data to suggest that anaerobic threshold is improved with beta-alanine supplementation (30, 31). According to research, beta-alanine helps to enhance performance under three conditions:

1. Single bouts of high-intensity exercise lasting 1–4 minutes
2. Multiple bouts of high-intensity training with short rest periods (think HIIT)
3. Single bouts of high-intensity training in the presence of fatigue

Specifically, it has been shown that 28 days of beta-alanine supplementation at a dosage of 4–6.4 grams per day increases carnosine levels in muscle by approximately 60 percent (32). Compared to creatine, where muscles can maximize storage capacity following a seven-day loading protocol, the upper limit to carnosine is unknown. In the previously mentioned study, the authors noted that some subjects continued to increase carnosine levels following 10 weeks of supplementation.

Beta-alanine supplementation does not appear to have a strong effect on endurance performance. While there are a couple of instances of increased aerobic capacity following supplementation, it appears that the exercise programs used in conjunction with the supplementation protocol were most likely responsible for the improvements (33, 34).

On the other hand, strong evidence suggests that beta-alanine affects anaerobic performance, including power output and fatigue threshold. In a classic study by Hoffman et al., college football players ingested 4.5 grams of beta-alanine or placebo for 30 days (28). Beta-alanine supplementation began 3 weeks before preseason training camp and continued for an additional nine days during camp. Anaerobic performance, training volume, and ratings of soreness and fatigue were assessed pre- and post-intervention. At the end of the 30-day investigative period, only the beta-alanine group showed a trend toward lower fatigue rates during the anaerobic performance test.

Additionally, greater training volumes were reported during all resistance training sessions for the beta-alanine group. Furthermore, feelings of fatigue were lower for the beta-alanine group versus the placebo group. In another study by Hoffman and colleagues, significant changes in lean body mass, percentage body fat, and strength were seen in college football players when beta-alanine and creatine supplementation were given during a 10-week resistance-training program (27).

Beta-alanine has also been reported to improve sport-specific measures. Soccer players who consumed 3.2 grams of beta-alanine per day for 12 weeks during a competitive soccer season significantly improved their performance by 34.3 percent during an intermittent running test, compared to a −7.6 percent change in those consuming a placebo (35). Similarly, researchers out of the UK presented evidence that just four weeks of beta-alanine (1.5 g, four times per day) increased the punch force and punch frequency of amateur boxers, as compared to a placebo (36).

3.3.4 MIXED MARTIAL ARTS (MMA)

Mixed martial arts (MMA) is a physically demanding combat sport involving three to five 5-minute rounds with short periods (6–14 seconds) of high-intensity explosive activity interspersed with longer (15–36 seconds) periods of rest or low-intensity movement (37). It is a hybrid combat sport using techniques from various striking and grappling arts such as Tae Kwon Do, kickboxing, Brazilian jujitsu, and wrestling. Mixed martial arts athletes compete in weight classes to gain an advantage over their opponents; they will often attempt to lose a large amount of weight in the days and weeks before "weighing in" for the event (colloquially termed "cutting weight"). Athletes then seek to regain the cut weight quickly before the competition (38). In the week before competition, MMA athletes have been reported to lose an average of 9% of body mass with a further 5% lost in the 24 hours before the weigh-in (39).

One of the most notable and negative effects of MMA is dehydration and fluid loss, and this is among the most common weight-loss methods in combat sports (40). Much of the science investigating the influence of acute dehydration on performance in combat sports has examined performance 2–5 hours after dehydration (40–43). These studies found dehydration to compromise lower- and upper-body anaerobic and aerobic performance (40, 41, 43) or to have no effect on combat sports-specific performance or repeat effort capacities (42). However, the majority of research examining acute dehydration either does not look at the effects after a sufficient recovery period to more accurately represent MMA competition or does not investigate the magnitude of dehydration likely used in MMA competitions (39). This is important because athletes are weighed 24 hours prior to professional combat sports events (boxing, kickboxing, judo, Thai boxing, and MMA). It is likely that performance is still compromised 24 hours after dehydration in combat athletes, with research indicating that dehydration can decrease and hinder total hemoglobin mass and blood volume for more than 24 hours (44, 45).

Specific Pre/Mid/Post Nutrition Strategy

Strength	Conditioning	Strength & Cond.
1:1 CHO/Pro	3:1 CHO/Pro	2:1 CHO/Pro
0.25g/lb CHO 0.25 g/lb Pro	0.75g/lb CHO 0.25 g/lb Pro	0.50g/lb CHO 0.25 g/lb Pro
Example: 175 lb 44g CHO 44g Pro	Example: 175 lb 135g CHO 44g Pro	Example: 175 lb 88g CHO 44g Pro

3.4 THE FIGHTER DIET PLAN

3.4.1 WAKE UP

16oz water with lemon

3.4.2 BREAKFAST (PRE-WORKOUT)

Green protein smoothie:
1–2 cups spinach, 1 banana, 1 serving of whey protein, sprouted brown rice or pea protein powder, blended with ice and water)
1 teaspoon of fish oil taken separately (or 2 capsules of krill oil)

3.4.3 Post-Workout

Organic plain nonfat Greek yogurt
2 tbs of chopped walnuts
1/2 cup organic blueberries

3.4.4 Lunch

Large green salad made up of 1 cup of baby romaine, 1 cup of spinach, 1 cup
of cabbage topped with cucumbers, tomatoes, mushroom
Protein can be mixed in: 1 can of wild river tuna, just tossed with vinegar,
mustard, green onions and celery
Dressing for salad can be *lightly* tossed with olive oil, lemon, and vinegar

3.4.5 Snack

1–2 red peppers and 1 sliced cucumber
3 hard-boiled eggs with 1 yolk

3.4.6 Dinner

1 bunch of grilled asparagus and zucchini lightly tossed in olive oil and
Himalayan pink salt
3–4 oz of organic chicken or turkey grilled, baked, or slow cooked
1/2 cup organic low-sodium black beans topped with pico de gallo

3.4.7 Evening Snack (Only If Hungry)

2 oz of organic chicken or turkey
Sliced cucumbers and celery

REFERENCES

1. Davis, P, Leithäuser, RM, and Beneke, R. The energetics of semicontact 3×2-min amateur boxing. *Int J Sports Physiol Perform* 9: 233–239, 2014.
2. Nassib, S, Hammoudi-Nassib, S, Chtara, M, Mkaouer, B, Maaouia, G, Bezrati-Benayed, I, and Chamari, K. Energetics demands, and physiological responses to boxing match and subsequent recovery. *J Sports Med Phys Fit* 57: 8–17, 2017.
3. Kerksick, CM, Arent, S, Schoenfeld, BJ, Stout, JR, Campbell, B, Wilborn, CD, Taylor, L, Kalman, D, Smith-Ryan, AE, Kreider, RB, Willoughby, D, Arciero, PJ, Van Dusseldorp, TA, Ormsbee, MJ, Wildman, R, Greenwood, M, Ziegenfuss, TN, Aragon, AA, and Antonio, J. International Society of Sports Nutrition position stand: Nutrient timing. *J Int Soc Sports Nutr* 14: 3, 2017.
4. Phillips, SM, Moore, DR, and Tang, JE. A critical examination of dietary protein requirements, benefits, and excesses in athletes. *Int J Sport Nutr Exerc Metab* 17(Suppl): S58–76, 2007.
5. Tipton, KD. Efficacy and consequences of very-high-protein diets for athletes and exercisers. *Proc Nutr Soc* 70: 205–214, 2011.

6. Sawka, MN, Burke, LM, Eichner, ER, Maughan, RJ, Montain, SJ, and Stachenfeld, NS. American College of Sports Medicine position stand: Exercise and fluid replacement. *Med Sci Sports Exerc* 39: 377–390, 2007.

7. Cheuvront, SN, Carter, R, Montain, SJ, and Sawka, MN. Daily body mass variability and stability in active men undergoing exercise heat stress. *Int J Sports Nutr Exerc Metab* 14: 532–540, 2004.

8. Edwards, AM, Mann, ME, Marfell-Jones, MJ, Rankin, DM, Noakes, TD, and Shillington, DP. The influence of moderate dehydration on soccer performance: Physiological responses to 45-min of performance of sport-specific and mental concentration tests. *Br J Sports Med* 41: 385–391, 2007.

9. Wilson, MM, and Morley, JE. Impaired cognitive function and mental performance in mild dehydration. *Eur J Clin Nutr* 57: S24–29, 2003.

10. Casa, DJ, Clarkson, PM, and Roberts, WO. American College of Sports Medicine roundtable on hydration and physical activity: Consensus statements. *Curr Sports Med Rep* 4: 115–127, 2005.

11. Casa, DJ, Armstrong, LE, Hillman, SK, Montain, SJ, Riff, RV, Rich, BS, Stone, JA, and Stone, JA. National Athletic Trainer's Association position statement: Fluid replacement for athletes. *J Athl Train* 35: 212–224, 2000.

12. Armstrong, LE. *Performing in Extreme Environments*. Champaign, IL: Human Kinetics, 2000.

13. Ouergui, I, Davis, P, Houcine, N, Marzouki, H, Zaouali, M, Franchini, E, Gmada, N, and Bouhlel, E. Hormonal, physiological and physical performance during simulated kickboxing combat: Differences between winners and losers. *Int J Sports Physiol Perform* 11: 425–431, 2016.

14. Ouergui, I, Hssin, N, Franchini, E, Gmada, N, and Bouhlel, E. Technical and tactical analysis of high level kickboxing matches. *Int J Perform Anal Sport* 13: 294–309, 2013.

15. Ouergui, I, Hssin, N, Haddad, M, Padulo, J, Franchini, E, Gmada, N, and Bouhlel, E. The effects of five weeks of kickboxing training on physical fitness. *Muscles Ligaments Tendons J* 4: 106–113, 2014.

16. Toskovic, NN, Blessing, D, and Williford, HN. The effect of experience and gender on cardiovascular and metabolic responses with dynamic Tae Kwon Do exercise. *J Strength Cond Res* 16: 278–285, 2002.

17. Kreider, RB. Effects of creatine supplementation on performance and training adaptations. *Mol Cell Biochem* 244: 89–94, 2003.

18. Buford, TW, Kreider, RB, Stout, JR, Greenwood, M, Campbell, B, Spano, M, Ziegenfuss, T, Lopez, H, Landis, J, and Antonio, J. International Society of Sports Nutrition position stand: Creatine supplementation and exercise. *J Int Soc Sports Nutr* 4: 6, 2007.

19. Escohotado, A, Symington, K, and Brief, A. *History of Drugs: From the Stone Age to the Stoned Age*. South Paris, ME: Park Street Press, 1999.

20. Rivers, WHR, and Webber, HN. The action of caffeine on the capacity for muscular work. *J Physiol* 36: 33–47, 1907.

21. Bonati, M, Latini, R, Galletti, F, Young, JF, Tognoni, G, and Garattini, S. Caffeine disposition after oral doses. *Clin Pharmacol Ther* 32: 98–106, 1982.

22. McLellan, TM, and Bell, DG. The impact of prior coffee consumption on the subsequent ergogenic effect of anhydrous caffeine. *Int J Sport Nutr Exerc Metab* 14: 698–708, 2004.

23. Astorino, TA, Martin, BJ, Schachsiek, L, Wong, K, and Ng, K. Minimal effect of acute caffeine ingestion on intense resistance training performance. *J Strength Cond Res* 25: 1752–1758, 2011.

24. Astorino, TA, and Roberson, DW. Efficacy of acute caffeine ingestion for short-term high intensity exercise: A systematic review. *J Strength Cond Res* 24: 257–265, 2010.

25. Duncan, MJ, and Oxford, SW. The effect of caffeine ingestion on mood state and bench press performance to failure. *J Strength Cond Res* 25: 178–185, 2011.

26. Hendrix, CR, Housh, TJ, Miekle, M, Zuniga, JM, Camic, CL, Johnson, GO, Schmidt, RJ, and Housh, DJ. Acute effects of caffeine containing supplement on bench press and leg extension strength and time to exhaustion during cycle ergometry. *J Strength Cond Res* 24: 859–865, 2010.

27. Hoffman, J, Ratamess, N, Kang, J, Mangine, G, Faigenbaum, A, and Stout, J. Effect of creatine and β-alanine supplementation on performance and endocrine responses in strength/power athletes. *Int J Sport Nutr Exer Metab* 16: 430–446, 2006.

28. Hoffman, JR, Ratamess, NA, Faigenbaum, AD, Ross, R, Kang, J, Stout, JR, and Wise, JA. Short-duration Beta-alanine supplementation increases training volume and reduces subjective feelings of fatigue in college football players. *Nutr Res* 28: 31–35, 2008.

29. Kendrick, IP, Harris, RC, Kim, HJ, Kim, CK, Dang, VH, Lam, TQ, Bui, TT, Smith, M, and Wise, JA. The effects of 10 weeks of resistance training combined with beta-alanine supplementation on whole body strength, force production, muscular endurance and body composition. *Amino Acids* 34: 547–554, 2008.

30. Stout, JR, Graves, BS, Smith, AE, Hartman, MJ, Cramer, JT, Beck, TW, and Harris, RC. The effect of beta-alanine supplementation on neuromuscular fatigue in elderly (55–92 years): A double-blind randomized study. *J Int Soc Sports Nutr* 5: 1–6, 2008.

31. Zoeller, RF, Stout, JR, O'Kroy, JA, Torok, DJ, and Mielke, M. Effects of 28 days of beta-alanine and creatine monohydrate supplementation on aerobic power, ventilatory and lactate thresholds, and time to exhaustion. *Amino Acids* 33: 505–510, 2007.

32. Hill, CA, Harris, RC, Kim, HJ, Harris, BD, Sale, C, Boobis, LH, Kim, CK, and Wise, JA. Influence of β-alanine supplementation on skeletal muscle carnosine concentrations and high intensity cycling capacity. *Amino Acids* 32: 225–233, 2007.

33. Smith, AE, Walter, AA, Graef, JL, Kendall, KL, Moon, JR, Lockwood, CM, Fukuda, DH, Beck, TW, Cramer, JT, and Stout, JR. Effects of β-alanine supplementation and high-intensity interval training on endurance performance and body composition in men; a double-blind trial. *J Int Soc Sports Nutr* 6: 1–9, 2009.

34. Kern, B, and Robinson, T. Effects of beta-alanine supplementation on performance and body composition in collegiate wrestlers and football players. *J Int Soc Sports Nutr* 6: 1–2, 2009.

35. Stout, JR, Cramer, JT, Zoeller, RF, Torok, D, Costa, P, Hoffman, JR, Harris, RC, and O'Kroy, J. Effects of beta-alanine supplementation on the onset of neuromuscular fatigue and ventilatory threshold in women. *Amino Acids* 32: 381–386, 2007.

36. Donovan, T, Ballam, T, Morton, JP, and Close, GL. B-alanine improves punch force and frequency in amateur boxers during a simulated contest. *Int J Sport Nutr Exer Metab* 22: 331–337, 2012.

37. Miarka, B, Coswig, VS, Vecchio, FB, Brito, CJ, and Amtmann, J. Comparisons of time-motion analysis of mixed martial arts rounds by weight divisions. *Int J Perform Anal Sport* 15: 1189–1201, 2015.

38. Franchini, E, Brito, CJ, and Artioli, GG. Weight loss in combat sports: Physiological, psychological and performance effects. *J Int Soc Sports Nutr* 9: 52, 2012.

39. Crighton, B, Close, GL, and Morton, JP. Alarming weight cutting behaviors in mixed martial arts: A cause for concern and a call for action. *Br J Sports Med* 50: 446–447, 2016.

40. Jetton, AM, Lawrence, MM, Meucci, M, Haines, TL, Collier, SR, Morris, DM, and Utter, AC. Dehydration and acute weight gain in mixed martial arts fighters before competition. *J Strength Cond Res* 27: 1322–1326, 2013.

41. Mendes, SH, Tritto, AC, Guilherme, JPL, Solis, MY, Vieira, DE, Franchini, E, Lancha, AH, and Artioli, GG. Effect of rapid weight loss on performance in combat sport male athletes: Does adaptation to chronic weight cycling play a role? *Br J Sports Med* 47: 1155–1160, 2013.

42. Artioli, GG, Iglesias, RT, Franchini, E, Gualano, B, Kashiwagura, DB, Solis, MY, Benatti, FB, Fuchs, M, and Lancha Junior, AH. Rapid weight loss followed by recovery time does not affect judo-related performance. *J Sports Sci* 28: 21–32, 2010.

43. Rankin, JW, Ocel, JV, and Craft, LL. Effect of weight loss and refeeding diet composition on anaerobic performance in wrestlers. *Med Sci Sports Exerc* 28: 1292–1299, 1996.

44. Reljic, D, Feist, J, Jost, J, Kieser, M, and Friedmann-Bette, B. Rapid body mass loss affects erythropoiesis and hemolysis but does not impair aerobic performance in combat athletes. *Scand J Med Sci Sports* 26: 507–517, 2015.

45. Reljic, D, Hässler, E, Jost, J, and Friedmann-Bette, B. Rapid weight loss and the body fluid balance and hemoglobin mass of elite amateur boxers. *J Athl Train* 48: 109–117, 2013.

4 An Overview on the Nutritional Requirements for Athletes Engaged in Extreme Endurance Events

Chad Kerksick

CONTENTS

4.1 Background 49
4.2 Extreme Endurance Events 50
    4.2.1 Running 50
    4.2.2 Cycling 50
    4.2.3 Triathlon 52
    4.2.4 Adventure Racing 53
    4.2.5 Swimming 53
    4.2.6 Ski Mountaineering 54
    4.2.7 Physiological Characteristics 55
4.3 Energy Considerations 55
4.4 Carbohydrate Considerations 57
4.5 Protein Considerations 60
4.6 Fat Considerations 62
4.7 Fluid, Hydration, and Micronutrient Considerations 62
4.8 Supplement Considerations 64
4.9 Other Considerations 64
4.10 Conclusions 65
Acknowledgments 66
References 66

4.1 BACKGROUND

Extreme endurance activities have grown in popularity across the world. While no consistent definition exists for what constitutes an extreme event, the majority of such designations occur when an event is of particular length or requires a substantial duration of time to complete. Today, extreme endurance competitions occur on each continent and require participants to complete a pre-determined distance or course (Table 4.1). Depending on the geographic location and the time of the year, the environmental conditions can pose as much, and oftentimes greater challenge to the participants than the physical effort of completing the activity. While running is easily the most common mode of exercise where extreme activity is completed, swimming, cycling, running, adventure racing, ski mountaineering, and trekking also have many different examples from which to observe. Due to the vast array of activities, it is challenging to universally set and define parameters upon which activities are discussed, particularly as it relates to the nutritional challenges and recommendations for such activities. For example, it is obvious to state that the energetic and feeding needs of a running event that spans 3–4 hours is different from an adventure race that takes 18–24 hours to complete. For this reason, the chapter has been organized to simply discuss the key nutritional considerations for these types of athletes and attempt to highlight as many practical and pragmatic considerations as possible.

4.2   EXTREME ENDURANCE EVENTS

4.2.1   RUNNING

Annually, hundreds of thousands of running events occur throughout the world. While events such as 5-kilometer (3.1-mile) and 10-kilometer (6.2-mile) runs are commonplace, the popularity of the half-marathon (13.1-mile) distance continues to grow in the United States and across the world. Due to the scope of this chapter being on extreme endurance events, the shortest running distance that will be discussed is the marathon distance (26.2 miles). Currently the world record for the men's marathon is 2:02:57, which was set by Dennis Kimetto from Kenya at the Berlin Marathon on September 28, 2014 while Paula Radcliffe set the women's marathon record of 2:15:25 on April 13, 2003 at the London Marathon. Beyond a simple marathon, many "ultra" events have been planned that require runners to traverse even greater distances, commonly 50 or 100 miles. From there, ultra-events have evolved into events that are completed in extreme terrain and environmental conditions (e.g., Antarctica marathon, cycling events across Alaska, Bad Water Marathon). In addition to individual events, several team events have also been organized that may require teams of 3–10 individuals to run in legs of varying distances (3–20 miles per individual and 50–500+ miles per team), again, oftentimes in select geographical locations and environmental conditions that further magnify the stress and physiological strain the event places on a participant's mind and body. For example, a simple Google search using the words "extreme running events" yields a wide variety of websites touting various races as the most challenging and the most extreme. It is beyond the scope of this chapter to attempt to highlight all such races.

4.2.2   CYCLING

Cycling events can span a wide variety of single-day distances ranging from 25 to 100 (and more) miles each day. At the professional level, cyclists can spend well

TABLE 4.1
Example Extreme Adventure Races

Name of Event	Location	Description	Source
Pikes Peak Marathon (Running)	Colorado Springs, CO USA	Single-day, marathon distance event traversing up Pikes Peak for the first 13.1 miles and then back down.	www.pikespeak marathon.org
Antarctic Ice Marathon (Running)	South Pole, Antarctica	The world's Southernmost marathon. Held in November on a glacier camp at the foot of the Ellsworth Mountains in Antarctica.	www.antarcticaice marathon.com
North Pole Marathon (Running)	North Pole Camp	A marathon distance covered on the Geographic North Pole. No single section is covered on land.	www.northpole marathon.com
Jungle Marathon (Running)	Floresta National de Tapajos, Amazon Rainforest, Brazil	Held in the Amazon rainforest in October. One can choose to cover 63 miles in four stages or 150 miles in two stages. Participants stay overnight in the jungle and bring their own provisions.	www.jungle marathon.com
Comrades Marathon (Running)	South Africa	A 56-mile road race from Durban to Pietermaritzburg. The course direction changes each year with the race broken up into cut-off points.	www.comrades.com
Chasqui Challenge (Running)	Andes Mountains, Perum	A 100-mile stage race in the Andes mountains. The race is comprised of a trail marathon, a 31-mile trek around Mt. Ausangate and other distance runs.	www.andes adventures.com
Race Across America (Cycling)	United States	A 3,000-mile, single-stage bike race that starts in California and ends in Maryland. The race course crosses 12 states and climbs over 175,000 feet. The race can be completed solo or in teams of 2, 4, or 8 people.	www.raceacross america.org
Ironman Triathlon (Swimming, Cycling, Running)	All over world	Classic triathlon consisting of a 2.4-mile (3.86-km) swim, a 112-mile (180.25-km) cycle ride and a 26.2-mile (42.2-km) run. Each event is completed in that order and without a break.	www.ironman.com
Badwater Ultramarathon (Running)	Death Valley (CA, USA) to Mt. Whitney, CA	Non-stop running race which covers 135 miles in temperatures that can get up to 130°F. Considered to be one of the most demanding and extreme ultra marathon running races in the world. Only 90 runners are allowed each year.	www.badwater.com
Patrouille des Glaciers' (Mountaineering Skiing)	Switzerland	Popular race held in Switzerland each year. Teams of three skiers complete one of two courses. Distances range from 26–53 km of varying degrees of incline and decline.	
FINA Open Water (Open Water Swimming)	Global	Series of open water swims held at locales all across the globe. The FINA World Championships include 5-, 10- and 25-kilometer individual events. The distance competed at the Olympic Games is 10 kilometers. The FINA Grand Prix is a series of events of varying distances.	www.fina.org

over all 100 days racing per year, oftentimes in multi-day, staged racing events. The most classic of these is the Tour de France, a 21-day stage that traverses over 2,200 miles in a 3-week time period. Other popular stage races include the Giro d'Italia, Vuelta a Espana, Paris-Nice and Criterium du Dauphine Libere. While professional road cycling is easily the most popular form of cycling worldwide, several extreme distance mountain biking races are completed each year as well. For example, the Trans Pyr (Spain) requires mountain bike riders to traverse parts of the Alps and Pyrenees mountains while covering distances that exceed 500 miles and over 66,000 feet of climbing. Additionally, events such as the Race Across America (a 3,000-mile race across the continental United States) serve as other unique examples of extreme endurance cycling. The Race Across America is approximately 1,000 miles longer than the Tour de France, with the winners covering the distance in less than two weeks. Of relevance to the chapter topic, it has been estimated that the winners of the Race Across America may burn more than 180,000 calories of energy on their trek. Finally, the Iditarod Invitational in Alaska asks bike riders to ride from Anchorage to Nome. The weather conditions are brutal and Fahrenheit temperatures can range from the low 30s to −50 or even −60°F). Average speeds are only 3 mph and only 42 people can call themselves "finishers".

Sanchez-Munoz et al. (2016) published a report that outlined the nutritional, physiological, and biochemical changes that occurred to six professional road cyclists throughout a four-day stage race. All participants in this study were elite male cyclists (24.8 ± 1.2 years) that trained, on average, 20–25 hours per week and typically accumulated 21,000–25,000 kilometers of cycling each year. The study followed them throughout completion of the Andalusia Tour, which covered a total distance of 647.6 kilometers over four days, with a temperature range of 6–20°C. Skinfolds and weighed food records were completed throughout completion of the activity. The cyclists were found to ingest, on average, 12.8 ± 1.7 g carbohydrates/ kg body mass/day (62.3% of daily kcals), 2.1 ± 0.2 g fat/kg body mass/day (23.2% of daily kcals), and 3.0 ± 0.3 g protein/kg body mass/day (14.5% of daily kcals). Total daily kcals were 5,644 ± 593 (~83.4 kcals/kg/day) (Sanchez-Munoz, Zabala, and Muros 2016).

4.2.3 TRIATHLON

While several multi-modal events exist combining a variety of activities, triathlons are easily the most popular of these events. Triathlons combine swimming, cycling, and running. Four common triathlon distances exist: sprint, Olympic, half-Ironman, and Ironman. A full Ironman requires the completion of a 3.0-kilometer swim, 180-kilometer cycle, and a 42.2-kilometer run. Depending on the distance and the ability of the athlete, these events can last between 1 and 17 hours. Due to the rapidly growing popularity of triathlons, the number of published reports has increased. For example, Speedy and colleagues (2001) highlighted that an athlete completing 12 hours of activity (a common duration required to prolonged triathlon) at 62% of their VO_2 max (4.5 L/min) will expend approximately 40,000 kJ (9,555 kcals) of energy. In addition, fluid loss throughout completion of an Ironman triathlon can be signifi- cant and is reported throughout this chapter. While swimming, biking, and running comprise the traditional triathlon, other modes of exercise (canoeing, kayaking, etc.) have been incorporated and in this respect, one could also point to various forms of biathlons (two disciplines) that are commonly created. Regardless of the type or number of events, the nutritional priorities and concerns these athletes employ should remain relatively consistent with those discussed in other sections. Certainly, as the duration of each event increases and the harshness of the weather conditions in which the event is taking place is considered, the individual requirements for energy, fluid and other nutritional considerations will be impacted.

4.2.4 Adventure Racing

While other extreme events challenge participants through the completion of often long-duration activities within a marked course under a wide range of grueling terrain and environmental conditions, adventure racing events are often much longer than other single-mode activities and require that more than one form of activity is completed. In this respect, adventure races commonly employ kayaking, canoeing, rafts, cycling, swimming, trekking, climbing, and orienteering. Adventure racing and triathlons are similar in that they both require the completion of multiple modes of exercise and typically require several hours to complete. A key point of separation between adventure racing and triathlons, however, is the multi-day aspect, potential to have team members, no typical "course" being mapped or marked, and the requirement to complete activities beyond swimming, running, and biking. Adventure races are typically non-stop or staged races that span several days and, uniquely, require the participants to be completely self-sufficient (i.e., no devices containing global positioning systems, motorized travel, support teams, and all participants must carry their gear and provisions). Adventure races can vary anywhere between two to five-person teams, with some solo events also being offered. The duration required to complete a race is largely predicated upon the distance, terrain, fitness status, navigation skills, sleep status, and environmental conditions where the race occurs.

4.2.5 Swimming

Extreme or ultra-endurance swimming events occur in sanctioned "open water" environments such as rivers, lakes, oceans, and water channels, and have progressively grown in popularity. Across the globe, events commonly range from 5–25 kilometers (3.1–15.5 miles). Hundreds of events occur worldwide with events being sanctioned by USA Swimming and other organizing groups. The FINA Marathon Swim World Series and FINA Open Water Grand Prix are international-caliber open water swimming events. Most events in the FINA Marathon Swim World Series are 10 kilometers in length while other Grand Prix events have ranged from 15–75+ kilometers. Swimming across the English Channel is widely considered to be the oldest form of endurance or open water swimming. Finally, the sport itself reached unprecedented exposure and popularity with its inclusion in the Olympic program of the 2008 Olympic Games in Beijing, China. Most open water swims are courses that span one, two, or six miles at one time with an estimated duration of four to six hours. At an estimated energy expenditure of 10 kcal/kg/hour and 3–12 hours in the pool, an estimated caloric expenditure might range from 2,500–4,000 kcals just during the race.

More so than other sports discussed throughout this chapter, very little research is available that has characterized the physiological and nutritional patterns of extreme endurance swimmers. For starters, actually getting the food and fluid to a swimmer can be challenging due to rough water while rough seas can lead to seasickness and vomiting. Within many sanctioned events, support kayaks or fueling boats are periodically spaced throughout the course. Here, a "feed" can be provided during the swim, which requires the swimmer to retrieve the provision and consume it while in the water (usually while treading on their back). Consequently, food and fluid delivery plans can be mapped, but are largely dependent upon how much of each feed is actually consumed and how much support is allowed by the event organizer or governing body.

In what remains as one of the only case studies to report on the nutritional practices of a competitive open water swimmer, Kumstat et al. (2016) tracked the nutritional intake of an elite female open water swimmer throughout part of the 2014 FINA Grand Prix. The day before the event the athlete strived to consumed 8–10 g of carbohydrate/kg/day and throughout several trial feeding tests, the athlete was able to report being able to ingest 60–90 grams of carbohydrates per hour of gels or beverages. In summary, the case study outlined the successful implementation of a feeding regimen that delivered ~80–90 grams of carbohydrate per hour (mixed carbohydrate sources), 400–450 milligrams of sodium per hour, and 3 mg/kg of caffeine. Protein intake did occur at times in the form of powdered whey protein concentrate and was delivered in amounts ranging from 8–165 grams, which was largely dependent upon the number of feeding stops throughout the monitored races (2–4 per hour or 5–30 stops throughout the race). Fat intake was negligible throughout each race.

4.2.6   SKI MOUNTAINEERING

Ski mountaineering is a popular leisure and competitive activity, particularly in alpine countries. The activity consists of ascending snow-covered slopes on skis resulting in periods of climbing, descending and skiing. Several types of races exist: individual, team (all members stay together), relay (team members relay each other), vertical, sprint, and long distance races. The primary difference between each type of event is the total vertical and horizontal distances traversed (Praz, Leger, and Kayser 2014). Team events alternate several steep ascents with downhill sections. Athletes are usually required to bring their own food and fluid. A characteristic race held in Switzerland each year in April called the Patrouille de Glaciers. This race involves up to 1,450 teams of three racers with two different race routes. One race (Zermat to Verbier) spans 53 kilometers, altitude differences of +3,994 and −4,090 meters and a maximum altitude of 3,650 meters. The absolute best time of this race was 2 hours, 55 minutes with the average time of finishers in Praz et al. (2014) was 5 hours, 7 minutes ± 44 minutes. Approximately 76 ± 1% of the race was uphill and 24 ± 1% was downhill. The other race (Arolla to Verbier) spans 26 kilometers, has altitude differences of 1,881 and −2,341 meters and a maximum altitude of 3,160 meters. The best time in this race was 3 hours 32 minutes with the average time for finishers in the Praz et al. (2014) report being 5 hours 51 minutes ± 53 minutes.

4.2.7 PHYSIOLOGICAL CHARACTERISTICS

Who does these events? Heydenreich and colleagues (2017) published one of the more extensive reports of energy balance on endurance athletes. This article included data from 1,674 endurance athletes with 71.4% being male and 28.6% female. In addition, 27.8% of the athletes were runners, 18.7% were cyclists, 16.4% were swimmers and the remaining 13.5% were endurance athletes participating in other sports. Table 4.2 outlines basic physiological characteristics of competitors in ultra-endurance running, cycling, swimming, adventure racing and other endurance events.

4.3 ENERGY CONSIDERATIONS

One of the most obvious but also most important nutritional challenges for any extreme or ultra-endurance event is to consume enough calories and fluid. This is no small task as events can range from a few hours (e.g., marathon, 100-mile cycle rides, half-Ironman triathlon) to several days (e.g., various disciplines of adventure racing). Regarding energy expenditure during the actual activity, Ranchordas (2012) indicated that adventure racers likely burn between 350–700 kcals/hour, Praz et al. (2014) reported that ski mountaineering athletes expend approximately 800–850 kcals/hour and Barrero et al. (2014) reported that triathletes completing an Ironman expended approximately 840 kcals/hour.

When considering ultra-endurance triathlons, a small number of studies have provided estimations of caloric expenditure rates throughout the event. Barrero et al. (2014) monitored the energy and fluid intake and estimated the energy expenditure of 11 male triathletes competing in an Ironman triathlon. The average time to complete the event was 755 ± 69 minutes. It was estimated using heart rate responses throughout the race (avg heart rate: 137 ± 6 beats/min) that 11,009 ± 664 kcals were expended (~840 kcals per hour). Energy intake was measured by weighing and recording all food and fluid provided to the athlete and was estimated to be 3,643 ± 1,219 kcals resulting in a negative energy balance of 7,365 ± 1,286 kcals (66.9 ± 11.7% of required kcals). Similar outcomes were found by Kimber et al. (2002) in male (~10,036 kcals expended) and female (~8,550 kcals expended) triathletes completing an ultra-endurance triathlon (Ironman), respectively. Using a combination of indirect calorimetry and doubly labeled water, Cuddy et al. (Cuddy et al. 2010) reported that approximately 9,000 kcals were expended by triathletes completing an Ironman triathlon. When considering cycling, Saris et al. (Saris et al. 1989) reported that professional cyclists participating in the Tour de France routinely achieved a daily energy expenditure of 25.4 MJ (~6,068 kcals) which reached up 32.7 MJ (7,812 kcals) on mountain stages.

Zimberg and colleagues (2008) had international caliber adventure racing athletes complete a simulated laboratory race while wearing heart rate monitors to assess energy expenditure. The stimulated race took 67 hours for the participants

TABLE 4.2

Physiological Characteristics of Extreme Endurance Participants

References	Sport/Event	# of Participants	Age (years)	Body Mass (kg)	Height (cm)	Adiposity	VO_2Peak
Barrero et al. (2014)	Ironman triathlon	11 M	36.8 ± 5.1	75.5 ± 6.4	174 ± 6		5.03 ± 0.4‡
Carlsohn and Muller (Burke et al. 2011)	Mountain runners	14 F	35.8 ± 9.3	54.8 ± 6.1	167 ± 4		64 (F) 66 (F)†
		48 M	37.7 ± 12.1	68.4 ± 6.9	178 ± 6		76 (M)†
Praz et al. (2014)	Mountaineer Skiing	3 F / 14 M	41 ± 6	69 ± 9	177 ± 6		60 ± 5†
Praz et al. (2014)	Mountaineer Skiing	11 M	30 ± 10	74 ± 8	178 ± 7		54 ± 5†
Stellingwerff (2016)	Ultramarathon	3 M	35.3 ± 1.5	59.5 ± 1.7	171.7 ± 3.2	–	–
Ranchordas (2012)	Adventure Racing	11 F	29.1 ± 6.4	69.9 ± 5.4	168 ± 7.3	**20.2 ± 5.7**	Cycling: 3.4 ± 0.2‡ Run: 3.4 ± 3.5‡
		61 M	31.5 ± 6.2	76.6 ± 7.2	177.3 ± 5.7	**13.1 ± 3.5**	Cycling: 4.6 ± 0.4‡ Run: 4.4 ± 0.4‡
Heydenreich et al. (2017)	Cyclists	37 F	24.2 ± 0.5	61.2 ± 1.1	166 ± 1	*22.1 ± 0.6 kg/m²*	55.8 ± 4.0†
		276 M	31.8 ± 5.6	74.4 ± 5.5	179 ± 3	*23.6 ± 1.6 kg/m²*	65.0 ± 4.8†
Heydenreich et al. (2017)	Runners	135 F	27.4 ± 6.7	55.6 ± 2.2	167 ± 3	*19.9 ± 1.0 kg/m²*	57.3 ± 5.8†
		330 M	31.4 ± 6.9	67.9 ± 5.5	175 ± 3	*20.6 ± 1.4 kg/m²*	64.3 ± 6.7†
Heydenreich et al. (2017)	Swimmers	134 F	19.4 ± 0.4	63.9 ± 2.5	170 ± 4	*22.0 ± 0.5 kg/m²*	–
		141 M	20.3 ± 1.9	74.3 ± 3.2	181 ± 3	*22.7 ± 0.7 kg/m²*	
Heydenreich et al. (2017)	Triathletes	68 M	25.8 ± 4.0	67.5 ± 1.8	176.0 ± 0	*21.8 ± 0.5 kg/m²*	65.3 ± 0.4†
Kumstat et al. (2016)	Open water Swimmer	1 F	28	60	171 cm	**16.0**	58.4†
VanHeest et al. (2004)	Open water Swimmers	4F	17.8	63.5 ± 5.8	168 ± 3	22.8 ± 2.3%	5.1 ± 0.6‡
		4M	18.6	71.3 ± 8.1	177 ± 7	9.8 ± 2.0%	5.5 ± 1.0‡

M = Male; F = Female; † = mL O$_2$/kg/min; ‡ = L O$_2$/min. In the adiposity and due to inconsistencies between what is presented in the literature, body fat percentage is provided in bold while body mass index is provided in italics.

to complete and of the original ten athletes, only seven completed the race. The athletes expended 365 kcals/hour or an estimated 24,455 kcals for the entire event; a total distance of 477.3 kilometers was covered throughout the simulation. Enqvist et al. (2010) completed a two-part investigation where the first part was a simulated ultra-endurance activity consisting of repeated blocks of kayaking, running, cycling (4 blocks of each discipline last 110 minutes per block). Throughout this simulation, the athletes expended an average of 750 kcal/hour. Nine months later the participants completed an actual adventure race and throughout the 800-kilometer race, the average energy expenditure was 500 kcal/hour.

Few published reports exist on ski mountaineering. Praz et al. (2014) reported on the energy expenditure of ski mountaineering athletes. Athletes who finished one race in 5 hours 7 minutes ± 44 minutes expended an estimated 4,588 ± 765 kcals (813 ± 120 kcals/hour) while athletes who finished a race in 5 hours 51 minutes ± 53 minutes expended 5,402 ± 693 kcals (837 ± 96 kcals/hour). In one of these races, the racers consumed a total of 1,052 ± 311 or approximately 20 ± 7% of the kcals that were expended during the race. When considered, food consumed immediately prior to and throughout the race, energy intake reached 35 ± 12% of the energy burned during the race (pre-race breakfast averaged 730 ± 253 kcals). During a 4-day period prior to the race, the ski mountaineering athletes consumed 2,533 ± 550 kcals/day. In an event most similar, but shorter in duration, Meyer et al. (2011) reported that cross-country skiers expend between 3,107–3,585 kcals for a 50-kilometer race.

While much debate exists surrounding the validity (or lack thereof) of performing simulated extreme endurance events, there is no doubt that the energy demands to complete such activities (irrespective of the mode) are some of the highest, if not the highest, for all forms of activity. As highlighted throughout the Hedenreich report and others (Heydenreich et al. 2017; Jeukendrup 2011; Praz, Leger, and Kayser 2014; Ranchordas 2012; Stellingwerff 2016), achieving a positive or even neutral energy balance is extremely challenging for these athletes. Due to its close association with an increase in overtraining, prevalence of injuries and disturbances to immune and endocrine functions, maintaining a negative energy balance and low energy availability is not advised irrespective of the sport (Mountjoy et al. 2014). For these reasons alone, one of the most important nutritional priorities for an extreme endurance athlete should be to minimize the magnitude of negative energy balance throughout periods of training and competing. While it is tempting to provide a recommendation of daily energy intake, the reality is that daily energy needs exhibit tremendous variability between athletes due to the known impact of body size, gender, training volume, and training intensity. Furthermore, the athlete and coach must also appreciate the vast differences in energy expenditure (and subsequently energy intake) that are reported within the same athletes whether they are in the preparation or competition phase of their training (Heydenreich et al. 2017).

4.4 CARBOHYDRATE CONSIDERATIONS

Put succinctly, carbohydrate needs for ultra-endurance leading up to and throughout training and competition are greatly increased and typically those endurance athletes who fail to achieve high intakes run the risk of not performing as well as they could.

On a daily basis, it is commonly recommended that athletes participating in intense, prolonged endurance activity should consume between 6–10 grams carbohydrate/kg/day (Rodriguez, Di Marco, and Langley 2009a; Rodriguez, Di Marco, and Langley 2009b), and when higher intensities and higher volumes are achieved, even greater amounts of daily carbohydrate (10–12+ grams carbohydrate/kg/day) may be needed (Burke et al. 2011; Coyle et al. 2001). In consideration of "eating fatigue", gastrointestinal complications and the sheer logistical challenge of providing the amount of carbohydrate, the athlete should understand that a point may exist where more carbohydrate may not yield greater performance outcomes. Certainly, the risks for not consuming enough carbohydrate seem to be far greater than exceeding amounts required to recover glycogen and promote performance. In this respect, Coyle et al. (2001) reported that while muscle glycogen levels did increase when daily carbohydrate intake was increased from 10 g/kg/day to 13 g/kg/day, endurance performance was not impacted. While many reasons may exist for this, the endurance athlete should understand that body mass does increase with increases in stored muscle glycogen, an outcome which may circumvent performance increases.

For all extreme endurance athletes, a pre-exercise meal that is high in carbohydrates (300–400 grams of carbohydrate) is an important consideration (Burke et al. 2011). In this respect, studies have indicated that muscle tissue with supercompensated glycogen levels typically perform 2–3% better than muscle with normal physiological glycogen levels in events lasting longer than 90 minutes (Hawley et al. 1997). Practically speaking, athletes and coaches must carefully consider the intensity and timing of the day's events against the athlete's individual tolerance to best understand what strategy works best for themselves (Kreider et al. 2010; Rodriguez, Di Marco, and Langley 2009a). Previous research has indicated that carbohydrate loading strategies can improve performance when longer distances are completed (Burke 2007; Sullo et al. 1998). As exercise duration extends beyond 90 minutes and gets into the second or third hour of activity, the importance of carbohydrate goes up (Kerksick et al. 2017). When considering multi-day events, the prolonged nature of the activity naturally lends itself to where the intensity of exercise is reduced to low, submaximal levels. At these intensities, the reliance upon endogenous glycogen stores goes down while energy production from gluconeogenesis and fat utilization increases (Lemon, and Mullin 1980; Romijn et al. 1993), a point discussed later in this chapter.

While it is widely accepted and recommended to ingest a high-carbohydrate meal containing 300–400 grams of carbohydrates 3–4 hours before the start of exercise (Hawley et al. 1997; Kerksick et al. 2017; Rodriguez, Di Marco, and Langley 2009a), much concern and debate exists surrounding the ingestion of carbohydrate within an hour before the start of exercise. Initial reports by Foster and colleagues (1979) that glucose ingestion in the hour before exercise can lead to hypoglycemia and reduced performance have permeated the endurance exercise community. While several physiological explanations exist for this response, a large number of studies since this initial publication have shown that, at worst, endurance performance is not impacted and, in many situations, performance is improved (Jeukendrup and Killer 2010). For these reasons, it is recommended that athletes do not avoid consuming carbohydrates in the hour before exercise. To this point, certain individuals do seem to be more sensitive to hypoglycemic responses and for these athletes, two common strategies are commonly recommended. First, the consumption of lower glycemic index carbohydrates can be considered. Second, studies have indicated that ingesting carbohydrates either continually throughout the hour prior to exercise or within the last 5–15 minutes (as opposed to 45–60 minutes prior) can effectively work to maintain glucose and insulin levels while also promoting favorable metabolic and performance outcomes (Moseley, Lancaster, and Jeukendrup 2003).

When considering carbohydrate ingestion during exercise, a common recommendation is to ingest 30–60 grams/hour ideally in a 6–8% glucose-electrolyte solution (Kerksick et al. 2017; Rodriguez, Di Marco, and Langley 2009a). In the past ten years, research has led to the understanding that carbohydrate oxidation in the muscle is limited to around one gram of carbohydrate per minute when a single type of carbohydrate is consumed. However, when different forms of carbohydrate are combined the oxidation rate of carbohydrate can increase markedly to levels that are well above the 1 g/min threshold (1.26 g/min). In summarizing a large number of studies in this area (Jeukendrup and Jentjens 2000), carbohydrate oxidation can be vastly improved when different forms of carbohydrate are provided and these higher rates can be achieved if administered as a beverage, gel, or bar (Pfeiffer et al. 2010a, 2010b). This latter development is quite significant for the ultra-endurance athlete who can suffer from carbohydrate fatigue throughout long bouts of training and competing. From a dose perspective during exercise, Smith et al. have determined first that higher doses of carbohydrate throughout a two-hour cycling performance more consistently improves performance (Smith et al. 2010), and second that a dose of 60–80 grams of carbohydrate per hour seems to be the dose that most consistently improves endurance performance (Smith et al. 2010).

Of the research available, several studies have reported on the carbohydrate intakes achieved both in the days leading up to the event and throughout the actual event. Throughout an ultra-endurance triathlon (Barrero, Erola, and Bescos 2014), participants ingested 89.9 ± 3.5% of their kcals from carbohydrates (6.2 ± 1.3 g/kg and 84 ± 18 grams/hour) with over three times this amount coming in solid forms. While more carbohydrate was ingested during the cycling portion, the rate of ingestion between cycling and running was similar. Kimber et al. (2002) reported that the average carbohydrate intake of female Ironman triathletes during the event was 1.0 g/kg/hour while male athletes achieved a rate of 1.1 g/kg/hour. Very large amounts (1.5 g/kg/hour) were ingested on the cycling portion, while one-third of that amount was ingested during the running portion. In the male athletes, carbohydrate intake was positively correlated with finishing time, but this was not confirmed in the female athletes. Carlsohn and Muller reported on the nutritional intake of six German mountain runners (five males, one female) throughout the completion of mountain running competitions that averaged 28.8 ± 15.0 kilometers and required 145 ± 67 minutes to complete. It was estimated that the athletes ingested 497 ± 128 grams of carbohydrate per day in their diet, which equated to 8.3 ± 1.8 g/kg/day.

During an ultra-endurance event held in Antarctica, 10 of the 17 competitors compiled dietary recall diaries every 24 hours for the duration of the event. The percentage contribution of macronutrients to daily energy intake for the entire group was CHO = 23.7% (221 ± 82 g.day−1), fat = 60.6% (251 ± 127 g.day−1) and protein = 15.7% (117 ± 52 g.day−1). There was a significant difference reported for energy intake between groups (faster finishers: 5,332 ± 469 vs. slower finishers: 3,048 ± 1,140 kcal.day−1; $p = 0.02$). The percentage contribution of macronutrients to daily energy intake for faster finishers was CHO = 17.4%, fat = 66.5% and protein = 16.1%. For the slower finishers, the percentage contribution of macronutrients was CHO = 28.6%, fat = 56.1% and protein = 15.3%. Mean fat and protein intakes were significantly different between faster and slower finishers (fat: 394 ± 1 vs. 190 ± 99 g.day−1 ($p = 0.02$) and protein: 172 ± 5 vs. 93 ± 34 g.day−1 ($p = 0.03$)). Carbohydrate intake was marginally higher in the faster finishers group (230 ± 61 g.day−1) compared to the slower finishers (217 ± 94 g. day−1), but was not statistically different ($p = 0.59$). Kumstat et al. (2016) reported that an elite open water swimmer ingested approximately of her energy from carbohydrates at a rate of approximately 60–80 grams of carbohydrate per hour.

An excellent resource regarding the carbohydrate intake of ultra-endurance athletes is a paper by Pfeiffer and colleagues (Pfeiffer et al. 2012) who surveyed 221 participants in events such as Ironman triathlons, marathons and 100–150 km cycle races. A post-race questionnaire was administered that quantified nutrient intake and found that carbohydrate ingestion rates varied greatly between competitors (6–136 g/hour). They found that individuals who consumed greater than the recommended 30–60 grams of carbohydrates per hour (Rodriguez, Di Marco, and Langley 2009a; Rodriguez, Di Marco, and Langley 2009b) performed significantly better. Unfortunately, and as highlighted throughout as a primary point to the chapter, the higher rates of carbohydrate ingestion were also associated with higher scores for nausea, flatulence, and symptoms of gastrointestinal distress.

Practically speaking, debate exists between the quality and quantity of various foods that should be considered during ultra-endurance events. While traditional carbohydrate-rich foods such as bananas, other fruits, granola bars, breads, bagels, honey, jam, biscuits, energy gels/bars and sports drinks are popular considerations, studies have indicated that in ultra-endurance events these foods and beverages become less appealing (Burke et al. 2001; Enqvist et al. 2010). The reasons for this shift is thought to be a combination of carbohydrate fatigue with taste sensation, natural utilization of more fat and protein as duration becomes more prolonged, and the likely occurrence that many forms of fat and protein may better survive the environmental elements while completing the event. Consequently, these athletes may be more prone to not consume as much of these foods and it may help to explain why energy expenditure exceeds energy intake. As explained in more detail later in the chapter, other practical considerations may offer valuable insight as to why carbohydrate needs are commonly not met by competing endurance athletes, particularly if they are female (Burke et al. 2001).

4.5 PROTEIN CONSIDERATIONS

There is no doubt that the primary fuel used by working muscle throughout ultra- or extreme endurance activities is carbohydrate. It is also well documented that protein oxidation increases throughout prolonged endurance exercise, particularly in those that extend well past two hours of activity (Burke and Deakin 2015). A review of the literature by Tarnopolsky (2004) concluded that dietary protein needs slightly above the RDA of 0.8 g/kg/day (~1.0 g/kg/day) are likely sufficient to meet the protein needs of endurance athletes completing low to moderate volumes of activity. Tarnopolsky also concluded that when daily activity and exercise volume reach a level that more closely matches those commonly seen in athletes completing extreme endurance activity, the maximal protein requirement was estimated to be 1.6 g/kg/day. However, studies directly investigating the protein needs of extreme endurance athletes are rare, which requires a reliance upon studies that have been completed using athletes who were completing higher volumes of training but were not necessarily ultra- or extreme bouts of endurance activity. Towards this end, Forslund et al. (Forslund et al. 1999) had athletes complete 90 minutes of exercise at 45–50% VO₂Max while consuming either 1.0 g/kg/day or 2.5 g/kg/day of protein. Nitrogen balance was negative at the lower dose and positive at the higher dose, suggesting that greater intakes of protein can better promote a positive nitrogen balance in athletes completing prolonged bouts of low to moderate intensity exercise. Other studies (Lamont, Patel, and Kalhan 1990, Meredith et al. 1989, Phillips et al. 1993) have also documented the failure to promote a positive nitrogen balance in endurance athletes completing moderate levels of training when consuming a daily protein intake of 0.86–1.0 g/kg/day. This is an important consideration for higher-level endurance athletes for a few key reasons. First, protein needs in those endurance athletes who are training and competing in much more prolonged activity seem to exhibit a greater daily need for dietary requirements. Second, overconsumption of protein, while not inherently dangerous, may displace the intake of valuable carbohydrates, which could undermine peak exercise performance. Of the few studies that have examined protein needs in high-level endurance athletes, a daily protein intake of 1.5–1.8 g/kg/day was suggested as the daily amount of protein required to maintain a positive nitrogen balance in the face of increased training volumes (Brouns et al. 1989; Friedman and Lemon 1989; Tarnopolsky, MacDougall, and Atkinson 1988).

In addition to daily dietary protein needs, several studies have investigated whether or not co-ingestion protein and carbohydrates can favorably impact recovery and exercise performance. In general, these studies have found that adding between 6.5–19.4 g of protein to carbohydrate drinks during exercise can improve various forms of endurance exercise performance (McLellan, Pasiakos, and Lieberman 2014; Osterberg, Zachwieja, and Smith 2008; Saunders et al. 2009; Saunders, Kane, and Todd 2004). Importantly, proper perspective must be used when considering this approach. For starters, the most common adverse event associated with extreme endurance activity is gastrointestinal-related, and consequently athletes are cautioned about introducing protein or amino acids into the body. However, several reports have indicated successful ingestion of protein-containing beverages, blocks, bars, or gels by various athletes participating in extreme endurance activity. As reported throughout, some athletes report "carbohydrate fatigue", and ingesting foods with protein or even fat can be welcomed. Another key point related to protein intake is the challenge of packing foods containing protein that do not need to be refrigerated or preserved during transport throughout the extreme endurance event. Finally, and as reported by Tarnopolsky (2004), a majority of endurance athletes do seem to be ingesting diets that can operate as a suitable starting point for daily protein

(Men: 1.8 ± 0.4 g/kg/day; Women: 1.2 ± 0.3 g/kg/day), but each athlete must be viewed individually as to ensure adequate protein is provided. Equally important is that these athletes avoid a scenario where adequate daily calories and carbohydrate intake is compromised, which will certainly negatively impact energy availability and exercise performance, in the pursuit of consuming greater amounts of daily protein.

4.6 FAT CONSIDERATIONS

For very prolonged events such as ultra-endurance activities, fat (lipid) intake becomes more important for two key reasons. First, as exercise duration extends beyond two hours, the likelihood that endogenous carbohydrate stores will become severely depleted is high resulting in the lack of a key fuel source for exercising muscle and other tissues that rely upon glucose as a fuel source. Second, as exercise duration increases the reliance upon fat as a fuel source increases markedly. Beyond acting as a fuel source, lipids also have several key functions inside the human body (i.e., essential elements of cell membranes, hormone production, storage of fat-soluble vitamins (Burke and Deakin 2015). In the past decade, interest in high-fat diets and even very-low carbohydrate, ketogenic diets as a dietary strategy to promote fuel utilization and endurance performance has exploded (Burke et al. 2000; Lambert et al. 1994; Muoio et al. 1994). While a number of studies have documented the ability of a high-fat diet to stimulate intramuscular adaptations that should shift fuel usage from carbohydrates to lipids during exercise, these adaptations have failed to consistently be translated to increases in performance (Burke et al. 2017; Burke 2015; Burke and Kiens 2006). What is consistently reported is that high-fat diets are associated with gut upset and gastrointestinal distress (Burke et al. 2007). While performance outcomes are mixed and adverse events are consistently reported, ultra-endurance athletes are strongly recommended to experiment with what diets, foods, and amount can be handled by one's gastrointestinal system, but the emphasis should remain on consuming enough carbohydrate in the diet. For these reasons, ultra-endurance athletes are generally recommended to adopt a diet that provides 25–35% of their calories from fat (Rodriguez, Di Marco, and Langley 2009a).

4.7 FLUID, HYDRATION, AND MICRONUTRIENT CONSIDERATIONS

Two primary nutritional concerns are present nearly every time an athlete attempts to train for or compete in an ultra-endurance exercise event: carbohydrate and fluid status. Dehydration can significantly impair exercise performance, stress the cardiovascular system and challenge one's health (Sawka et al. 2007). As dehydration progresses its impact on various types of performance is evident and for this reason, a primary nutritional goal should be to minimize major dehydration. Several factors work together (sweat rate, ambient temperate, humidity, wind currents, etc.) to impact how much an individual will sweat (McDermott et al. 2017; Sawka et al. 2007). It is important to note that if exercise duration is long enough and the environmental conditions are hot and humid, the onset of dehydration is viewed by many to be inevitable. For these reasons, endurance athletes are strongly advised to develop a hydration plan and monitor their fluid balance throughout workouts as to devise a plan that will help limit losses of body water to no more than 2–3% of body mass (Sawka et al. 2007; Shirreffs and Sawka 2011).

Prior to exercise, athletes are generally recommended to consume 5–7 mL of fluid per kilogram of body mass at least four hours prior to the training or competition. If urine production is very low or its color is dark gold or has a brownish tint, then an additional 3–5 mL/kg can be considered. Practically, for many athletes, this translates into ingesting 350–600 mL of fluid at least four hours before and another 150–400 mL of fluid in closer proximity to the event. For those athletes who struggle with maintaining fluid balance or are competing in very long events in hot and humid environmental conditions, "hyper-hydration" strategies might be considered. While these strategies do increase body water levels and can improve thermoregulation (van Rosendal et al. 2010), some concerns regarding these approaches should be discussed. For starters, the urgency to void your bladder during competition will be increased, hyperhydration can lead to dilution of one's blood resulting in reduced blood sodium levels and increase the risk of developing hyponatremia (Montain, Cheuvront, and Sawka 2006) and finally, many hyperhydrating agents and strategies are banned for competition. In considering the maintenance of fluid levels throughout competition, it should be highlighted again that athletes are strongly encouraged to plan strategically. Simply recommending that an athlete should ingest 1.5–2 cups of a 6–8% carbohydrate/electrolyte solution every 10–15 minutes throughout exercise may not be realistic in all situations. While this recommendation does serve as an excellent goal and foundation from which all endurance athletes can strive to maintain fluid balance and deliver adequate carbohydrate (Sawka et al. 2007), other practical factors such as individual sweat rates, environmental conditions, race distances, and course profiles must be considered. Drink composition can significantly impact the rate at which fluid is released from the gut, with hypertonic solutions exhibiting slow gastric release and subsequent fluid absorption (Brouns et al. 1995; Noakes, Rehrer, and Maughan 1991). In this respect, consuming a drink that contains multiple forms of carbohydrate can help athletes achieve higher rates of fluid delivery with greater gastrointestinal tolerance when compared to ingestion of single carbohydrates at higher ingestion rates (Jeukendrup and Moseley 2010). Finally, all such drinks should contain sodium (10–30 mM) as a strategy to help drive fluid ingestion, promote optimal fluid absorption and minimize risk of hyponatremia.

In what can be confusing for athletes, consuming excessive amounts of water can increase the risk of developing hyponatremia, low blood sodium levels, which can lead to initial side effects very similar to dehydration (mental confusion, weakness, and fainting). These symptoms commonly (but not always) begin when serum sodium reaches 126–130 mEq/L while values below 126 mEq/L can lead to very serious side effects such as seizures, coma, and death. Normal blood sodium levels have a range of 135–145 mEq/L. It is important for athletes to recognize the symptoms, but they should understand that not all people who develop hyponatremia will present with classical symptoms. While some people view that adding sodium to beverages will best prevent hyponatremia, other reports have suggested that an emphasis should be made on simply avoiding purposeful over-consumption of fluid.

Multiple studies have assessed fluid intake in different extreme endurance scenarios. For example, Barrero et al. (2014) assessed fluid balance during an ultra-endurance triathlon in ten participants. Slightly over four liters of fluid (4,188 ± 1837 mL) were consumed at an average rate of 366.6 ± 146.9 mL/hour. Additionally, approximately 2,152 ± 1124 mg of sodium were ingested. As part of an elite ski mountaineering race, Praz et al. (2014) indicated that competitive ski mountaineering athletes consumed 1.8 ± 0.7 L throughout a race that required them between 5–6 hours to complete. Additionally, the average body weight loss throughout the race 1.5 ± 1.1 kg (2 ± 1% of body mass). In a simulated 160-kilometer adventure race, Zimberg and investigators (2008) reported that those who were able to finish the simulated race ($n = 13$) consumed higher amounts of fluid (19.4 ± 8.1 L) and sodium (16.4 ± 9.5 g) than non-finishers ($n = 10$). Finally and as reported by Stellingwerff (2016) three elite ultramarathoners reported ingesting 6,907 ± 2,426 mg of sodium for an average of 426 ± 176 mg sodium/hour of activity.

4.8   SUPPLEMENT CONSIDERATIONS

Overwhelmingly, it should be clear that the primary nutritional considerations for an athlete participating in any form of extreme endurance activity should be adequate energy and carbohydrate intake. The most commonly reported nutritional supplement in extreme endurance athletes is caffeine. A robust literature base has documented caffeine's ability to operate in an ergogenic fashion, particularly during endurance exercise (Glade 2010; Goldstein et al. 2010; Graham 2001). Common dosages range from 3–6 mg/kg body mass taken approximately one hour prior to exercise, however, studies involving prolonged exercise has also indicated the smaller doses (1–2 mg/kg body mass) can also serve an ergogenic role, even if ingested late in the exercise bout (Cox et al. 2002). Pharmacokinetically, caffeine reaches peak concentrations within 30–90 minute with a half-life of five hours. Notably, Cox et al. (Cox et al. 2002) recommended a dose of 3 mg/kg body mass approximately one hour prior to starting and then an additional 1 mg/kg body mass every two hours after starting exercise. In reviewing the dietary intake of three elite ultramarathoners, Stellingwerff (2016) reported an average caffeine intake of 912 ± 322 mg (55 ± 22 mg/hour). While considered a high intake, one must realize the average duration of events for these athletes was 16.7 ± 2.5 hours.

A clear pattern exists between the incidence of stomach upset and gastric distress in endurance athletes. For these reasons, ultra-endurance athletes have reported consuming ginger throughout prolonged bouts of exercise. For example, ultra-marathoners reported ingesting 12.5 grams of ginger throughout a 19.5-hour race while another ingested 4.2 grams while completing a 14.88-hour event (Stellingwerff 2016). Due to known individualized responses to ingestion of ginger and other supplements, all athletes are encouraged to experiment prior to competition.

4.9   OTHER CONSIDERATIONS

As highlighted throughout this chapter, the extended duration of many ultra-endurance events brings forth many challenges. The most notable of these challenges is gastrointestinal problems. Previously, Rehrer et al. (1992) reported that, depending on the event, the prevalence of gastrointestinal complaints ranges from 10–95% while Pfeiffer et al. (Pfeiffer et al. 2012) indicated severe gastrointestinal distress occurred from 4% in marathon running and up to 32% in Ironman triathlon races. Furthermore, evidence exists to suggest that some people are more predisposed to developing gastrointestinal distress with common symptoms being dizziness, nausea, cramps (stomach or intestinal), vomiting, and diarrhea. While optimal nutrition is an important factor, various foods have been linked to a greater likelihood of gastrointestinal problems and for these reasons should be avoided prior to and throughout completion of prolonged endurance exercise. In this respect, Rehrer et al. (1992) identified a link in reported gastrointestinal problems and the intake of foods containing fiber, fat, protein, and concentrated carbohydrate solutions throughout a triathlon. This is particularly perplexing for athletes as extremely high rates of carbohydrate intake are needed to modulate performance, but reports linked greater incidence of nausea, flatulence, loose stool, and leaky gut with higher amounts of carbohydrate intake (Pfeiffer et al. 2012).

To avoid gastrointestinal complications, it is recommended (Jeukendrup 2011; Rodriguez, Di Marco, and Langley 2009a) that athletes develop and outline a feeding regimen to best understand what form (liquid, gel, or solid) of food and what amounts will predict the smallest number of complications. While pragmatic and strongly recommended, the reader must realize this suggestion might be a challenge (or downright impossible) for some activities. For example, in reviewing the dietary practice of three elite ultramarathoners, Stellingwerff (2016) highlighted the challenge of truly practicing race-day nutrition because their typical training runs likely don't exceed 30 miles, while their events might span 50–100 miles.

Several best-case scenarios and recommendations have been presented for athletes participating in an array of endurance and ultra-endurance events. When these events are completed over the course of several days on unmarked trails, in extreme cold or extreme heat, in mountains, or require brief periods of swimming, several pragmatic challenges arise that cannot be overlooked. For example, the ability to appropriately pack necessary items and the subsequent bulk, weight, and shift in biomechanics that results from carrying them, all work to make the event more challenging. In addition, the challenge of maintaining a supply of clean drinking water and avoidance of subsequent gastrointestinal distress all work to impact these athlete's health and performance throughout these events.

4.10 CONCLUSIONS

In conclusion, training for and competing in prolonged, extreme, or ultra-endurance events requires remarkable expenditure of energy and exerts a physical and mental toll on the athlete. Currently, such events are seemingly growing in number each year, with each one requiring more distance and more fuel, oftentimes in harsh, extreme environmental conditions. In preparing for these events, the athlete must focus on three primary goals: consume enough calories, ingest enough carbohydrate and maintain hydration levels. Undoubtedly, on the day of competition, the likelihood an athlete will reach a negative energy balance, often of extremely large magnitudes, is high, which requires significant planning and preparation. These planning efforts should seek not to avoid deficiencies altogether but should work to minimize them on competition days and throughout training. Carbohydrate needs should take priority with a broad recommendation of 6–10 g/kg/day and the athlete should strive to be consume carbohydrate at all points in time throughout their days. Protein needs are also increased and while distinct recommendations for extreme endurance athletes, a recommended daily protein intake of 1.4–1.8 g/kg/day has been suggested to be a reasonable starting point. High-fat, ketogenic, and fat supplementation have been purported to offer distinct intramuscular metabolic adaptations and advantages, but consistent reports of gastrointestinal upset and no change or a decrease in performance continue to preclude their recommendation. Maintaining necessary hydration levels should be viewed with the highest level of importance as the completion of long and prolonged bouts of endurance exercise can result in significant dehydration, which will decrease exercise performance, increase thermal load and strain on the cardiovascular system. Finally, nutritional supplementation of caffeine in dosages ranging from 3–6 mg/kg is the most common and has been shown to yield positive ergogenic physical outcomes related to exercise, but may also help with substrate utilization during exercise, and improve perceptions of effort and cognition.

ACKNOWLEDGMENTS

The author would like to acknowledge his previous mentors, students, and colleagues for providing continual inspiration and motivation to complete projects such as these. Special thanks are extended to Jeff Rothschild, MS, RD, CSSD, CSCS, for his valuable insight.

REFERENCES

Barrero, A., P. Erola, and R. Bescos. 2014. "Energy balance of triathletes during an ultra-endurance event". *Nutrients* 7 (1):209–22. doi:10.3390/nu7010209.

Brouns, F., W. H. Saris, J. Stroecken, E. Beckers, R. Thijssen, N. J. Rehrer, and F. ten Hoor. 1989. "Eating, drinking, and cycling. A controlled Tour de France simulation study, Part I". *Int J Sports Med* 10 (Suppl 1):S32–40. doi:10.1055/s-2007-1024952.

Brouns, F., J. Senden, E. J. Beckers, and W. H. Saris. 1995. "Osmolarity does not affect the gastric emptying rate of oral rehydration solutions". *JPEN J Parenter Enter Nutr* 19 (5):403–6. doi:10.1177/0148607195019005403.

Burke, L. M. 2007. "Nutrition strategies for the marathon: fuel for training and racing". *Sports Med* 37 (4–5):344–7.

Burke, L. M. 2015. "Re-examining high-fat diets for sports performance: did we call the 'Nail in the Coffin' too soon?". *Sports Med* 45 (S1):S33–49. doi:10.1007/s40279-015-0393-9.

Burke, L. M., D. J. Angus, G. R. Cox, N. K. Cummings, M. A. Febbraio, K. Gawthorn, J. A. Hawley, M. Minehan, D. T. Martin, and M. Hargreaves. 2000. "Effect of fat adaptation and carbohydrate restoration on metabolism and performance during prolonged cycling". *J Appl Physiol* 89 (6):2413–21.

Burke, L. M., G. R. Cox, N. K. Culmmings, and B. Desbrow. 2001. "Guidelines for daily carbohydrate intake: do athletes achieve them?". *Sports Med* 31 (4):267–99.

Burke, L. M., and V. Deakin, eds. 2015. *Clinical Sports Nutrition*. Australia: McGraw Hill Education.

Burke, L. M., J. A. Hawley, S. H. Wong, and A. E. Jeukendrup. 2011. "Carbohydrates for training and competition". *J Sports Sci* 29 (Suppl 1):S17–27. doi:10.1080/02640414.2011.585473.

Burke, L. M., and B. Kiens. 2006. "'Fat adaptation' for athletic performance: The nail in the coffin?" *J Appl Physiol* 100 (1):7–8. doi:10.1152/japplphysiol.01238.2005.

Burke, L. M., G. Millet, M. A. Tarnopolsky, and Federations International Association of Athletics. 2007. "Nutrition for distance events". *J Sports Sci* 25 (Suppl 1):S29–38. doi:10.1080/02640410701607239.

Burke, L. M., M. L. Ross, L. A. Garvican-Lewis, M. Welvaert, I. A. Heikura, S. G. Forbes, J. G. Mirtschin, L. E. Cato, N. Strobel, A. P. Sharma, and J. A. Hawley. 2017. "Low carbohydrate, high fat diet impairs exercise economy and negates the performance benefit from intensified training in elite race walkers". *J Physiol* 595 (9):2785–807. doi:10.1113/jp273230.

Cox, G. R., B. Desbrow, P. G. Montgomery, M. E. Anderson, C. R. Bruce, T. A. Macrides, D. T. Martin, A. Moquin, A. Roberts, J. A. Hawley, and L. M. Burke. 2002. "Effect of different protocols of caffeine intake on metabolism and endurance performance." *J Appl Physiol* 93 (3):990–9. doi: 10.1152/japplphysiol.00249.2002.

Coyle, E. F., A. E. Jeukendrup, M. C. Oseto, B. J. Hodgkinson, and T. W. Zderic. 2001. "Low-fat diet alters intramuscular substrates and reduces lipolysis and fat oxidation during exercise". *Am J Physiol Endocrinol Metab* 280 (3):E391–8.

Cuddy, J. S., D. R. Slivka, W. S. Hailes, C. L. Dumke, and B. C. Ruby. 2010. "Metabolic profile of the Ironman World Championships: a case study". *Int J Sports Physiol Perform* 5 (4):570–6.

Enqvist, J. K., C. M. Mattsson, P. H. Johansson, T. Brink-Elfegoun, L. Bakkman, and B. T. Ekblom. 2010. "Energy turnover during 24 hours and 6 days of adventure racing". *J Sports Sci* 28 (9):947–55. doi:10.1080/02640411003734069.

Forslund, A. H., A. E. El-Khoury, R. M. Olsson, A. M. Sjodin, L. Hambraeus, and V. R. Young. 1999. "Effect of protein intake and physical activity on 24-h pattern and rate of macronutrient utilization". *Am J Physiol* 276 (5): E964–76.

Foster, C., D. L. Costill, and W. J. Fink. 1979. "Effects of preexercise feedings on endurance performance". *Med Sci Sports Exerc* 11:1–5.

Friedman, J. E., and P. W. Lemon. 1989. "Effect of chronic endurance exercise on retention of dietary protein". *Int J Sports Med* 10 (2):118–23. doi:10.1055/s-2007-1024886.

Glade, M. J. 2010. "Caffeine-not just a stimulant". *Nutrition* 26 (10):932–8. doi:10.1016/j.nut.2010.08.004.

Goldstein, E. R., T. Ziegenfuss, D. Kalman, R. Kreider, B. Campbell, C. Wilborn, L. Taylor, D. Willoughby, J. Stout, B. S. Graves, R. Wildman, J. L. Ivy, M. Spano, A. E. Smith, and J. Antonio. 2010. "International society of sports nutrition position stand: caffeine and performance". *J Int Soc Sports Nutr* 7 (1):5. doi:10.1186/1550-2783-7-5.

Graham, T. E. 2001. "Caffeine and exercise: metabolism, endurance and performance". *Sports Med* Sports Med 31 (11):785–807.

Hawley, J. A., E. J. Schabort, T. D. Noakes, and S. C. Dennis. 1997. "Carbohydrate-loading and exercise performance. An update". *Sports Med* 24 (2):73–81.

Heydenreich, J., B. Kayser, Y. Schutz, and K. Melzer. 2017. "Total energy expenditure, energy intake, and body composition in endurance athletes across the training season: a systematic review". *Sports Med Open* 3 (1):8. doi:10.1186/s40798-017-0076-1.

Jeukendrup, A. E. 2011. "Nutrition for endurance sports: marathon, triathlon, and road cycling". *J Sports Sci* 29 (Suppl 1):S91–9. doi:10.1080/02640414.2011.610348.

Jeukendrup, A. E., and R. Jentjens. 2000. "Oxidation of carbohydrate feedings during prolonged exercise: current thoughts, guidelines and directions for future research". *Sports Med* 29 (6):407–24.

Jeukendrup, A. E., and S. C. Killer. 2010. "The myths surrounding pre-exercise carbohydrate feeding". *Ann Nutr Metab* 57 (Suppl 2):18–25. doi:10.1159/000322698.

Jeukendrup, A. E., and L. Moseley. 2010. "Multiple transportable carbohydrates enhance gastric emptying and fluid delivery". *Scand J Med Sci Sports* 20 (1):112–21. doi:10.1111/j.1600-0838.2008.00862.x.

Kerksick, C. M., S. Arent, B. J. Schoenfeld, J. R. Stout, B. Campbell, C. D. Wilborn, L. Taylor, D. Kalman, A. E. Smith-Ryan, R. B. Kreider, D. Willoughby, P. J. Arciero, T. A. VanDusseldorp, M. J. Ormsbee, R. Wildman, M. Greenwood, T. N. Ziegenfuss, A. A. Aragon, and J. Antonio. 2017. "International society of sports nutrition position stand: nutrient timing". *J Int Soc Sports Nutr* 14 (1):33. doi:10.1186/s12970-017-0189-4.

Kimber, N. E., J. J. Ross, S. L. Mason, and D. B. Speedy. 2002. "Energy balance during an ironman triathlon in male and female triathletes". *Int J Sport Nutr Exerc Metab* 12 (1):47–62.

Kreider, R. B., C. D. Wilborn, L. Taylor, B. Campbell, A. L. Almada, R. Collins, M. Cooke, C. P. Earnest, M. Greenwood, D. S. Kalman, C. M. Kerksick, S. M. Kleiner, B. Leutholtz, H. Lopez, L. M. Lowery, R. Mendel, A. Smith, M. Spano, R. Wildman, D. S. Willoughby, T. N. Ziegenfuss, and J. Antonio. 2010. "ISSN exercise & sports nutrition review: research & recommendations". *J Int Soc Sports Nutr* 7 (1). doi:10.1186/1550-2783-7-7.

Kumstat, M., S. Rybarova, A. Thomas, and J. Novotny. 2016. "Case study: competition nutrition intakes during the open water swimming grand prix races in elite female swimmer". *Int J Sport Nutr Exerc Metab* 26 (4):370–6. doi:10.1123/ijsnem.2015-0168.

Lambert, E. V., D. P. Speechly, S. C. Dennis, and T. D. Noakes. 1994. "Enhanced endurance in trained cyclists during moderate intensity exercise following 2 weeks adaptation to a high fat diet". *Eur J Appl Physiol Occup Physiol* 69 (4):287–93.

Lamont, L. S., D. G. Patel, and S. C. Kalhan. 1990. "Leucine kinetics in endurance-trained humans". *J Appl Physiol* 69 (1):1–6.

Lemon, P. W., and J. P. Mullin. 1980. "Effect of initial muscle glycogen levels on protein catabolism during exercise". *J Appl Physiol Respir Environ Exer Physiol* 48 (4):624–9.

McDermott, B. P., S. A. Anderson, L. E. Armstrong, D. J. Casa, S. N. Cheuvront, L. Cooper, W. L. Kenney, F. G. O'Connor, and W. O. Roberts. 2017. "National Athletic Trainers' Association position statement: fluid replacement for the physically active". *J Athl Train* 52 (9):877–95. doi:10.4085/1062-6050-52.9.02.

McLellan, T. M., S. M. Pasiakos, and H. R. Lieberman. 2014. "Effects of protein in combination with carbohydrate supplements on acute or repeat endurance exercise performance: a systematic review." *Sports Med* 44 (4):535–50. doi:10.1007/s40279-013-0133-y.

Meredith, C. N., M. J. Zackin, W. R. Frontera, and W. J. Evans. 1989. "Dietary protein requirements and body protein metabolism in endurance-trained men". *J Appl Physiol* 66 (6):2850–6.

Meyer, N. L., M. M. Manore, and C. Helle. 2011. "Nutrition for winter sports". *J Sports Sci* 29 (Suppl 1):S127–36. doi:10.1080/02640414.2011.574721.

Montain, S. J., S. N. Cheuvront, and M. N. Sawka. 2006. "Exercise associated hyponatraemia: quantitative analysis to understand the aetiology". *Br J Sports Med* 40 (2):98–105; discussion 98–105. doi:10.1136/bjsm.2005.018481.

Moseley, L., G. I. Lancaster, and A. E. Jeukendrup. 2003. "Effects of timing of pre-exercise ingestion of carbohydrate on subsequent metabolism and cycling performance". *Eur J Appl Physiol* 88 (4–5):453–8. doi:10.1007/s00421-002-0728-8.

Mountjoy, M., J. Sundgot-Borgen, L. Burke, S. Carter, N. Constantini, C. Lebrun, N. Meyer, R. Sherman, K. Steffen, R. Budgett, and A. Ljungqvist. 2014. "The IOC consensus statement: beyond the Female Athlete Triad – Relative Energy Deficiency in Sport (RED-S)". *Br J Sports Med* 48 (7):491–7. doi:10.1136/bjsports-2014-093502.

Muoio, D. M., J. J. Leddy, P. J. Horvath, A. B. Awad, and D. R. Pendergast. 1994. "Effect of dietary fat on metabolic adjustments to maximal VO_2 and endurance in runners". *Med Sci Sports Exerc* 26 (1):81–8.

Noakes, T. D., N. J. Rehrer, and R. J. Maughan. 1991. "The importance of volume in regulating gastric emptying". *Med Sci Sports Exerc* 23 (3):307–13.

Osterberg, K. L., J. J. Zachwieja, and J. W. Smith. 2008. "Carbohydrate and carbohydrate + protein for cycling time-trial performance". *J Sports Sci* 26 (3):227–33. doi:10.1080/02640410701459730.

Pfeiffer, B., T. Stellingwerff, A. B. Hodgson, R. Randell, K. Pottgen, P. Res, and A. E. Jeukendrup. 2012. "Nutritional intake and gastrointestinal problems during competitive endurance events". *Med Sci Sports Exerc* 44 (2):344–51. doi:10.1249/MSS.0b013e31822dc809.

Pfeiffer, B., T. Stellingwerff, E. Zaltas, and A. E. Jeukendrup. 2010a. "CHO oxidation from a CHO gel compared with a drink during exercise". *Med Sci Sports Exerc* 42 (11):2038–45. doi:10.1249/MSS.0b013e3181e0efe6.

Pfeiffer, B., T. Stellingwerff, E. Zaltas, and A. E. Jeukendrup. 2010b. "Oxidation of solid versus liquid CHO sources during exercise". *Med Sci Sports Exerc* 42 (11):2030–7. doi:10.1249/MSS.0b013e3181e0efc9.

Phillips, S. M., S. A. Atkinson, M. A. Tarnopolsky, and J. D. MacDougall. 1993. "Gender differences in leucine kinetics and nitrogen balance in endurance athletes". *J Appl Physiol* 75 (5):2134–41.

Praz, C., B. Leger, and B. Kayser. 2014. "Energy expenditure of extreme competitive mountaineering skiing". *Eur J Appl Physiol* 114 (10):2201–11. doi:10.1007/s00421-014-2939-1.

Ranchordas, M. K. 2012. "Nutrition for adventure racing". *Sports Med* 42 (11):915–27. doi:10.2165/11635130-000000000-00000.

Rehrer, N. J., F. Brouns, E. J. Beckers, W. O. Frey, B. Villiger, C. J. Riddoch, P. P. Menheere, and W. H. Saris. 1992. "Physiological changes and gastro-intestinal symptoms as a result of ultra-endurance running.". *Europ J Appl Physiol* 64 (1):1–8.

Rodriguez, N. R., N. M. Di Marco, and S. Langley. 2009a. "American College of Sports Medicine position stand. Nutrition and athletic performance". *Med Sci Sports Exerc* 41 (3):709–31. doi:10.1249/MSS.0b013e31890eb86.

Rodriguez, N. R., N. M. DiMarco, S. Langley, American Dietetic Association, Dietitians of Canada, and American College of Sports Medicine: Nutrition and Athletic Performance. 2009b. "Position of the American Dietetic Association, Dietitians of Canada, and the American College of Sports Medicine: nutrition and athletic performance". *J Am Diet Assoc* 109 (3):509–27.

Romijn, J. A., E. F. Coyle, L. S. Sidossis, A. Gastaldelli, J. F. Horowitz, E. Endert, and R. R. Wolfe. 1993. "Regulation of endogenous fat and carbohydrate metabolism in relation to exercise intensity and duration". *Am J Physiol Endocrinol Metab* 265 (3): E380–91.

Sanchez-Munoz, C., M. Zabala, and J. J. Muros. 2016. "Nutritional intake and anthropometric changes of professional road cyclists during a 4-day competition". *Scand J Med Sci Sports* 26 (7):802–8. doi:10.1111/sms.12513.

Saris, W. H., M. A. van Erp-Baart, F. Brouns, K. R. Westerterp, and F. ten Hoor. 1989. "Study on food intake and energy expenditure during extreme sustained exercise: the Tour de France". *Int J Sports Med* 10 (Suppl 1):S26–31. doi:10.1055/s-2007-1024951.

Saunders, M. J., M. D. Kane, and M. K. Todd. 2004. "Effects of a carbohydrate-protein beverage on cycling endurance and muscle damage". *Med Sci Sports Exerc* 36 (7):1233–8.

Saunders, M. J., R. W. Moore, A. K. Kies, N. D. Luden, and C. A. Pratt. 2009. "Carbohydrate and protein hydrolysate coingestions improvement of late-exercise time-trial performance". *Int J Sport Nutr Exerc Metab* 19 (2):136–49.

Sawka, M. N., L. M. Burke, E. R. Eichner, R. J. Maughan, S. J. Montain, and N. S. Stachenfeld. 2007. "American College of Sports Medicine position stand. Exercise and fluid replacement". *Med Sci Sports Exerc* 39 (2):377–90. doi:10.1249/mss.0b013e31802ca597.

Shirreffs, S. M., and M. N. Sawka. 2011. "Fluid and electrolyte needs for training, competition, and recovery". *J Sports Sci* 29 (Suppl 1):S39–46. doi:10.1080/02640414.2011.614269.

Smith, J. W., J. J. Zachwieja, F. Peronnet, D. H. Passe, D. Massicotte, C. Lavoie, and D. D. Pascoe. 2010. "Fuel selection and cycling endurance performance with ingestion of [13C]glucose: Evidence for a carbohydrate dose response". *J Appl Physiol* 108 (6):1520–9. doi:10.1152/japplphysiol.91394.2008.

Speedy, D. B., T. D. Noakes, N. E. Kimber, I. R. Rogers, J. M. Thompson, D. R. Boswell, J. J. Ross, R. G. Campbell, P. G. Gallagher, and J. A. Kuttner. 2001. "Fluid balance during and after an ironman triathlon". *Clin J Sport Med* 11 (1):44–50.

Stellingwerff, T. 2016. "Competition nutrition practices of elite ultramarathon runners". *Int J Sport Nutr Exerc Metab* 26 (1):93–9. doi:10.1123/ijsnem.2015-0030.

Sullo, A., M. Monda, G. Brizzi, V. Meninno, A. Papa, P. Lombardi, and B. Fabbri. 1998. "The effect of a carbohydrate loading on running performance during a 25-km treadmill time trial by level of aerobic capacity in athletes". *Eur Rev Med Pharmacol Sci* 2 (5-6):195–202.

Tarnopolsky, M. 2004. "Protein requirements for endurance athletes". *Nutrition* 20 (7–8): 662–8. doi:10.1016/j.nut.2004.04.008.

Tarnopolsky, M. A., J. D. MacDougall, and S. A. Atkinson. 1988. "Influence of protein intake and training status on nitrogen balance and lean body mass". *J Appl Physiol* 64 (1):187–93.

van Rosendal, S. P., M. A. Osborne, R. G. Fassett, and J. S. Coombes. 2010. "Guidelines for glycerol use in hyperhydration and rehydration associated with exercise". *Sports Med* 40 (2):113–29. doi:10.2165/11530760-000000000-00000.

VanHeest, J. L., C. E. Mahoney, and L. Herr. 2004. "Characteristics of elite open-water swimmers". *J Strength Cond Res* 18 (2):302–5. doi:10.1519/R-13513.1.

Zimberg, I. Z., C. A. Crispim, C. R. Juzwiak, H. K. Antunes, B. Edwards, J. Waterhouse, S. Tufik, and M. T. de Mello. 2008. "Nutritional intake during a simulated adventure race". *Int J Sport Nutr Exerc Metab* 18 (2):152–68.

Section III

Overview of Food and
Nutritional Requirements for
Diverse Extreme Sports

5 Functional Foods
Role in Endurance Sports

Kamesh Venkatakrishnan and Chin-Kun Wang

CONTENTS

5.1 Introduction 74
5.2 Sports Nutrition 75
5.3 Endurance Sports.. 75
5.4 Bioenergetics (Energy Flow) 76
5.5 Evaluating Caloric/Energy Needs for Athletes 77
5.6 Total Energy Expenditure (TEE).. 77
5.7 Total Energy Intake (TEI) 78
5.8 Muscle Metabolism.. 78
5.9 The Myth about Lactic Acid and Muscle Pain (Sensor of Pain) 79
5.10 Role of Macro and Micronutrients for Endurance Sports 79
    5.10.1 Macronutrients... 79
        5.10.1.1 Carbohydrates 79
        5.10.1.2 Importance of Carbohydrates on Physical or Athletic
                 Performance 80
        5.10.1.3 Proteins (Amino Acids) 80
        5.10.1.4 Importance of Proteins on Physical or Athletic
                 Performance 81
        5.10.1.5 Recommendation of Carb and Protein for Endurance
                 Athletes Weighing 85 kg (before and after Exercise/
                 Training Based on the Reports of Rasmussen, 2008).......... 81
        5.10.1.6 Fats/Lipids 82
        5.10.1.7 Fat Requirement for Athletes...82
    5.10.2 Micronutrients 83
        5.10.2.1 Vitamins..83
5.11 Role of Vitamins for Improving Performance in Athletes (Endurance) 83
5.12 Minerals (Electrolytes) 84
    5.12.1 Macrominerals..84
    5.12.2 Microminerals/Trace Elements 85
5.13 Ergogenic Drugs or Agent 85
5.14 Popular Ergogenic Compounds 85
    5.14.1 Caffeine 85
    5.14.2 L-Creatine...86
    5.14.3 Taurine 86
    5.14.4 L-Carnitine 87

        5.14.5 β-Hydroxy-β-Methyl Butyrate (HMB) 87
        5.14.6 Sodium Bicarbonate/Citrate 87
        5.14.7 β Alanine 87
5.15 Nutritional Aid...88
        5.15.1 Ergogenic Herbs 88
                5.15.1.1 *Panax ginseng* (Chinese/Asian Ginseng–Saponins:
                            Ginsenoside)...88
                5.15.1.2 *Eurycoma longifolia* Jack (Malaysian Ginseng)................89
                5.15.1.3 *Eleutherococcus senticosus* or *Acanthopanax*
                            senticosus (Siberian Ginseng)....................................89
                5.15.1.4 *Paullinia cupana* (Guarana) 90
                5.15.1.5 *Withania somnifera* (Indian Ginseng–Relaxing)...............90
                5.15.1.6 *Schisandra chinensis* 91
                5.15.1.7 *Rhodiola rosea* (Vitality; Rhodioloside–Bitter Flavor
                            Added to Salads) 91
                5.15.1.8 *Cordyceps sinensis* (Tibetan Mushroom–Fungi)...............92
        5.15.2 Ephedrine (Banned in Most Countries)..92
5.16 Role of Ergogenic Functional Food/Nutraceuticals on Endurance
        Sports/Athletes..93
        5.16.1   *Allium sativum* (Garlic)...93
        5.16.2   *Zingiber officinale* (Ginger) 93
        5.16.3   Green Tea (EGCG) 94
        5.16.4   *Beta vulgaris* (Beetroots)..94
        5.16.5   *Citrullus vulgaris/lanatus* (Watermelon) 95
        5.16.6   *Prunus cerasus* (Tart Cherry/Sour Cherry)..................................96
        5.16.7   *Citrus aurantium* (Bitter Orange) 96
        5.16.8   *Garcinia* (Hydroxycitric Acid) 97
        5.16.9   Quercetin..97
        5.16.10 Resveratrol..97
        5.16.11 Tapioca (Starch; Amylopectin) 98
5.17 Mechanism of Ergogenic (Adaptogenic) Herbs for Biochemical
        Tuning for Athletes 99
5.18 Conclusion 99
References..99

5.1 INTRODUCTION

Nutrition plays a crucial role in athlete health, fitness and training ability and thus has a direct impact on athlete performance. The purpose of this chapter is to address the roles of various functional foods/nutraceuticals (nutritional supplements) for endurance athletes to ensure the maximum benefits regarding athletic performance (training), body composition and optimal health status. Numerous studies have demonstrated that endurance athletes can improve their training period/duration and performance by properly scheduling their training plans with taking balanced nutrients (Bridge and Jones, 2006; Saunders et al., 2004). Since athletes (especially endurance sportsmen) do extensive workout/training or exercise, they are highly prone to nutritional deficiency (especially micronutrients) than the general population and hence consumption of a proper diet (balanced diet) with sufficient micro- and macronutrients will boost their performance by helping them avoid illness or injury (Lundy, 2011; Snell et al., 2010).

5.2 SPORTS NUTRITION

Sports nutrition is a field of study dealing with proper training and a sensible approach to nutrition (diet plan) to ensure the maximum benefits regarding athletic performance, body composition and optimal health and wellness (Fink, 2017). It is impossible to recommend a single diet plan for all athletes; it varies in each individual and the type of sport. However, following the planned diet pattern (eating regularly, especially breakfast, with a balanced diet and plenty of water/electrolytes) with regular training could considerably improve sports performance. Therefore, it is essential for all members of the athlete's team, especially the trainer/coach/sports nutritionist, to have a good knowledge about different diets (nutrients or supplements) and their metabolic properties to ensure the maximum return from training (to enhance performance). The types of food and their route of administration, as well as the timing of nutrient intake to avoid gastric discomfort, are crucial for athletes to get the maximum benefits. In addition, athletes must know the factors (lack of nutrients or electrolytes) that contribute to muscle weakness/soreness or fatigue, which result in reduced performance. Hence, a proper nutritional regimen with an appropriate scheduled exercise program is the key to success, resulting in enhanced performance and function (Eberle, 2018).

5.3 ENDURANCE SPORTS

Endurance sports are a collection of many competitive sports in which each athlete exercises or works out his crucial muscles at submaximal intensity for long periods of time. The term includes cycling, swimming, running (marathon/triathlon-combination), wrestling, weightlifting, etc. Endurance athletes need additional nutritional strategies (nutritional/sports supplements) with proper training to maximize their performance by combating certain factors that might limit the performance (Ryan, 2012). The common problem faced by endurance athletes includes maintaining adequate calories with lean body mass (LBM), particularly for weight-related endurance sports athletes (due to eating disorder), while they must also make sure to intake a sufficient amount of micronutrients (minerals and vitamins) and macronutrient (protein (ptn), carbohydrates (carb), and fats). Muscle cramp and heat shock are also frequent events that might hamper the endurance capacity. Hence, sufficient electrolytes should be consumed during and after workout or training (electrolyte replenishment). Endurance sportspersons are highly prone to exercise-induced oxidative stress, as intense aerobic exercise would facilitate the production of excessive free radicals (nullifying antioxidants) and result in oxidative stress (an imbalance between oxidant and antioxidant), which in turn triggers inflammatory response and eventually resulting in muscle damage or fatigue (physiological stress). It is better to maintain both physical and emotional health status through the training and competition period to get better results or performance in the competition.

As mentioned above, endurance athletes' teams (especially the sports nutritionist and coach/trainer) must have a good knowledge of the factors that might enhance or suppress the athletic performance. The primary limiting factors include depletion of muscle glycogen contents (lacto-acidosis), decreased blood and muscle glucose level, central and muscular fatigue, illness or injury, dehydration (sweat/evaporation/gas exchange-fluid loss) which leads to imbalance in cardiac output and lack of proper sleep or rest due to emotional problems (stress). Hormonal fluctuation associated with menopause (physical and emotional changes) would significantly limit the performance in female endurance athletes (Kellmann, 2010). Meanwhile, the major enhancing factors include consistent training with a balanced diet and supplementation of ergogenic agents to maintain adequate muscle glycogen content (glycogen replenishment) after exercise (Fullagar et al., 2015; Thibault, 2006). The better nutrient supplements for endurance athletes include meal replacement powders (MRP), energy bars, energy drinks (glucose-electrolyte solution), energy gels and water. Liquid supplements are highly preferred during thermal stress-related endurance sports (to avoid nausea and gastric discomfort). For a further understanding of endurance sports nutrition, a basic knowledge of the primary energy system is a must. Therefore, the author would like to give a brief note on bioenergetics (energy or calorie requirement/expenditure) followed by muscle metabolism, the importance of different nutrients (macro and micronutrients) and finally focus on functional foods in endurance sports.

5.4 BIOENERGETICS (ENERGY FLOW)

Bioenergetics is the study of energy production and expenditure (exchange in the form of heat) in a living organism performing different biological functions. Energy exchange takes place through aerobic (with oxygen) and anaerobic (without oxygen) conditions through the multi-step enzymic pathway. In humans, the oxidation of macromolecules like carbohydrates (glucose), fats (fatty acids) and proteins (amino acids) results in adenosine triphosphate (ATP) production via cellular respiration (redox) including glycolysis, citric acid or tricarboxylic acid (TCA) cycle and electron transport chain (ETC) and oxidative phosphorylation. Combustion is a well-known energy exchange process which occurs when energy fuel (molecules) with a proton (H^+) and electron (e^-) readily liberates oxygen. Higher proton and electron donation or transfer would yield higher energy (heat). Similarly, glucose and fatty acids (energy is held within the molecular bonds) undergoes oxidation (based on ATP turnover) in the presence of molecular oxygen to yield ATP and CO_2 (Volkov, 2010).

Carb are considered the primary energy source, and one gram of carb will yield 4 kcal of energy. If one molecule of glucose undergoes cellular respiration, it will yield 36–38 ATP molecules under aerobic conditions (with O_2), whereas only 2 ATP molecules will be produced during anaerobic conditions (without O_2). The reserve energy source glucose is stored in the liver and muscles as glycogen (by glycogenesis) and plays a crucial role in endurance exercise. Ptn are considered the tertiary energy source, and one gram of ptn yields 4 kcal of energy. Ptn cannot be stored in the body and also contributes to ATP production via gluconeogenesis (carbohydrate production from non-carbohydrate substances like proteins (aa) and fats). Fat is considered the secondary energy source, and one gram of fat yields 9 kcal of energy, which is double the amount of carb or ptn. However, fats are not considered as a primary energy source, as energy generation from fat is a time-consuming complicated process which involves numerous enzymes, and hence carb (glucose) is preferred (Bagchi et al., 2018).

5.5   EVALUATING CALORIC/ENERGY NEEDS FOR ATHLETES

Before determining the caloric requirement of each athlete, it is essential to know about their energy requirement and expenditure (energy homeostasis). Energy homeostasis is the balance between total energy intake (TEI) or consumption and total energy expenditure (TEE) and plays a major role in athletic performance. The caloric requirement (dietary intake) of each athlete (especially an endurance sportsman) differs based on the type of sport (energetic demands–sport specific eating), types of training (amount of energy requirement), body mass index (BMI), age, gender and environment (temperature-aerobic or anaerobic workouts). Therefore, each athlete must balance the TEI:TEE ratio; however, if the TEI value is slightly higher than TEE (TEI > TEE), it could help in improving physical and training performance (Greenwood et al., 2015; Thivel et al., 2011).

5.6   TOTAL ENERGY EXPENDITURE (TEE)

TEE is determined based on factors like resting metabolic rate (RMR), thermogenesis and physical activity level (PAL), which includes exercise energy expenditure (EEE) and energy required for daily living. RMR is the main component of TEE (accounting for about 60–70%), and is corroborated by the body mass and size (Black et al., 1996). The best method to assess RMR is chamber-indirect calorimetry (with metabolic chart and RMR software), but this is expensive and not suitable for most athletes. RMR is also calculated by the Harris and Benedict equation (1919) using the formulae:

Male: RMR (kcal/day) = 66.47 + 13.75 (wt in kg) + 5 (ht in cm) − 6.76 (age in years)

Female: RMR (kcal/day) = 655.1 + 9.56 (wt in kg) + 1.85 (ht in cm) − 4.68 (age in years)

The above equations are only used to predict RMR within 200 kcal/day in endurance athletes, as it is an inexpensive and very convenient method (Thompson and Manore, 1996). Thermogenesis is related to the thermic effect of food and accounts for about 5–10% of TEE. Thermogenesis plays a vital role for sportspersons, especially in weight dependent sports like wrestling boxing and bodybuilding to maintain constant body weight. Finally, PAL, which includes EEE and energy for daily activities such as walking, running, climbing upstairs, etc., is calculated by the energy expenditure kcal/min by body weight (kg), based on Black and others' (1996) formulation:

A normal person (PAL range from 1 to 1.8) (Calorie requirement: 1800–2400 kcal)

Athletes (PAL range from 1.9 to 2.4) (Calorie requirement: 2500–8000 kcal)

5.7   TOTAL ENERGY INTAKE (TEI)

For most athletes, the preferred portion of macromolecules includes 60% of carbohydrates, 15% of protein and 25% of fat. The above composition may vary from person to person and type of sport. Previous studies have shown that a combination of different macromolecules (with the above combination) are shown to be effective for endurance sports (Muoio et al., 1994; Pendergast et al., 1996). Adequate energy (requirement) is the ratio of daily food intake to daily activities, and hence each athlete must monitor their food intake using diet charts and calorimetry as well as energy expenditure. Based on the caloric requirement, each endurance athlete could determine the nutrients requirement (macronutrients). However, based on the type of endurance sports and their training pattern, the athlete can modify the intake of macro and micronutrients to enhance their performance. For better performance results, each athlete must intake sufficient food or supplements to replace the energy immediately after exercise to overcome the loss during exercise, but also need to be cautious about becoming overweight (Greenwood et al., 2015).

5.8   MUSCLE METABOLISM

Muscle metabolism includes the bioenergetics (energy consumption and expenditure) of muscle tissue in contracting and relaxing. Major sources of ATP (energy currency) in muscle are glucose (glycogenolysis), fatty acids (FA) and creatine phosphate (CP) for muscle contraction. Where glucose can be metabolized in muscle aerobically or anaerobically, FA can be metabolized only aerobically. The energy requirement for the muscle tissue varies based on the type of exercise or sports. In this section, the author would like to give an outline of muscle metabolism in different conditions.

During resting/full fed state (ATP are stored): free FAs (from plasma) undergo oxidation (β-oxidation) to yield acetyl co-A as well as NADH and $FADH_2$, which enters TCA and ETC to produce ATP. These ATPs are used for storing excess glucose to glycogen by the process called glycogenesis. Moreover, these ATP were also used for converting creatine to creatine phosphate as a phosphate reserve to aid in ATP production (phosphagen system) during intense or strenuous exercise (Greenhaff, 1997). The remaining ATP is used for the regular (normal) contraction and relaxation process.

During moderate workout state (ATP is the major and creatine phosphate the minor energy source): the glycogen reserve is broken down into glucose (glycogenolysis). The glucose and fatty acid undergo catabolism in a moderate amount to yield ATP via aerobic glycolysis (utilized for muscle contraction).

During heavy or intense workout state (ATP by anaerobic glycolysis and creatine phosphate are the primary energy sources): the glycogen reserve is broken down to glucose and undergoes catabolism to yield ATP via anaerobic glycolysis in excessive amounts (utilized for muscle contraction), while creatine phosphate is converted to creatine to aid in ATP production. During anaerobic glycolysis, further amounts of lactic acid are produced and should reach the liver (via blood) to convert back to glucose (gluconeogenesis). Once the glycogen reserve is depleted, the free fatty acid (fatty reserve) again becomes a primary energy source (Tesch et al., 1986).

5.9 THE MYTH ABOUT LACTIC ACID AND MUSCLE PAIN (SENSOR OF PAIN)

Excessive production of lactic acid (after intense workout) in muscle cells, which triggers pain/fatigue (due to reduced pH and increased K^+) and indicates to our system (sensor) that increased lactic acid content in blood (more than 20 mM) needs to be metabolized by our liver cells; however, too much lactic acid would burden the liver cells which leads (increased lactic acid builds up in muscle) to fatigue and lactic acidosis. However, recent studies have documented that even the lactic acid levels are less in the muscle cell after endurance training (adaption on ion handling) but still the athlete experiences fatigue or pain (Allen et al., 2008; Hostrup and Bangsbo, 2017). Another study also suggests that accumulation of lactic acid did not induce fatigue, but instead protected against muscle fatigue (Nielsen et al., 2001). Hence, it is clear that the elevated lactic acid level (blood and muscle) is not the sole reason for muscular fatigue or pain.

5.10 ROLE OF MACRO AND MICRONUTRIENTS FOR ENDURANCE SPORTS

Macronutrients (>1 g/day)

- Carbohydrate (Primary energy fuel; 1 g = 4 kcal; Consume 55–60%)
- Protein (Tertiary energy fuel; 1 g = 4 kcal; Consume 15–20%)
- Fat (Secondary energy fuel; 1 g = 9 kcal; Consume 25–30%)

Micronutrients (<1 g/day)

- Minerals (electrolytes)
- Vitamins

5.10.1 MACRONUTRIENTS

5.10.1.1 Carbohydrates

Carbohydrates (carb) are the primary energy source, and hence are highly concentrated on by athletes and sports nutritionists. Also, carbohydrates maintain cellular homeostasis and thereby regulate cellular respiration (ATP production) and overall health status. Major types of carbohydrates are mono-, oligo- and polysaccharides. Monosaccharides are simple sugars, including glucose (dextrose), fructose and galactose, whereas oligo and polysaccharides are complex sugars, which contain many monosaccharides. Glycemic index (GI) is a score assigned to food (carbohydrate) based on how quickly or slowly they increase the blood glucose levels (Baynes, 2018). Glycogen is a type of polysaccharide made of high numbers of glucose, which is the stored form of glucose in our body (liver and skeletal muscles). Glycogen is the major source of energy for endurance athletes.

5.10.1.2 Importance of Carbohydrates on Physical or Athletic Performance

High carbohydrate availability (store more creatine phosphate and glycogen) would provide adequate fuel (energy) and spare muscle protein for training and thereby optimize performance (Burke et al., 2011). Moreover, high carb consumption during exercise could spare muscle glycogen stores and delay the onset of fatigue during exercise as well as prevent ketosis (ketone bodies as fuel). High glycaemic index (GI) foods (dextrin/maltose/glucose and sucrose) are recommended after exercise as replenishment or to restore normal glucose and glycogen level. However, low- or moderate GI food is recommended before exercise to avoid gastric discomfort (delayed gastric emptying). Most athletes have about 2 hours' worth of energy stored as muscle glycogen. For effective absorption of glucose, it should be taken together with minerals like sodium to deliberately change the pattern of carbohydrate intake based on the individual and the type of endurance sport (Bartlett et al., 2015; Stellingwerff, 2013). Overall, carbohydrate requirement for a light trainer would need between 350–500 g/day, while the heavy trainer would need between 500–700 g/day and the extreme trainer between 700–830 g/day for a healthy 70 kg (154.3 lbs) man. Endurance athletes are recommended to consume 7–12 g of carbohydrates/kg/day (follow high carbohydrate availability pattern).

- 7 g/kg/day for 1 h training
- 8 g/kg/day for 2 h training
- 10 g/kg/day for 3–4 h training
- 10–12 g/kg/day for 5–6 h training

5.10.1.3 Proteins (Amino Acids)

Proteins are the nitrogen-containing molecules composed of many amino acids (AA). AA are joined together by a peptide bond to form polypeptide, and this polypeptide chain binds together to form a protein. Protein is mainly classified as simple or conjugated. Simple protein has only AA and its derivatives, whereas conjugated proteins contain non-protein molecules like carbohydrates and lipids. Hence, for athletes, these conjugated proteins are highly recommended. Proteins are the building block of the body (muscle) and play various functions as a structural unit and functional unit and therefore are highly important for athletes (Chen et al., 2014b). A complete protein is recommended for athletes, as it contains all types of essential AA, in particular the branched chain amino acids (BCAAs), including leucine, isoleucine and valine, which can be directly utilized by muscle cells (Jafari et al., 2016).

5.10.1.4 Importance of Proteins on Physical or Athletic Performance

Proteins are required before, during and after exercise to decrease muscle damage (early fatigue) as well as for recovery (protein turnover-balance). Whey, ova, soy or casein proteins are the best proteins for the ordinary person. However, whey protein is highly recommended for athletes (due to its rapid absorption rate with high percentage of BCAAs like leucine, isoleucine, and valine and glutamine) (Dangin et al., 2001). BCAAs help in maintaining the immune system and muscle activity and thus avoid muscle soreness/fatigue or overtraining syndrome (Shimomura et al., 2010). Essential amino acids (EAA) aid in glycogen synthesis (upregulating insulin synthesis) and muscle formation, thereby enhancing endurance capacity. Supplemented protein helps in maintenance, repair and new synthesis of muscle protein. Athletes involved in regular resistance training are encouraged to intake higher amounts of protein to maintain the anabolic environment and muscle mass/size. Protein balance (breakdown and synthesis) is a crucial factor for improving health status and performance in endurance athletes (Phillips and Van Loon, 2011). The International Society of Sports Nutrition (ISSN) recommended a protein intake of the range between 1.4 to 2 g/kg/day for all types of athletes. However, endurance athletes are advised to consume around 1.2–1.6 g of protein/kg/day from balanced proteins or complete proteins (essential AA like BCAAs) which might delay the muscle fatigue (Moore et al., 2005; Shimomura et al., 2010). Overall, light and moderate trainers would need between 88–120 g/day, heavy or endurance trainers would need between 90–115 g/day and extreme young trainers would need 100–140 g/day for a healthy 70 kg (154.3 lbs) man.

5.10.1.5 Recommendation of Carb and Protein for Endurance Athletes Weighing 85 kg (before and after Exercise/ Training Based on the Reports of Rasmussen, 2008)

Pre-exercise meals (3–4 h before exercise): endurance athletes should consume 120–280 g of carb (starch, sucrose, maltodextrin-with moderate or low GI) with 20–30 g of proteins (BCAAs) to enhance glycogen content (carb level) for more extended training sessions. Other than macromolecules, electrolytes and vitamins are recommended with the pre-exercise meal to maintain the optimal psycho-physical function. It is also important to avoid high fiber and fatty foods, which might delay gastric emptying (and lead to gastric discomfort).

Pre-exercise snack (15–60 min before exercise): endurance athletes should consume 50–80 g of carb (glucose/dextrose with moderate GI to avoid gastric discomfort) to maintain glycogen content (carb level). Make sure that you are fully fuel and hydrated before exercise. During exercise (every h) endurance athletes are requested to consume 40–70 g of carb (glucose with high GI) in liquid or bar form to maintain carb level (normoglycemia).

Post-exercise snack (20–40 min after exercise): endurance athletes are requested to consume 120–340 g of carb (glucose/sucrose or starch with moderate or high GI) with 20–30 g of proteins (BCAAs) to replenish glycogen content (glycogen recovery) to avoid fatigue. Rehydrate with mineral water to avoid thermal stress.

Post-exercise meal (2 h after exercise): endurance athletes are requested to consume 80–140 g of carb (starch) with 10–20 g of proteins to continuously maintain glycogen content (glycogen recovery). Make sure that every day you are fully recovered and ready for the next day's training (deep sleep). As mentioned previously, the requirement of each athlete varies based on various factors including the type of endurance sports, types of training/exercise, BMI, age, sex and environment.

An ample number of researchers demonstrated that a combination of protein (hydrolysate) and carbohydrate supplementation would considerably improve performance in endurance athletes by reducing cortisol production and enhancing glycogen (insulin) and protein synthesis (Luden et al., 2007; McLellan et al., 2014; Moore, 2015). Hence most of the nutritional guidelines focus on carbohydrates and proteins. However, some reports indicate the importance of fat for endurance athletes (Volek et al., 2015), but to date, no scientific evidence to proves its significant impact in endurance athletes (Burke, 2015; Burke and Kiens, 2006). Also, fat-rich diets are associated with insulin resistance, which hampers glycogen synthesis and hence might decrease performance. However, it is recommended that all types of athletes consume 20–25% of calories from fats, as this promotes numerous biological functions (Kreider et al., 2010).

5.10.1.6   Fats/Lipids

Lipids or fats comprise water-insoluble molecules. Lipids include fats (triacylglycerol), oils and fatty substances like sterols and phospholipids. Lipids can maintain optimal health condition as they serve several functions including fat-soluble vitamins, cell membrane formation, bile formation, signal transduction, insulation of visceral organs and secondary energy sources. Fatty acids (muscle) are the one major energy source for skeletal muscle during intense training/endurance sports (Greenwood et al., 2015). Triglyceride (TG) is made of fatty acid and glycerol and is stored in adipose tissue as a fat reserve (ATP production). Fatty acids are classified as saturated (no double bond) and unsaturated (many double bonds) based on the presence of double bonds. Further, unsaturated fatty acids are classified as mono-unsaturated fatty acids (MUFA) and polyunsaturated fatty acids (PUFA). PUFA includes ω-3 FA including arachidonic acid, docosahexaenoic acid (DHA) and eicosapentaenoic acid (EPA), and has been reported to exhibit numerous pharmacological properties including anti-inflammatory, anti-oxidant, anti-fatigue, analgesic and anti-rheumatoid arthritis (Simopoulos, 2007). Fat/lipids have a high energy value (25% of body needs), and they provide more energy per gram (9 kcal/gm) than carbohydrates and proteins (4 kcal/gm). Even one fatty acid that has undergone beta oxidation will yield more ATP (129–147) than glucose (38 ATP). However, fat metabolism is a complicated and time-consuming process, and hence carbohydrates (instance ATP producer) are recommended as a primary energy source (Greenwood et al., 2015). No substantial scientific evidence is available to showcase the importance of a diet rich in fat for athletes (Burke, 2015; Burke and Kiens, 2006). However, fats have glycogen sparing activity and increase intramyocellular lipids during endurance sports (Knechtle et al., 2003).

5.10.1.7   Fat Requirement for Athletes

Athletes require 20–30% of total energy (Nutrition and Athletic Performance; NAP, 2009); out of that 10% is from saturated fat, 10% from monosaturated and 10% from poly-saturated sources. This 20–30% of fats are required by all type of people to maintain various metabolic functions to maintain optimal health (Rodriguez et al., 2009). Overall, the fat requirement for a light or moderate trainer would need to be between 45–60 g/day, a heavy or endurance trainer 50–75 g/day and an extreme young trainer 55–80 g/day for a healthy 70 kg (154.3 lbs) man. Endurance athletes are recommended to consume around 0.8–1.1 g of fat/kg/day.

5.10.2 MICRONUTRIENTS

Micronutrients include vitamins (fat soluble and water soluble), and minerals/electrolytes play a crucial role in maintaining optimal health status without providing any measurable energy. Micronutrients exhibit several biological properties in our body including maintaining the immune system (defense and recovery), bone density, muscle contraction and relaxation, blood and fluid homeostasis, and helping in transportation and absorption of macronutrients; they are thereby indirectly involved in energy metabolism or cellular respiration to maintain optimal physical and mental status. To ensure the optimal effects of micronutrients, they should be supplemented in highly absorbable form, while dosage (based on recommended daily allowance; RDA/daily value; DV) of micronutrients is essential (Lukaski, 2004). Furthermore, dietary reference intakes (DRIs) have recommended the intake of all types of micronutrients to prevent deficiency. DRIs include many categories of reference values, such as adequate intake (AI), recommended daily allowance (RDA) and estimated average requirement (EAR). RDA ensure a sufficient dietary intake of 98% required for a healthy person. AI is used if no RDA value has been determined and the EAR is employed to satisfy 50% of the needs of each person in the specific group (Trumbo et al., 2002).

5.10.2.1 Vitamins

Vitamins are organic compounds with an amine group and naturally found in various food products. Vitamins are essential micronutrients as they cannot be synthesized by our body in sufficient amounts to exhibit the normal physiological function and hence must be supplied through food. Vitamins are classified as water soluble (Vit B complex, Vit C) and fat-soluble (Vit A, D, E and K) vitamins.

5.11 ROLE OF VITAMINS FOR IMPROVING PERFORMANCE IN ATHLETES (ENDURANCE)

Thiamine (B1) acts as a coenzyme precursor for most of the enzymes involved in carbohydrate metabolism especially in the TCA cycle. Thiamine supplementation (100 ng/day) significantly lowers muscle fatigue as compared to a placebo group after 30 min on a bicycle ergometer (Suzuki and Itokawa, 1996). Riboflavin (B2) is required for the flavoenzymes involved in ETC and thereby supports energy metabolism. Niacin (B3) is involved in the synthesis of a reduced form of nicotinamide adenine dinucleotide (NADH) acts as a proton supplier or carrier in ETC and thus plays a pivotal role in energy production. It is also involved in the production of neurotransmitters like dopamine, nor-epinephrine and serotonin. Murray et al. (1995) indicated that niacin supplementation would improve physical performance during exercise. Pyridoxine (B6) is a crucial coenzyme involved in protein (amino acid), lipid and carbohydrate metabolism, while it also plays a vital role in red blood cell (RBC) production with Vitamin B12 and is directly involved in RNA and DNA synthesis. Folic acid (B9) and cyanocobalamin (B12) also have a direct role in erythrocyte production, and hence might enhance athletic or physical performance. Results of one study showed that although folate supplementation in an athletic population did significantly increase circulating levels of serum folate, this increase did not translate into improved performance (Matter et al., 1987). Some studies indicated indirect benefits to physical performance after supplementation with ascorbic acid (Vit C) by decreasing body temperature (Kotze et al., 1977) and enhanced immune function (Peters et al., 1993). Vitamin A and E are recommended to attenuate oxidative stress and hence are beneficial for exercising induced-oxidative stress, while vitamins D and K are involved in bone formation and might indirectly beneficial for athletes. However, there is no evidence or study to prove the direct effects of various vitamins on improving athletic performance.

5.12 MINERALS (ELECTROLYTES)

Minerals are the chemical agents required by the living organism to maintain an optimal health condition. Minerals exert numerous biological functions, including nerve function, acid–base balance, cellular growth and enzyme regulation (Anderson, 2000). Minerals are subdivided into macro- and microminerals based on body requirement.

5.12.1 MACROMINERALS

Macrominerals include magnesium, calcium, phosphorous, chloride, sulfur, sodium and potassium and more than 100 mg/day are required. Calcium (Ca^{2+}) and phosphorous (p) are reported to play a vital role in bone mineralization (density), vitamin D production and the improvement of oxygen release in muscle cells, and have a moderate influence on athletic or sports performance. Magnesium (mg) acts as a co-factor and helps in Vit D metabolism as well as in energy generation. Brilla and Haley (1992) concluded that supplementation with mg significantly increased quadriceps torque and leg press count in strength training athletes. Potassium (k^+) is reported to improve muscle strength (enhance contraction and relaxation by increased nerve excitation). A double-blind trial conducted by Goss and his colleagues (2001) demonstrated that the overall rating of perceived exertion (RPE) was significantly lowered after administration with potassium phosphate in endurance runners. Sodium (Na^{2+}) and chloride (Cl^-) both are major electrolytes used for maintaining acid–base balance and thus indirectly contribute to muscle strength. During strenuous activity or exercise in a hot environment, high sweat losses may result in increased dietary requirements of sodium and chloride and result in exercise-induced hyponatremia (decreased blood Na^{2+} concentration), which is the leading cause for muscle cramps in endurance athletes. Therefore, rehydration with an electrolyte-rich drink would improve athletic performance (Noakes et al., 2005; Von Dullivard et al., 2004). Nevertheless, well-nourished athletes being supplemented with macrominerals has no significant improvement in athletic performance (Williams, 2005).

5.12.2 Microminerals/Trace Elements

Microminerals include zinc, iron, copper, iodine, selenium, chromium, fluoride, manganese and boron, and less than 100 mg/day are required. Iron (Fe) is critical for endurance athlete due to its role in oxygen transport, energy metabolism and acid–base balance (Hinton, 2014). Oxidative stress and inflammatory response in endurance athletes would impede iron absorption by modulating iron regulatory protein and hepcidin and thus lower the levels of iron in endurance athletes, hence limiting their performance (Dahlquist et al., 2017). There is no strong evidence to prove the involvement of other microminerals in athletic performance (Williams, 2015).

5.13 ERGOGENIC DRUGS OR AGENT

Ergogenic drugs or agents are substances used to enhance or improve athletic performance or recovery and are marketed as nutritional or dietary supplements. Recently, even general people (not only athletes or sportsmen) are consuming nutritional/dietary supplements with ergogenic properties to enhance their health status or improve their working ability (Yeh et al., 2011). Therefore, this nutritional supplement market is booming considerably throughout the world. In sports arenas and scientific publications, the usage of words or terms like dietary or sport or nutritional supplements, nutraceuticals, functional foods and ergogenic aid are interchangeable (Lanham-New et al., 2011). Commonly used ergogenic agents include steroid precursors (dehydroepiandrosterone and androstenedione), androgenic steroids and growth hormones (those mentioned agents are to be taken cautiously, as they are reported with severe adverse effects, also abusive); also included are compounds like caffeine, creatine, taurine, HMB and carnitine (less adverse effects), but all these ergogenic agents are combined with macro or micronutrients for better functionality (Calfee and Fadale, 2006).

5.14 POPULAR ERGOGENIC COMPOUNDS

Currently, many types of commercial ergogenic agents (both synthetic and natural) are available on the market, but only a few ergogenic agents are quite popular, as they are scientifically proven. These include caffeine, L-creatine, taurine, L-carnitine, β-hydroxy-β-methyl butyrate (HMB), sodium bicarbonate/citrate and β alanine.

5.14.1 Caffeine

Caffeine (1,3,7-trimethylxanthine; alkaloid derivative) is the primary component of beverages like coffee and tea. It is commonly used for its ergogenic properties (increase heart rate) as well as a central nervous system (CNS) stimulant, as it is an adenosine receptor antagonist (Jones, 2008; Keisler and Armsey, 2006). Thus, it increases the levels of awareness or alertness (arousal), informational processing and control-oriented mechanisms by increased release of epinephrine. Caffeine (adrenaline) mobilizes fat stores (TG breaks into FFA and glycerol, then FFA to b oxidation) and thus triggers the myocytes to utilize fat as a fuel, which delays the depletion of muscle glycogen (glycogen sparing activity) and allows for prolonged exercise (Schneiker et al., 2006). It also maintains water level by regulating the kidneys (diuretic effect) and thus maintains blood pressure and physical performance by increasing VO_2 max. In addition, it increases intracellular Ca^{2+} release (SR) in skeletal muscle, resulting in a muscle contraction. A review by Ganio and his co-workers (2009) concluded that caffeine consumption (in a moderate amount) would considerably improve the performance in endurance athletes (aerobic) when taken before or during exercise. Studies have shown that a combination of caffeine with ephedrine (caffeine-ephedrine mixture) or bicarbonate displayed better ergogenic properties via improving muscle metabolism (Christensen et al., 2017; Keisler and Armsey, 2006). The adverse effect of caffeine increases cardiac output/blood pressure and addiction, and hence its use is considerably limited by athletes (Burke, 2008). Therefore, caffeine is included in the 2015 monitoring program of the World Anti-Doping Agency (WADA). However, it is not prohibited or banned (Hughes, 2015).

5.14.2 L-Creatine

Creatine is one of the popular ergogenic aids, which is formed from amino acids like methionine, glycine and arginine in the liver, pancreas and kidneys and is transported to muscles, heart and brain; however, it is transported mostly to the muscles and stored as creatine phosphate (phosphagen system), an energy reserve, with the help of enzyme creatine phosphokinase (CPK). Creatine (creatine monohydrate) is supplemented with carbohydrates for better absorption, especially for endurance athletes (Theodorou et al., 2017; Wall et al., 2011). Creatine supplementation enhances the plasma creatine level and thus improves the intramuscular creatine level and can improve training adaptation and physical performance. Creatine is beneficial for short training, while studies with creatine (clinical trial) on endurance athletes did not show significant improvement in performance (Stuessi et al., 2005). Scientific evidence has shown that ingestion of creatine would increase LBM, improve muscle mass (strength) as well as increase water retention and thereby improve sports performance (Kreider et al., 2017; Panjwani et al., 2007).

5.14.3 Taurine

Taurine (2-aminoethyl sulfonic acid) is a sulfonic amino acid which cannot be synthesized by our body and hence must be supplemented through diet. Taurine does not contribute to protein synthesis. Taurine may considerably alter the skeletal muscle contractile function and thus attenuate exercise-induced oxidative stress (DNA damage), with lipolysis activity thereby improving endurance capacity and athletic performance (Imagawa et al., 2009; Rutherford et al., 2010; Zhang et al., 2004). It also improves cognitive function (neurotransmitters), increasing alertness and lowering depression. It exhibits antioxidant, anti-inflammatory and lipolysis activities and thus protects the muscles from fatigue or injury or pain and thus aids athletic performance especially for endurance athletes (De Carvalho et al., 2017; De Carvalho et al., 2018).

5.14.4 L-CARNITINE

Carnitine (L-trimethyl-3-hydroxy-ammoniobutanoate) is a naturally occurring amino acid made by the liver and kidneys from lysine and methionine. It does affect energy levels (ergogenic aid-anaerobic cycling sprints) by enhancing lipolysis (long chain fatty acids undergoing β-oxidation) to produce ATP (glycogen sparing property). The primary function of carnitine in muscle is to alleviate pain and muscle damage with high lactic acid clearing property, while it also scavenges free radicals (antioxidant/anti-inflammatory activities) and thus lowers the risk of muscle fatigue or exercise-induced oxidative stress and enhances the post-exercise muscle recovery (Pandareesh and Anand, 2013; Sung et al., 2016). Moreover, it improves cognitive function (elevate dopamine level) and reduces anxiety and depression in endurance athletes (Orer and Guzel, 2014). Several human studies have confirmed the ergogenic property of L-carnitine, which thus has a direct impact on endurance athletes (Guzel et al., 2015; Lee et al., 2007; Orer and Guzel, 2014).

5.14.5 β-HYDROXY-β-METHYL BUTYRATE (HMB)

HMB is a principal metabolite of leucine (BCAA). Both leucine and its metabolite HMB (free form, highly absorbable) are reported to play a crucial role in muscle protein metabolism (preferably anabolism–protein synthesis) in an insulin-independent manner (without triggering insulin as like leucine), which also increases ATP and glycogen content in muscles and thereby improves aerobic physical performance (Lamboley et al., 2007; Wilkinson et al., 2013). Other studies also highlighted that HMB supplementation would considerably attenuate muscle damage (recovery) as well as maintain LBM (decrease fat) and thus improve endurance/stamina in athletes (Wilson et al., 2013; Zanchi et al., 2011). HMB is highly recommended as an ergogenic aid among strength/power athletes and bodybuilders, who might improve skeletal muscle hypertrophy more than endurance athletes (Wilson et al., 2008). Only a few studies have shown the impact of HMB on endurance athletes. Vukovich and Adams (1997), as well as Vukovich and Dreifort (2001), hinted that HMB supplementation increased the time to reach VO_2 peak more than leucine or placebo in endurance-trained cyclists.

5.14.6 SODIUM BICARBONATE/CITRATE

Sodium bicarbonate/citrate creates resistance against muscle fatigue by modulating the acid–base balance in myocytes (buffering agent). For short and moderate training, the ergogenic effects of sodium bicarbonate/citrate are well documented (Goldfinch et al., 1988; Lindh et al., 2008). However, the results with sodium bicarbonate/citrate in endurance athletes are not that convincing. Moreover, sodium bicarbonate/citrate are reported to elicit gastric discomfort and elevate blood pressure (hyperhydration) (McNaughton et al., 2008; Price and Simons, 2010).

5.14.7 β ALANINE

β alanine is a non-essential amino acid synthesized by the liver. With histidine, it is the building block for carnosine (a muscle pH regulator and excellent antioxidant) and hence helps in maintaining muscle pH (buffering system), thereby lowering muscle fatigue and improving muscle performance (Artioli et al., 2010). β alanine is also recommended with sodium bicarbonate for endurance athletes for better performance (de Salles Painelli et al., 2013). Researchers have supported the use of β alanine to improve training adaptations (increase training ability-tolerance) through high-intensity training (Hill et al., 2007). Some studies suggested that β alanine supplementation would increase muscle carnosine and thus stabilize the intramuscular pH (lowering H^+) during intense training and thereby lower or delay muscular fatigue (Harris et al., 2006; Stout et al., 2007). Hoffman and his co-workers (2007) reported that β alanine consumption might allow for higher intense training volume (stimulus) and eventually result in increased LBM and lower fatigue. Smith et al. (2009) concluded that chronic supplementation of β alanine with high-intensity interval training could significantly increase VO_2 peak and LBM due to decreased anaerobic ATP production and thereby improve the endurance performance in a double-blind clinical trial.

Other minor ergogenic drugs are glycerol (banned), while amino acids like arginine, glutamine and nitrate can peak the athletic performance. However, only some data are available to support their ergogenic properties.

5.15   NUTRITIONAL AID

5.15.1   ERGOGENIC HERBS

Natural ergogenic herbs need to be consumed by individuals for many years to optimize the health status with improved energy metabolism and muscular hypertrophy/strength to thereby improve performance without any adverse effects. Some ergogenic herbs are classified as adaptogen (used to lower body stress), since exercise can induce physiological stress; adaptogens are hence recommended to overcome exercise-induced stress by preventing fatigue as well as improving mental capacity via lowering cortisol production (acting antioxidant and anti-inflammatory agent) and thus improving physical performance (Bucci, 2000; Molinos, 2013). In this chapter, the author only concentrates on popular ergogenic/adaptogenic herbs including *Panax ginseng, Eurycoma longifolia, Eleutherococcus senticosus, Schisandra chinensis, Withania somnifera, Paullinia cupana* (Guarana), *Rhodiola rosea* and *Cordyceps sinensis.*

5.15.1.1   *Panax ginseng* (Chinese/Asian Ginseng–Saponins: Ginsenoside)

Panax ginseng (*P. ginseng*) is a perennial plant with fleshy roots and belongs to the Araliaceae family. *P. ginseng* is a popular Chinese herb and commonly called the king of herbs due to its numerous pharmacological properties including antioxidant, anti-inflammatory, anti-microbial, anti-stress and anti-cancerous, as well as neuroprotective, cardioprotective and hepatoprotective (Chan, 2012; Nuri et al., 2016). Scientific investigation showed that ginsenoside (saponin) of red *P. ginseng* (roots) is the primary contributor for most biological functions (Shergis et al., 2013) and is safe for human consumption. *P. ginseng* is commonly prescribed for all types of health issues owing to its adaptogenic property (anti-stress/anti-depressant).

P. ginseng efficiently blocks the adrenocorticotropic hormone (ACTH) and thus suppresses the production of the glucocorticoid steroid hormone (cortisol, the stress hormone) as well as reduces the production of nor-adrenalin and serotonin (stress responders) and thereby is an effective natural adaptogen. *P. ginseng* directs the free fatty acids to β-oxidation (ATP production) and maintains the glucose/glycogen level and thereby improves aerobic exercise performance. It also improves cognitive function, relieves pain (anti-analgesic and anti-inflammatory) and chronic muscle fatigue with enhanced lipolysis, thus promoting physical activity (Ma et al., 2017; Rai et al., 2003). A recent study conducted by Alsmadi and his colleagues (2018) demonstrated that consumption of Asian ginseng (Panax) at a dose of 1 g/day for six weeks would considerably increase quadriceps and pectoral muscle strength even in the non-exercising individual. Several other clinical trials also supported its usage for endurance training with lesser muscle fatigue due to enhanced anabolic properties (Liang et al., 2005; Wong et al., 2011).

5.15.1.2 *Eurycoma longifolia* Jack (Malaysian Ginseng)

Eurycoma longifolia (*E. longifolia*) Jack is a famous tropical medicinal plant and commonly called Tongkat Ali or Malaysian ginseng. *E. longifolia* (roots/stem) belongs to the family Simaroubaceae and has been used traditionally for aphrodisiac, anti-anxiety, anti-aging, anti-fatigue and anti-microbial qualities. Several alkaloids, flavonoids, saponins and terpenoids (quassinoids) are isolated from the roots of *E. longifolia* and reported to have many beneficial properties including anti-inflammation, anti-oxidant, anti-pyretic, anti-microbial, anti-fatigue and anti-aging (Bhat and Karim, 2010; Khanijo and Jiraungkoorskul, 2016). Quassinoids (eurycomalacton, eurycomanol, eurycomanon) of *E. longifolia* are reported to enhance muscle strength (endurance) as well as reduce stress and anxiety by balancing the production of testosterone and cortisol hormone. A clinical trial conducted by Hamzah and Yusof (2003) demonstrated that more extended supplementation (5 weeks) of *E. longifolia* could significantly improve muscle strength, size and mass (LBM) and thus infer its ergogenic property. However, Muhamad and his co-workers (2010) concluded that acute supplementation of *Eurycoma longifolia* (capsule for 7 days) did not improve the endurance running capacity performance in 12 young athletes. Likewise, Khanijo and Jiraungkoorskul (2016) in their review also concluded that consumption of *Eurycoma longifolia* for a longer period would elicit benefits on endurance performance and physiological performance. Nevertheless, more studies are needed to confirm its mechanism behind the ergogenic property.

5.15.1.3 *Eleutherococcus senticosus* or *Acanthopanax senticosus* (Siberian Ginseng)

Eleutherococcus senticosus (*E. senticosus*) is a woody shrub belonging to Araliaceae family, commonly called Siberian ginseng or *Acanthopanax senticosus* or ciwujia. *E. Senticosus'* roots and stem (barks) have been used in traditional Chinese medicine (TCM) for curing various illness as it is a potent adaptogen (anti-stress). The roots of *E. senticosus* contain several major phytocomponents including sesamin, lignans, coumarin, β-sitosterol and syringaresinol, eleutherosides which contribute to various biological properties (Bai et al., 2011). It exhibits many pharmacological activities including anti-inflammatory, anti-oxidant and anti-microbial (Kimura and Sumiyoshi, 2004; Sumiyoshi and Kimura, 2016). *E. senticosus* has been suggested to improve cardiorespiratory fitness and endurance performance due to lipolytic and anti-fatigue activity (Goulet and Dionne, 2005; Zhang et al., 2010). Copious numbers of clinical and pre-clinical studies demonstrated that administration of *E. senticosus* increased VO_2 max (exercise tolerance), glycogen contents, β-oxidation of FA (lipolysis) with decreased lactate (upregulating the expression of LDH), BUN and cortisol levels thereby improving athletic performance in different endurance sports (Huang et al., 2011; Kuo et al., 2010; Sumiyoshi and Kimura, 2016).

5.15.1.4 *Paullinia cupana* (Guarana)

Guarana is the extract from the fruits/berries of the Amazon plant called *Paullinia cupana,* which belongs to the Sapindaceae family, and is used in folk medicine for treating dysentery, fever, headache, rheumatism and sexual dysfunction (Hamerski et al., 2013). Guaranine is the major compound, also called caffeine, which acts as CNS/PNS stimulant (Burke et al., 2011). Guaranine is the only plant with high contents of caffeine (4–6%), twice the amount of coffee beans. Owing to the high content of caffeine, guarana is the primary natural stimulant for most energy or sports drinks (Kennedy et al., 2008). Other than its stimulant property, it also exhibits other biological functions such as anti-fatigue, anti-inflammatory, immunomodulatory as well as neuroprotective (Kennedy et al., 2004). In addition, it contains theobromine and theophylline, which also act as CNS stimulant and lipolytic properties (Weckerle et al., 2003). Studies have indicated that guarana supplemented with multivitamins and mineral contributed to better athletic and cognitive performance (Scholey et al., 2013; Veasey et al., 2015). Overall, guarana is used to enhance physical and mental functions owing to its lipolytic, anti-inflammatory, antioxidant and anti-fatigue properties.

5.15.1.5 *Withania somnifera* (Indian Ginseng–Relaxing)

Withanias somnifera (*W. somnifera*), or Indian ginseng or Ashwagandha, belongs to the Solanaceae family. It is a well-known medicinal herb in India with numerous medicinal benefits including vitality (endurance/stamina), longevity, adaptogenic (anti-stress) and immunomodulatory activities owing to the presence of alkaloids, steroidal lactones and glycosides. Therefore, *W. somnifera* is marketed as a rejuvenator or vitality supplement. It helps the body adapt to stressful situations, owing to the regulating of cortisol and testosterone hormones as well as improving RBC count, and thus improving both aerobic and anaerobic endurance capacity or physical performance (Choudhary et al., 2015; Sandhu et al., 2010). The anabolic property of *W. somnifera* is due to increased secretion of testosterone which, in turn, helps in the build-up of various macromolecules especially carbohydrates and proteins, thereby avoiding fatigue and improving power and strength (Shenoy et al., 2012; Srinivas-Shanker et al., 2010). Shenoy and others (2012) concluded that 8 weeks of administration with *W. somnifera* leads to significant improvement in anaerobic capacity (watts/peak power) in elite cyclists. Similarly, Choudhary and others (2015) demonstrated that 12 weeks of supplementation with *Withania sominfera* greatly improved VO_2 max and thus increased energy levels by improving cardiorespiratory and cognitive (neuro-muscular co-ordination) functions in healthy athletes. A recent study also reported that treatment with *Withania sominfera* significantly increased muscle strength and size with reduced exercise-induced muscle damage markers (recovery) in resistance-training men (Wankhede et al., 2015). However, no studies have been conducted with *W. somnifera* on endurance performance.

5.15.1.6 *Schisandra chinensis*

Schisandra chinensis (*S. chinensis*) is a climbing plant and belongs to the Schisandraceae family. The *S. chinensis* fruit has been commonly used in TCM for many years especially for anti-aging and as a rejuvenating tonic. The lignans (dibenzocyclooctadiene-Schisandrol) are the major ingredients of *S. chinensis* with various biological properties (Chan, 2012; Chun et al., 2014). *S. chinensis* blocks the ACTH and thus suppresses the cortisol production as well as reduces the production of noradrenalin and serotonin (stress responders) and thus acts as an adaptogen. Moreover, *S. chinensis* is reported to exhibit antioxidant and anti-inflammatory activities and therefore abolishes exercise-induced muscle fatigue (injury) and eventually increases endurance and physical performance (Dilshara et al., 2013; Panossian and Wikman, 2009). The anti-athletic effect of *Schisandra chinensis* was demonstrated by escalating hemoglobin concentration and swimming time with decreased blood lactate level in mice model (Cao et al., 2009). Zhang and Xu (2012) concluded that polysaccharide present in the *S. chinensis* is the major contributor to anti-fatigue property and thus increases physical performance.

5.15.1.7 *Rhodiola rosea* (Vitality; Rhodioloside–Bitter
Flavor Added to Salads)

Rhodiola rosea (*R. rosea*) belongs to the Crassulaceae family. Its roots were mostly used by the Chinese, Tibetans and Russians for several years for treating fatigue and mood-related disorders and hence were called golden root (Chan, 2012). Literature indicates that *R. rosea* exhibits numerous pharmacological properties including anti-inflammation, anti-oxidant, anti-fatigue, anti-aging, anti-stress as well as neuroprotective and hepatoprotective (De Bock et al., 2004; Xu and Li, 2012). Salidroside/rhodioloside is the main active component of *R. rosea* with numerous biological activities especially anti-fatigue (Mao et al., 2010; Wu et al., 2009; Xu and Li, 2012). *R. rosea* is a Himalayan root used to adapt to the stress of living (suppress cortisol production) as well as stimulate the production of dopamine and serotonin and thus lower stress (thus, acting as an anti-depressant). *R. rosea* also effectively burns fat and helps to improve oxygen transfer (via upregulating the production of erythropoietin, EPO) and enhance cognitive function, therefore possessing ergogenic properties as well (Walker and Roberds, 2006). A study conducted by De Bock and his colleagues (2004) found that ingestion of *R. rosea* extended the time to exhaustion during bicycle ergometer tests. Noreen et al. (2013) concluded that acute supplementation of *R. rosea* significantly decreases heart rate (due to increased endogenous opioids production) and the perception of effort (Borg scale) and thus improves the exercise performance in athletes. Many clinical trials and animal studies have also confirmed that consumption of *R. rosea* could improve sports performance by reducing lactate level and muscle weakness (Duncan et al., 2016; Parisi et al., 2010; Shanely et al., 2014). Furthermore, it is used to treat anxiety and depression but increases excessive opioid production and EPO, and hence the FDA did not approve it.

5.15.1.8 *Cordyceps sinensis* (Tibetan Mushroom–Fungi)

Cordyceps sinensis (*C. sinensis*) is an annual Ascomycetes fungus related to the mushroom. It is a rare combination of caterpillar and fungus and commonly found in higher altitudes especially in Tibet, India, Nepal and China. *C. sinensis* is a famous Chinese traditional/Tibetan medicine used to improve strength (endurance), sleep, sexuality and longevity (Panda and Swain, 2011), and is commonly recognized for many beneficial effects including anti-fatigue, anti-aging, anti-insomnia, anti-diabetic as well as cardioprotective, hepatoprotective and renoprotective properties. Polysaccharides of *C. sinensis* are the major contributor for the various pharmacological effects mainly related to endurance/stamina by stimulating energy metabolism (ATP production), improving cardiorespiratory function and enhancing erythropoiesis (increase RBC count). Studies have hinted that the fermentable strain of the mycelia could enhance fat metabolism (β-oxidation) and thus regulate blood glucose and insulin level during prolonged or endurance sports or training (Yan et al., 2014, 2012). Kumar and others (2011), confirmed the mechanism behind the anti-fatigue and ergogenic properties of *Cordyceps sinensis* through upregulation of 5' AMP-activated protein kinase (AMPK), peroxisome proliferator-activated receptor delta (PPAR-δ) and the nuclear factor-erythroid derived-2-antioxidant response element (NRF-2-ARE) signaling pathway to suppress the exercise-induced oxidative stress. Clinical studies also confirmed that supplementation of *Cordyceps sinensis* results in significant improvements in oxygen uptake with decreased muscle fatigue and endurance exercise performance (Chen et al., 2010). Researchers also indicated that a combination of *Cordyceps sinensis* with other herbs like *Rhodiola crenulate* or *Ginkgo biloba* could considerably improve the endurance performance by elevating oxygen consumption as well as having controlled regulation of PNS activity (Chen et al., 2014a; Zhang et al., 2009).

5.15.2 Ephedrine (Banned in Most Countries)

Ephedrine (alkaloid) is derived from the ephedra herb (Chinese herb *ma hung*) and acts as a CNS stimulant by acting as an agonist on α and β adrenergic receptor and thus releasing nor-epinephrine (Ma et al., 2007). It aids in lipolysis and therefore possesses glycogen sparing properties and thus prolongs the glycogen availability and performance or exercise (Bell et al., 2002; Gill et al., 2000). Mostly ephedrine is combined with caffeine or other herbs like guarana (which is rich in caffeine) and showed significant improvement in athletic performance; however, ephedrine displayed numerous adverse effects including arrhythmias, ischemic stroke, hypertension, tremors, insomnia and myocardial infarction, and rarely death (Haller and Benowwitz, 2000; Shekelle et al., 2003). It was banned by FDA in the 1980s.

Other than the above mentioned ergogenic/adaptogenic herbs, others are available like holy basil (*Ocimum sanctum*) and *Gingko biloba*, but these herbs did not have sufficient evidence to showcase their ergogenic properties in endurance athletes. Sometimes these ergogenic herbs are also used as food especially for salads and as a spice to enhance the flavor.

5.16   ROLE OF ERGOGENIC FUNCTIONAL FOOD/ NUTRACEUTICALS ON ENDURANCE SPORTS/ATHLETES

Even in the olden days (300 BCE), natural foods and beverages were used as ergogenic agents to improve athletic performance. Recently, many scientists from the sports nutrition field focus on functional foods/nutraceuticals (food with health-promoting or beneficial properties) with antioxidant properties to overcome exercise-induced oxidative stress and fatigue. Moreover, the major advantage of preferring functional foods/nutraceuticals for athletic performance is due to less or no adverse effects as well as the synergistic effect of various components in food improving post-workout muscle recovery and enhanced performance (Levers et al., 2016). Therefore, the production and commercialization of ergogenic functional foods have gained massive momentum as they not only provide the nutritional value but also enhance overall health status (without any adverse effects) in athletes and thereby improve the athletic or physical performance (Corbo et al., 2014; Eussen et al., 2011). Currently, several sport supplement products are available as a single ergogenic compound or in combinations with micro or macronutrients. However, only a few natural ergogenic agents are supported by scientific evidence while others are still under scientific investigation. Some of the major ergogenic functional foods/nutraceuticals are garlic, ginger, quercetin (onion/grape), green tea (EGCG), beetroot, watermelon, tart cherry, bitter or sour orange, *Garcinia* (Hydroxycitric acid), resveratrol (grapes/berries) and tapioca starch.

5.16.1   *Allium sativum* (Garlic)

Garlic is commonly known as a flavoring agent with numerous medicinal values. Garlic (especially aged) has a long history as a remedy for improving strength (oxygen supply), reducing fatigue, and increasing immunity and is reported to reduce corticosterone concentration owing to the presence of various active phytocomponents including allicin (lignans) and s-alyl-cysteine (Oi et al., 2001; Seo et al., 2014). Aged garlic extract is shown to decrease blood viscosity (improve blood fluidity) and thus increase O_2/nutrient supply to the muscles and thus improve physical performance. It is also reported to enhance the turnover of aerobic glucose metabolism (more ATP), which decreases oxidative stress and inflammation (Damirichi et al., 2015; Ince Di et al., 2000; Morris et al., 2013). Morihara and his co-workers (2006) demonstrated that supplementation of aged garlic extract would significantly increase the succinate dehydrogenase (SDH) enzyme activity by 40% and thus improve aerobic energy metabolism of skeletal muscle during exercise with increased VO_2 max value in a rat model.

5.16.2   *Zingiber officinale* (Ginger)

Zingiber officinale is a flowering plant belonging to the Zingiberaceae family. Its rhizome or root is called ginger. Ginger is a popular spice and used commonly in food to give flavor (due to volatile oil) with various biological properties including antioxidant, anti-inflammation, anti-aging, anti-microbial, anti-obesity, anti-cancer, and anti-diabetic, hence it is used as a dietary supplement. Zingerone and gingerols are the two major active components of ginger (Srinivasan, 2017). Furthermore, ginger is shown to display both analgesics (pain killer-inhibit prostaglandins synthesis) and ergogenic properties owing to its bronchodilatory and gastroprotective properties, along with antioxidant, anti-inflammatory (inhibit COX and iNOS expression) and anti-emetic activities; hence it is effective against exercise-induced fatigue and pain (Anosike et al., 2009; Wilson, 2015; Wilson et al., 2015). Zehsaz and his colleagues (2014) concluded that consumption of dried ginger powder by runners would significantly suppress the pro-inflammatory markers and thus indirectly lower the pain in their randomized, double-blind, parallel trial. Nevertheless, there was no significant evidence to showcase the direct ergogenic property of ginger.

5.16.3 GREEN TEA (EGCG)

Green tea is made of the leaves of *Camellia sinensis* by the mild oxidation process. Green tea is one of the most widely consumed beverages globally. Studies have reported that the catechins, especially epigallocatechin-3-gallate (EGCG), are the major contributors for most of the biological properties including antioxidant, anti-inflammatory, anti-fatigue, anti-cancer as well as cardioprotective, neuroprotective (Malaguti et al., 2013; Venkatakrishnan et al., 2018). Ample amount of studies also indicated that green tea catechin (EGCG) exhibits thermogenic/lipogenic activities (fat oxidation-increase hormone-sensitive lipase; HSL) as well as that it increases maximal oxygen uptake (VO_2 max) and thus improves exercise/sports performance (Richards et al., 2010; Wang et al., 2010). Healthy males ($n = 14$) who have a habit of regular treadmill exercise were supplemented with green tea extract beverages rich in catechin for 2 months and a 24% increase in fat oxidation was found as compared to placebo (Ota et al., 2005). A clinical trial conducted by Ichinose and others (2011) found that consumption of green tea extract by healthy men who underwent endurance training (Cycling for 60 min) every day would considerably decrease in the respiratory exchange ratio (RER) with increased fat oxidation during exercise compared to the placebo. Moreover, green tea also contains caffeine which might also be the reason for maintaining LBM via enhancing lipolysis by acting along with other catechins (Hursel et al., 2009; Phung et al., 2010). Green tea polyphenols are found to improve cognitive and cardiorespiratory functions and thus physical and mental health for athletes (Babu et al., 2008; Park et al., 2011). Many studies also highlighted that the intake of green tea extract can protect from exercise-induced oxidative stress and muscle damage by upregulating the antioxidant defense system (Jowko et al., 2011, 2015).

5.16.4 *BETA VULGARIS* (BEETROOTS)

Beta vulgaris (beetroot) is a common vegetable used globally. *B. vulgaris* belongs to the Amaranthaceae family and is called sugar beet. Both its root (tuber) and leaves are used in folk medicine to treat a broad range of ailments, especially fever, constipation, and blood-related disorders. The active ingredients of *B. vulgaris* are betaine and betalain, which are responsible for the various biological properties of beetroot (Georgiev et al., 2010) and are the best natural sources of nitrate (nitric oxide) to enhance sports or training performance without any adverse effects (Jones, 2014). Nitrate in beetroot is converted to nitrite and finally to nitric oxide (NO), which affects vasodilation, enhances mitochondrial biogenesis (ATP production), increases muscle contraction ability and glucose uptake, thereby exhibiting its ergogenic property. The major reason for improved athletic or sports performance by beetroot (nitrate) is due to increased blood volume (erythropoiesis, high hemoglobin production and RBC) with increased oxygenation (oxygenated blood); improved blood flow to muscles results in bulk muscle mass and increased exercise tolerance (anti-fatigue) and performance (Zafeiridis, 2014). A clinical trial in trained cyclists with supplementation of beetroot juice considerably improved their performance in a 10-kilometer cycle test (Cermak et al., 2012). Bailey and others (2009) indicated that ingestion of beetroot juice (500 mL) for 6 days could significantly increase plasma nitrate levels with decreased blood pressure and thus improved physical performance. Another study by Bailey and others (2010) confirmed that consumption of beetroot juice could alter maximum oxygen uptake (VO_2 max) by 5% in low-intensity exercise, but alter maximum oxygen uptake (VO_2 max) by 25% in high-intensity exercise as compared to the placebo group. Moreover, pre-supplementation of beetroot juice (60 min-single dose) before training could markedly lower oxygen utilization and improve exercise tolerance after 150 min of consumption to prove the effect of absorbed nitrates (Muggeridge et al., 2014). Better ergogenic effects of beetroot juice are mostly noted after 6 days of consumption in endurance athletes (Hoon et al., 2013).

5.16.5 *Citrullus vulgaris/lanatus* (Watermelon)

Citrullus vulgaris/lanatus or watermelon is a vine belonging to Cucurbitaceae. Watermelon is a sweet summer fruit, used in fruit salads and its juice is consumed for re-hydration (91% water). It contains many minerals and vitamins with rich carbohydrate and water content (carbohydrate-electrolyte) and hence is commonly recommended for athletes and sportsperson (Erhirhie and Ekene, 2013). Watermelon is the richest source of L-citrulline (non-essential amino acid). Ingestion of watermelon juice could significantly increase the plasma L-citrulline, L-arginine and thus favors the synthesis of nitric oxide (NO-Vasodilator) (Mandel et al., 2005). We already indicated the importance of NO in *Beta vulgaris* (section above) on endurance sports. Studies have suggested that L-citrulline (watermelon) possesses an ergogenic property by improving muscle oxygenation, fatigue resistance and oxidative metabolism (Martinez-Sanchez et al., 2017b; Sureda et al., 2009). Watermelon intake can efficiently attenuate muscle fatigue/soreness after intense exercise (Tarazona-Diaz et al., 2013). Watermelon (L-citrulline) also possesses antioxidant and anti-inflammatory qualities and thus aids in attenuating exercise-induced oxidative stress (Glenn et al., 2017; Sureda et al., 2009). Martinez-Sanchez (2017a) concluded that supplementation of watermelon juice rich in citrulline with pomegranate juice rich in ellagitannins showed the potent ergogenic effect of lowering muscle soreness (fatigue) and muscle damage markers. Previous studies have shown a positive impact of watermelon on athletic performance only after low or moderate intensity exercise, not after endurance or high-intensity exercise (Bailey et al., 2016; Suzuki et al., 2016). Therefore, more trials or experiments are required to check whether watermelon enhances the athletic performance in intense training athletes.

5.16.6 *Prunus cerasus* (Tart Cherry/Sour Cherry)

Prunus cerasus or tart cherry belongs to the Rosaceae family and is native to Europe and South-western Asia. Tart cherry is commonly used for baking owing to its unique taste and is also used for making soup and desserts. Tart cherry is rich in polyphenolic compounds, anthocyanins (cyanidin 3-glucosyl-rutinoside) and melatonin with dietary fibers (Chaovanalikit and Wrolstad, 2004; Kirakosyan et al., 2009). As tart cherries are rich in polyphenolic compounds, they exhibit numerous pharmacological properties including antioxidant, anti-inflammatory, anti-fatigue, anti-cancer and anti-arthritis (Schumacher et al., 2013). Kuehl and others (2010) have reported that consumption of tart cherry juice for 8 days can significantly lower the post-run muscle pain (faster recovery) in healthy runners. Two more trials were conducted to further explore the benefits of tart cherry juice on cyclists and runners (endurance sport). Some experiments have shown that intake of tart cherry juice (polyphenols and anthocyanins) can notably reduce muscle damage markers and inflammation with enhanced antioxidant activity and thereby assist muscle recovery (delayed onset of muscle soreness; DOMS) and physical performance (Bell et al., 2014; Howatson et al., 2010). Bell and his co-workers (2016) carried out another clinical trial by supplementing tart cherry concentrate to soccer players (semi-professional) and inferred that tart-supplemented players could recover from muscle pain faster than the placebo group. Lately, Levers et al. (2016) concluded that acute supplementation of powdered tart cherry effectively abolishes the markers of muscle catabolism and inflammatory markers, while also balancing redox status and thus escalating endurance exercise performance.

5.16.7 *Citrus aurantium* (Bitter Orange)

Bitter or soar orange refers to a small citrus tree. Its peel and fruits are used for various biological benefits including antioxidant, anti-cancer, anti-obesity and anti-microbial properties (Allison et al., 2005). Active components are synephrine and octopamine, which are similar to epinephrine and nor-epinephrine and affect the β-3 receptor (CNS stimulant) and thereby stimulate lipolysis (Bent et al., 2004; Fugh-Berman and Myers, 2004). Allison and his co-workers (2005) indicated that bitter orange contains both p- and m-synephrine, which are responsible for lipolysis and can be recommended for obesity and to improve LBM. Mostly, bitter orange juice was combined with caffeine diet to maintain LBM and lose excessive fat and thereby enhance athletic performance (Colker et al., 1999; Haaz et al., 2006). However, bitter orange is mostly recommended with other herbal extracts (CNS stimulant) like green tea and guarana (caffeine) as a weight management supplement to reduce excessive fat (Sale et al., 2006).

5.16.8 GARCINIA (HYDROXYCITRIC ACID)

Garcinia plant genus belongs to Clusiaceae family, which includes *Garcinia cambogia, Garcinia indica Garcinia mangosteen* and has been used a flavoring agent for many years in Asia. Garcinia contains a significant amount of Hydroxycitric acid (HCA), which is highly recommended to lose excessive fat (anti-obesity). HCA is reported to enhance fat oxidation (β-oxidation) by reducing cytosolic malonyl-CoA (Semwal et al., 2015). A clinical trial has proved that HCA supplementation could mitigate the de-novo lipogenesis process and thus decrease the lipid profile (Westernterp-Plantenga and Kovacs, 2002). HCA has been recognized for its ergogenic property owing to its lipolysis or fat oxidation activity (glycogen sparing property) and thus improve the endurance capacity in athletes. Lim and his co-workers (2002) demonstrated that intake of HCA would lead to a marked decrease in RQ and energy expenditure during moderate exercise. Similarly, another study also showed that ingestion of HCA in athletes can significantly improve the fat oxidation and thus reduce RQ with increased VO_2 max level (Tomita et al., 2003). However, more studies are required to confirm or support the ergogenic property of HCA on endurance athletes.

5.16.9 QUERCETIN

Quercetin is a flavonol (flavonoid) that constitutes the aglycone of rutin and is commonly found in fruits and vegetable like onion, grapes, apple and berries. Enhanced mitochondrial biogenesis (ATP production) acts as a potent antioxidant and anti-inflammatory agent (Davis et al., 2009; Lagouge et al., 2006). Quercetin glycoside has a best absorbable form with a longer half-life of 6–9 h and hence it gets more attention from researchers especially in exercise-related studies (Kresslers et al., 2011). Studies have shown that quercetin possesses antioxidant, anti-inflammatory, anti-fatigue, anti-cancer, anti-microbial as well as cardioprotective, neuroprotective and hepatoprotective properties (Lu et al., 2015). Kresslers and his co-workers (2011) conducted a meta-analysis study that included 8 studies and summarized that administration of quercetin provides a significant benefit in endurance exercise capacity by modulating oxygen consumption (VO_2 max) and mitochondrial biogenesis as compared to a placebo group. Most of the clinical trial conducted to assess athletic performance in athletes and sportspersons with quercetin showed no or small significance (Casuso et al., 2013; Ganio et al., 2010; Nieman et al., 2010); however, a small number of studies showed high importance on athletic or physical performance (Askari et al., 2013; Davis et al., 2010). The above controversial results are due to different doses, durations and types of sports or the routes of intervention (quercetin). Another study conducted by Nieman et al. (2009) also concluded that supplementation of quercetin and epigallocatechin gallate (EGCG) on trained cyclists could significantly lower the inflammatory markers and thus aid in fast muscle recovery.

5.16.10 RESVERATROL

Resveratrol is a naturally occurring non-flavonoid polyphenolic compound (stilbene class) belonging to the phytoalexin superfamily. The major dietary sources (food) of RESV are red wine/red grapes, berries, soybeans and pomegranates (Liu et al., 2007).

RESV has been used to treat various ailments including diabetes, cardiovascular diseases, cancers and neurological diseases (Berman et al., 2017). Previous studies have demonstrated that resveratrol consumption could enhance exercise performance (endurance capacity) by upregulating the Sirtuin-1 (SIRT-1) pathway in the mitochondria (ATP production) of myocytes as well as improving fatty oxidation in various animal models, thus indicating its ergogenic properties (Menzies et al., 2013; Wu et al., 2013). Mostly, animal studies showed positive results on exercise performance (Dolinsky et al., 2012; Wu et al., 2013) owing to anti-oxidant, anti-inflammatory, and hypolipidemic activities, but no clinical trial has been conducted to date. Hence, more studies are required before recommending resveratrol as an ergogenic aid for humans.

5.16.11 Tapioca (Starch; Amylopectin)

Tapioca is extracted from the cassava plant (*Manihot esculenta*). It has a neutral taste with low osmotic pressure in the stomach and hence prevents nausea or bloating. Tapioca starch has less GI value with the slow and steady release of glucose into the bloodstream, which is ideal for endurance athletes as it does not cause an immediate insulin response and reduces hunger during prolonged exercise. Tapioca has a denser packing structure than other types of starch and thereby results in the delivery of high levels of energy that are major criteria for endurance athletes during prolonged workout or exercise (Thompson, 2015). There are some studies that indicated the importance of tapioca-based sports drinks (from cassava) for endurance sportsman (Earnest and Rasmussen, 2015; Haramizu et al., 2012).

Another non-popular ergogenic function foods/nutraceuticals is pomegranate juice (anthocyanins/proanthocyanidins), and it has been proven that its consumption for 21 days improved antioxidant status and thus aids in protecting against exercise-induced oxidative stress (Fuster-Munoz et al., 2016). Another study also indicated that supplementation of pomegranate juice rich in ellagitannins and watermelon juice rich in citrulline showed the potent ergogenic effect by lowering muscle soreness (fatigue) and muscle damage markers (Martinez-Sanchez 2017a). Coconut water (tender) is rich in electrolytes and carbohydrates (Carbohydrate-electrolyte) and is used as a natural sports drink (alternative to artificial sports drink). It is good for rehydration, but there is no reliable evidence for its involvement in endurance or physical performance (Kalman et al., 2012). Capsaicin from red pepper is a major pungent element that contributes to spicy taste and hence is used in many dishes in most Asian countries. Many animal and human studies have proven that it has a thermogenic/lipolysis effect and thus lowers glycogen utilization, RQ during exercise and increases the plasma catecholamine as well as alertness, similar to caffeine (Kim et al., 2016; Oh and Ohta, 2003). In addition, some foods including banana, avocado, lemon and orange, berries, kale, oats, sweet potatoes, raisins, walnut, cashew nut and milk (probiotics) are used to improve training/sports performance, but these functional foods lack scientific evidence/proof of such.

5.17 MECHANISM OF ERGOGENIC (ADAPTOGENIC) HERBS FOR BIOCHEMICAL TUNING FOR ATHLETES

- CNS/PNS–stimulant (improves cognitive function)
- Enhances ATP production in muscle (mitochondria) with glucose utilization
- Increases insulin, pCr and Na^{2+} production
- Glycogen/protein sparing function
- Adaptogenic property (anti-stress or anti-depressant)–suppresses corticosteroid hormones
- Increases blood fluidity (lower viscosity, less fibrinogen) thus increasing VO_2 max (increase oxygen efficiency), thus contributing to muscle growth (mass)
- Elevated erythropoiesis by increasing erythropoietin (EPO) production
- Bronchodilators (increased oxygenated blood) and vasodilator (lowers blood pressure)
- Antioxidant and anti-inflammatory property (reduces free radicals and muscle injury)

5.18 CONCLUSION

The role of functional foods in endurance sports is a new approach in the nutritional sport arena, but studies conducted so far show that supplementation of functional foods/ nutraceuticals in various forms, durations and doses could significantly improve the athletic performance by lowering muscle weakness (fatigue), oxygen consumption as well as increasing mitochondrial biogenesis with antioxidant, anti-stress (adaptogenic) and anti-inflammatory activities, thereby abolishing exercise-induced fatigue or oxidative stress and bringing about prolonged physical performance. However, the effects of functional food on endurance athletes are sparse and hence more studies are required to prove its importance. Nevertheless, the individual effects of functional foods on endurance sports are significantly fewer but the mixing of various functional foods would maximize ergogenic properties with other biological properties.

REFERENCES

Allen DG, Lamb GD, Westerblad H. Skeletal muscle fatigue: Cellular mechanisms. *Physiological Reviews*. 2008;88(1):287–332.

Allison DB, Cutter G, Poehman ET, Moore DR, Barnes S. Exactly which synephrine alkaloids does citrus aurantium (bitter orange) contain? *International Journal of Obesity (Lond)*. 2005;29(4):443–6.

Alsmadi AM, Tawalbeh LI, Gammoh OS, Shawagfeh MQ, Zalloum W, Ashour A, Attarian H. The effect of Ginkgo biloba and psycho-education on stress, anxiety and fatigue among refugees. *Proceedings of Singapore Healthcare*. 2018;27: 26–32.

Anderson JJB. Minerals. In: Mahan KL, Escott-Stump S (eds) *Krause's Food, Nutrition, & Diet Therapy* (pp. 110–52). Saunders, Philadelphia; 2000.

Anosike CA, Obidoa O, Ezeanyika LU, Nwuba MM. Antiinflammatory and anti-ulcerogenic activity of the ethanol extract of ginger (Zingiber officinale). *African Journal of Biochemistry Research*. 2009;3: 379–84.

Artioli GG, Gualano B, Smith A, Stout J, Lancha Jr AH. Role of beta-alanine supplementation on muscle carnosine and exercise performance. *Medicine and Science in Sports and Exercise*. 2010;42(6):1162–73.

Askari G, Ghiasvand R, Paknahad Z, Karimian J, Rabiee K, Sharifirad G, Feizi A. The effects of quercetin supplementation on body composition, exercise performance and muscle damage indices in athletes. *International Journal of Preventive Medicine*. 2013;4(1):21.

Babu A, Pon V, Liu D. Green tea catechins and cardiovascular health: An update. *Current Medicinal Chemistry*. 2008;15(18):1840–50.

Bagchi D, Nair S, Sen CK, editors. *Nutrition and Enhanced Sports Performance: Muscle Building, Endurance, and Strength*, 2nd edition. Academic Press, London; 2013.

Bai Y, Tohda C, Zhu S, Hattori M, Komatsu K. Active components from Siberian ginseng (Eleutherococcus senticosus) for protection of amyloid β 25–35-induced neuritic atrophy in cultured rat cortical neurons. *Journal of Natural Medicines*. 2011;65(3–4):417–23.

Bailey SJ, Blackwell JR, Williams E, Vanhatalo A, Wylie LJ, Winyard PG, Jones AM. Two weeks of watermelon juice supplementation improves nitric oxide bioavailability but not endurance exercise performance in humans. *Nitric Oxide*. 2016;59:10–20.

Bailey SJ, Fulford J, Vanhatalo A, Winyard PG, Blackwell JR, DiMenna FJ, Wilkerson DP, Benjamin N, Jones AM. Dietary nitrate supplementation enhances muscle contractile efficiency during knee-extensor exercise in humans. *Journal of Applied Physiology*. 2010;109(1):135–48.

Bailey SJ, Winyard P, Vanhatalo A, Blackwell JR, DiMenna FJ, Wilkerson DP, Tarr J, Benjamin N, Jones AM. Dietary nitrate supplementation reduces the O_2 cost of low-intensity exercise and enhances tolerance to high-intensity exercise in humans. *Journal of Applied Physiology*. 2009;107(4):1144–55.

Bartlett JD, Hawley JA, Morton JP. Carbohydrate availability and exercise training adaptation: Too much of a good thing? *European Journal Sports Science*. 2015;15(1):3–12.

Baynes JW. Carbohydrates and lipids. In Baynes JW, Dominiczak M, editors, *Medical BioChemistry* (pp. 23–32). Elsevier, Amsterdam; 2018.

Bell DG, McLellan TM, Sabiston CM. Effect of ingesting caffeine and ephedrine on 10 km run performance. *Medicine and Science in Sports and Exercise*. 2002;34(2):344–9.

Bell PG, Stevenson E, Davison GW, Howatson G. The effects of Montmorency tart cherry concentrate supplementation on recovery following prolonged, intermittent exercise. *Nutrients*. 2016;8(7):441.

Bell PG, Walshe IH, Davison GW, Stevenson E, Howatson G. Montmorency cherries reduce the oxidative stress and inflammatory responses to repeated days high-intensity stochastic cycling. *Nutrients*. 2014;6(2):829–43.

Bent S, Padula A, Neuhaus J. Safety and efficacy of citrus aurantium for weight loss. *The American Journal of Cardiology*. 2004;94(10):1359–61.

Berman AY, Motechin RA, Wiesenfeld MY, Holz MK. The therapeutic potential of resveratrol: A review of clinical trials. *NPJ Precision Oncology*. 2017;1(1):35.

Bhat R, Karim AA, Ali T. Tongkat Ali (Eurycoma longifolia Jack): A review on its ethnobotany and pharmacological importance. *Fitoterapia*. 2010;81(7):669–79.

Black AE, Coward WA, Cole TJ, Prentice AM. Human energy expenditure in affluent societies: An analysis of 574 doubly-labelled water measurements. *European Journal of Clinical Nutrition*. 1996;50:72–92.

Bridge CA, Jones MA. The effect of caffeine ingestion on 8 km run performance in a field setting. *Journal of Sports Sciences*. 2006;24(4):433–9.

Brilla LR, Haley TF. Effect of magnesium supplementation on strength training in humans. *Journal of the American College of Nutrition*. 1992;11(3):326–9.

Bucci LR. Selected herbals and human exercise performance. *The American Journal of Clinical Nutrition*. 2000;72(2):624S–36S.

Burke LM. Caffeine and sports performance. *Applied Physiology, Nutrition, and Metabolism.* 2008;33(6):1319–34.

Burke LM. Re-examining high-fat diets for sports performance: Did we call the 'nail in the coffin' too soon? *Sports Medicine.* 2015;45(1):33–49.

Burke LM, Hawley JA, Wong SH, Jeukendrup AE. Carbohydrates for training and competition. *Journal of Sports Sciences.* 2011;29(sup1):S17–27.

Burke LM, Kiens B. "Fat adaptation" for athletic performance: The nail in the coffin? *Journal of Applied Physiology.* 2006;100(1):7–8.

Calfee R, Fadale P. Popular ergogenic drugs and supplements in young athletes. *Pediatrics.* 2006;117(3):e577–89.

Cao S, Shang H, Wu W, Du J, Putheti R. Evaluation of anti-athletic fatigue activity of Schizandra chinensis aqueous extracts in mice. *African Journal of Pharmacy and Pharmacology.* 2009;3(11):593–7.

Casuso RA, Martinez-Amat A, Martinez-Lopez EJ, Camiletti Moiron D, Porres JM, Aranda P. Ergogenic effects of quercetin supplementation in trained rats. *Journal of the International Society of Sports Nutrition.* 2013;10(1):3.

Cermak N, Gibala M, Van Loon J. Nitrate supplementation's improvement of 10-km time-trial performance in trained cyclists. *International Journal of Sport Nutrition and Exercise Metabolism.* 2012;22(1):64–71.

Chan SW. Panax ginseng Rhodiola rosea and Schisandra chinensis. *International Journal of Food Sciences and Nutrition.* 2012;63(sup1):75–81.

Chaovanalikit A, Wrolstad RE. Total anthocyanins and total phenolics of fresh and processed cherries and their antioxidant properties. *Journal of Food Science.* 2004;69(1):67–72.

Chen CY, Hou CW, Bernard JR, Chen CC, Hung TC, Cheng LL, Liao YH, Kuo CH. Rhodiola crenulata-and Cordyceps sinensis-based supplement boosts aerobic exercise performance after short-term high-altitude training. *High Altitude Medicine and Biology.* 2014a;15(3):371–9.

Chen WC, Huang WC, Chiu CC, Chang YK, Huang CC. Whey protein improves exercise performance and biochemical profiles in trained mice. *Medicine and Science in Sports and Exercise.* 2014b;46(8):1517–24.

Chen S, Li Z, Krochmal R, Abrazado M, Kim W, Cooper CB. Effect of Cs-4® (Cordyceps sinensis) on exercise performance in healthy older subjects: A double-blind, placebo-controlled trial. *The Journal of Alternative and Complementary Medicine.* 2010;16(5):585–90.

Choudhary B, Shetty A, Langade DG. Efficacy of Ashwagandha (Withania somnifera [L.] Dunal) in improving cardiorespiratory endurance in healthy athletic adults. *Ayu.* 2015;36(1):63.

Christensen PM, Shirai Y, Ritz C, Nordsborg NB. Caffeine and bicarbonate for speed. A meta-analysis of legal supplements potential for improving intense endurance exercise performance. *Frontiers in Physiology.* 2017;8:240.

Chun JN, Cho M, So I, Jeon JH. The protective effects of Schisandra chinensis fruit extract and its lignans against cardiovascular disease: A review of the molecular mechanisms. *Fitoterapia.* 2014;97:224–33.

Colker CM, Kalman DS, Torina GC, Perlis T, Street C. Effects of Citrus aurantium, caffeine, and St. John's wort on body fat loss, lipid levels, and mood states, in overweight healthy adults. *Current Therapeutic Research.* 1999;60(3):145–52.

Corbo MR, Bevilacqua A, Petruzzi L, Casanova FP, Sinigaglia M. Functional beverages: The emerging side of functional foods. *Comprehensive Reviews in Food Science and Food Safety.* 2014;13(6):1192–206.

Dahlquist DT, Stellingwerff T, Dieter BP, McKenzie DC, Koehle MS. Effects of macro-and micronutrients on exercise-induced hepcidin response in highly trained endurance athletes. *Applied Physiology, Nutrition, and Metabolism.* 2017;42(10):1036–43.

Damirchi A, Zareei AS, Sariri R. Salivary antioxidants of male athletes after aerobic exercise and garlic supplementation on: A randomized, double blind, placebo-controlled study. *Journal of Oral Biology and Craniofacial Research*. 2015;5(3):146–52.

Dangin M, Boirie Y, Garcia-Rodenas C, et al. The digestion rate of protein is an independent regulating factor of postprandial protein retention. *American journal of Physiology. Endocrinology and Metabolism*. 2001;280:E340–348.

Davis JM, Carlstedt CJ, Chen S, Carmichael MD, Murphy EA. The dietary flavonoid quercetin increases VO$_2$max and endurance capacity. *International Journal of Sport Nutrition and Exercise Metabolism*. 2010;20:5662.

Davis JM, Murphy EA, Carmichael MD, Davis B. Quercetin increases brain and muscle mitochondrial biogenesis and exercise tolerance. *American Journal of Physiology. Regulatory Integrative and Comparative Physiology*. 2009;296(4):R10717.

De Bock K, Eijnde BO, Ramaekers M, Hespel P. Acute Rhodiola rosea intake can improve endurance exercise performance. *International Journal of Sport Nutrition and Exercise Metabolism*. 2004;14(3):298–307.

De Carvalho FG, Barbieri RA, Carvalho MB, Dato CC, Campos EZ, Gobbi RB, Papoti M, Silva AS, de Freitas EC. Taurine supplementation can increase lipolysis and affect the contribution of energy systems during front crawl maximal effort. *Amino Acids*. 2018;50(1):189–98.

De Carvalho FG, Galan BS, Santos PC, Pritchett K, Pfrimer K, Ferriolli E, Papoti M, Marchini JS, de Freitas EC. Taurine: A potential ergogenic aid for preventing muscle damage and protein catabolism and decreasing oxidative stress produced by endurance exercise. *Frontiers in Physiology*. 2017;8:710.

de Salles Painelli V, Roschel H, De Jesus F, Sale C, Harris RC, Solis MY, Benatti FB, Gualano B, Lancha Jr AH, Artioli GG. The ergogenic effect of beta-alanine combined with sodium bicarbonate on high-intensity swimming performance. *Applied Physiology, Nutrition, and Metabolism*. 2013;38(5):525–32.

Dilshara MG, Jayasooriya RGPT, Kang C, Lee S, Park SR, Jeong J, Choi YH, Seo YT, Jang YP, Kim G. Downregulation of pro-inflammatory mediators by a water extract of Schisandra chinensis (Turcz.) Baill fruit in lipopolysaccharide-stimulated RAW 264.7 macrophage cells. *Environmental Toxicology and Pharmacology*. 2013;36(2):256–64.

Dolinsky VW, Jones KE, Sidhu RS, Haykowsky M, Czubryt MP, Gordon T, Dyck JR. Improvements in skeletal muscle strength and cardiac function induced by resveratrol during exercise training contribute to enhanced exercise performance in rats. *The Journal of Physiology*. 2012;590(11):2783–99.

Duncan MJ, Tallis J, Wilson S, Clarke ND. The effect of caffeine and Rhodiola rosea, alone or in combination, on 5-km running performance in men. *Journal of Caffeine Research*. 2016;6(1):40–8.

Earnest CP, Rasmussen C. Nutritional Supplements for Endurance Athletes. In Greenwood M, Cooke MB, Ziegenfuss T, Kalman DS, Antonio J, editors, *Nutritional Supplements in Sports and Exercise* (pp. 253–72). Springer, Cham; 2015.

Eberle SG. *Endurance Sports Nutrition*, 3rd edition. Human Kinetics, Champaign, IL; 2013.

Erhirhie EO, Ekene NE. Medicinal values on Citrullus lanatus (watermelon): Pharmacological review. *International Journal of Research in Pharmaceutical and Biomedical Sciences*. 2013;4(4):1305–12.

Eussen SR, Verhagen H, Klungel OH, Garssen J, van Loveren H, van Kranen HJ, Rompelberg CJ. Functional foods and dietary supplements: Products at the interface between pharma and nutrition. *European Journal of Pharmacology*. 2011;668:S2–9.

Fink HH. *Practical Applications in Sports Nutrition*, 5th edition (pp. 330–337). Jones & Bartlett Learning, Sudbury, MA; 2017.

Fugh-Berman A, Myers A. Citrus aurantium, an ingredient of dietary supplements marketed for weight loss: Current status of clinical and basic research. *Experimental Biology and Medicine*. 2004;229(8):698–704.

Fullagar HH, Skorski S, Duffield R, Hammes D, Coutts AJ, Meyer T. Sleep and athletic performance: The effects of sleep loss on exercise performance, and physiological and cognitive responses to exercise. *Sports Medicine*. 2015;45(2):161–86.

Fuster-Muñoz E, Roche E, Funes L, Martínez-Peinado P, Sempere JM, Vicente-Salar N. Effects of pomegranate juice in circulating parameters, cytokines, and oxidative stress markers in endurance-based athletes: A randomized controlled trial. *Nutrition*. 2016;32(5):539–45.

Ganio MS, Armstrong LE, Johnson EC, Klau JF, Ballard KD, Michniak-Kohn B, Kaushik D, Maresh CM. Effect of quercetin supplementation on maximal oxygen uptake in men and women. *Journal of Sports Sciences*. 2010;28(2):201–8.

Ganio MS, Klau JF, Casa DJ, Armstrong LE, Maresh CM. Effect of caffeine on sport-specific endurance performance: A systematic review. *The Journal of Strength and Conditioning Research*. 2009;23(1):315–24.

Georgiev VG, Weber J, Kneschke EM, Denev PN, Bley T, Pavlov AI. Antioxidant activity and phenolic content of betalain extracts from intact plants and hairy root cultures of the red beetroot Beta vulgaris cv. Detroit dark red. *Plant Foods for Human Nutrition*. 2010;65(2):105–11.

Gill ND, Shield A, Blazevich AJ, Zhou S, Weatherby RP. Muscular and cardiorespiratory effects of pseudoephedrine in human athletes. *British Journal of Clinical Pharmacology*. 2000;50(3):205–13.

Glenn JM, Gray M, Wethington LN, Stone MS, Stewart RW, Moyen NE. Acute citrulline malate supplementation improves upper-and lower-body submaximal weightlifting exercise performance in resistance-trained females. *European Journal of Nutrition*. 2017;56(2):775–84.

Goldfinch J, McNaughton LR, Davies P. Bicarbonate ingestion and its effects upon 400-m. *European Journal of Applied Physiology and Occupational Physiology*. 1988;57:45–48.

Goss F, Robertson R, Riechman S, Zoeller R, Dabayebeh I, Moyna N, Boer N, Peoples J, Metz K. Effect of potassium phosphate supplementation on perceptual and physiological responses to maximal graded exercise. *International Journal of Sport Nutrition and Exercise Metabolism*. 2001;11(1):53–62.

Goulet ED, Dionne IJ. Assessment of the effects of eleuterococcus senticosus on endurance performance. *International Journal of Sport Nutrition and Exercise Metabolism*. 2005;15(1):75–83.

Greenhaff P. The nutritional biochemistry of creatine. *The Journal of Nutritional Biochemistry*. 1997;11(11):610–8.

Greenwood M, Cooke MB, Ziegenfuss T, Kalman DS, Antonio J, editors. *Nutritional Supplements in Sports and Exercise*, 2nd edition. Humana Press, New York; 2015.

Guzel NA, Orer EG, Bircan SF, Cevher CS. Effects of acute L-carnitine supplementation on nitric oxide production and oxidative stress after exhaustive exercise in young soccer players. *The Journal of Sports Medicine and Physical Fitness*. 2015;55:9–15.

Haaz S, Fontaine KR, Cutter G, Limdi N, PerumeanChaney S, Allison DB. Citrus aurantium and synephrine alkaloids in the treatment of overweight and obesity: An update. *Obesity Reviews*. 2006;7(1):79–88.

Haller CA, Benowitz NL. Adverse cardiovascular and central nervous system events associated with dietary supplements containing ephedra alkaloids. *New England Journal of Medicine*. 2000;343(25):1833–88.

Hamerski L, Somner GV, Tamaio N. Paullinia cupana Kunth (Sapindaceae): A review of its ethnopharmacology, phytochemistry and pharmacology. *Journal of Medicinal Plants Research*. 2013;7(30):2221–9.

Hamzah S, Yusof A. The ergogenic effects of Eurycoma longifolia jack: A pilot study. *British Journal of Sports Medicine.* 2003;37:464–70.

Haramizu S, Shimotoyodome A, Fukuoka D, Murase T, Hase T. Hydroxypropylated distarch phosphate versus unmodified tapioca starch: Fat oxidation and endurance in C57BL/6J mice. *European Journal of Applied Physiology.* 2012;112(9):3409–16.

Harris JA, Benedict FG. *A Biometric Study of Basal Metabolism in Man.* Vol 279. Carnegie Institute, Washington, DC; 1919.

Harris RC, Tallon MJ, Dunnett M, Boobis L, Coakley J, Kim HJ, Fallowfield JL, Hill CA, Sale C, Wise JA. The absorption of orally supplied beta-alanine and its effect on muscle carnosine synthesis in human vastus lateralis. *Amino Acids.* 2006;30(3):279–89.

Hill CA, Harris RC, Kim HJ, Harris BD, Sale C, Boobis LH, Kim CK, Wise JA. Influence of beta-alanine supplementation on skeletal muscle carnosine concentrations and high intensity cycling capacity. *Amino Acids.* 2007;32(2):225–33.

Hinton PS. Iron and the endurance athlete. *Applied Physiology, Nutrition, and Metabolism.* 2014;39(9):1012–8.

Hoffman J, Ratamess N, Faigenbaum A, Ross R, Kang J, Stout J, Wise JA. Short-duration beta-alanine supplementation increases training volume and reduces subjective feelings of fatigue in college football players. *Nutrition Research.* 2007;28(1):31–5.

Hoon MW, Johnson NA, Chapman PG, Burke LM. The effect of nitrate supplementation on exercise performance in healthy individuals: A systematic review and meta-analysis. *International Journal of Sport Nutrition and Exercise Metabolism.* 2013;23(5):522–32.

Hostrup M, Bangsbo J. Limitations in intense exercise performance of athletes–effect of speed endurance training on ion handling and fatigue development. *The Journal of Physiology.* 2017;595(9):2897–913.

Howatson G, McHugh MP, Hill JA, Brouner J, Jewell AP, Van Someren KA, Shave RE, Howatson SA. Influence of tart cherry juice on indices of recovery following marathon running. *Scandinavian Journal of Medicine and Science in Sports.* 2010;20(6):843–52.

Huang LZ, Huang BK, Yea Q, Qina LP. Bioactivity-guided fractionation for anti-fatigue property of Acanthopanax senticosus. *Journal of Ethnopharmacology.* 2011;133(1):213–9.

Hughes D. The World Anti-Doping Code in sport: Update for 2015. *Australian Prescriber.* 2015;38(5):167–70.

Hursel R, Viechtbauer W, Westerterp-Plantenga MS. The effects of green tea on weight loss and weight maintenance: A meta-analysis. *International Journal of Obesity.* 2009;33(9):956–61.

Ichinose T, Nomura S, Someya Y, Akimoto S, Tachiyashiki K, Imaizumi K. Effect of endurance training supplemented with green tea extract on substrate metabolism during exercise in humans. *Scandinavian Journal of Medicine and Science in Sports.* 2011;21(4):598–605.

Imagawa TF, Hirano I, Utsuki K, Horie M, Naka A, Matsumoto K, Imagawa S. Caffeine and taurine enhance endurance performance. *International Journal of Sports Medicine.* 2009;30(7):485–8.

İnce Dİ, Sönmez GT, İnce ML. Effects of garlic on aerobic performance. *Turkish Journal of Medical Sciences.* 2000;30(6):557–61.

Jafari H, Ross JB, Emhoff CA. Effects of branched-chain amino acid supplementation on exercise performance and recovery in highly endurance-trained athletes. *The FASEB Journal.* 2016;30:1s.

Jones AM. Dietary nitrate supplementation and exercise performance. *Sports Medicine.* 2014;44(1):35–45.

Jones G. Caffeine and other sympathomimetic stimulants: Modes of action and effects on sports performance. *Essays in Biochemistry.* 2008;44(1):109–23.

Jówko E, Długołęcka B, Makaruk B, Cieśliński I. The effect of green tea extract supplementation on exercise-induced oxidative stress parameters in male sprinters. *European Journal of Nutrition*. 2015;54(5):783–91.

Jówko E, Sacharuk J, Balasińska B, Ostaszewski P, Charmas M, Charmas R. Green tea extract supplementation gives protection against exercise-induced oxidative damage in healthy men. *Nutrition Research*. 2011;31(11):813–21.

Kalman DS, Feldman S, Krieger DR, Bloomer RJ. Comparison of coconut water and a carbohydrate-electrolyte sport drink on measures of hydration and physical performance in exercise-trained men. *Journal of the International Society of Sports Nutrition*. 2012;9(1):1.

Keisler BD, Armsey TD. Caffeine as an ergogenic aid. *Current Sports Medicine Reports*. 2006;5(4):215–9.

Kellmann M. Preventing overtraining in athletes in high-intensity sports and stress/recovery monitoring. *Scandinavian Journal of Medicine and Science in Sports*. 2010;20:95–102.

Kennedy DO, Haskell CF, Robertson B, Reay J, Brewster-Maund C, Luedemann J, Maggini S, Ruf M, Zangara A, Scholey AB. Improved cognitive performance and mental fatigue following a multi-vitamin and mineral supplement with added guarana (Paullinia cupana). *Appetite*. 2008;50(2–3):506–13.

Kennedy DO, Haskell CF, Wesnes KA, Scholey AB. Improved cognitive performance in human volunteers following administration of guarana (Paullinia cupana) extract: Comparison and interaction with panax ginseng. *Pharmacology, Biochemistry and Behavior*. 2004;79(3):401–11.

Khanijo T, Jiraungkoorskul W. Review ergogenic effect of long jack, Eurycoma longifolia. *Pharmacognosy Reviews*. 2016;10(20):139.

Kim J, Park J, Lim K. Nutrition supplements to stimulate lipolysis: A review in relation to endurance exercise capacity. *Journal of Nutritional Science and Vitaminology*. 2016;62(3):141–61.

Kimura Y, Sumiyoshi M. Effects of various Eleutherococcus senticosus cortex on swimming time, natural killer activity and corticosterone level in forced swimming stressed mice. *Journal of Ethnopharmacology*. 2004;95(2–3):447–53.

Kirakosyan A, Seymour EM, Llanes DE, Kaufman PB, Bolling SF. Chemical profile and antioxidant capacities of tart cherry products. *Food Chemistry*. 2009;115(1):20–5.

Knechtle B, Zapf J, Zwyssig D, Lippuner K, Hoppeler H. Energieumsatz und muskelstruktur bei Langzeitbelastung: Eine Fallstudie. *Schweizerische Zeitschrift für Sportmedizin und Sporttraumatologie*. 2003;51(4):180–7.

Kotze HF, van derWalt WH, Rogers GG, Strydom NB. Effects of plasma ascorbic acid levels on heat acclimatization in man. *Journal of Applied Physiology*. 1977;42(5):711–6.

Kreider RB, Kalman DS, Antonio J, Ziegenfuss TN, Wildman R, Collins R, Candow DG, Kleiner SM, Almada AL, Lopez HL. International Society of Sports Nutrition position stand: Safety and efficacy of creatine supplementation in exercise, sport, and medicine. *Journal of the International Society of Sports Nutrition*. 2017;14(1):18.

Kreider RB, Wilborn CD, Taylor L, Campbell B, Almada AL, Collins R, Cooke M, Earnest CP, Greenwood M, Kalman DS, Kerksick C. ISSN exercise & sport nutrition review: Research & recommendations. *Journal of the International Society of Sports Nutrition*. 2010;7(1):1–7.

Kressler J, Millard-Stafford M, Warren GL. Quercetin and endurance exercise capacity: A systematic review and meta-analysis. *Medicine and Science in Sports and Exercise*. 2011;43(12):2396–404.

Kuehl KS, Perrier ET, Elliot DL, Chesnutt JC. Efficacy of tart cherry juice in reducing muscle pain during running: A randomized controlled trial. *Journal of the International Society of Sports Nutrition*. 2010;7(1):17.

Kumar R, Negi PS, Singh B, Ilavazhagan G, Bhargava K, Sethy NK. Cordyceps sinensis promotes exercise endurance capacity of rats by activating skeletal muscle metabolic regulators. *Journal of Ethnopharmacology*. 2011;136(1):260–6.

Kuo J, Chen KW, Cheng IS, Tsai PH, Lu YJ, Lee NY. The effect of eight weeks of supplementation with Eleutherococcus senticosus on endurance capacity and metabolism in human. *The Chinese Journal of Physiology*. 2010;53(2):105–1.

Lagouge M, Argmann C, Gerhart-Hines Z, Meziane H, Lerin C, Daussin F, Messadeq N, Milne J, Lambert P, Elliott P, Geny B. Resveratrol improves mitochondrial function and protects against metabolic disease by activating SIRT1 and PGC-1alpha. *Cell*. 2006;127:1109–22.

Lamboley CR, Royer D, Dionne IJ. Effects of β-hydroxy-β-methylbutyrate on aerobic-performance components and body composition in college students. *International Journal of Sport Nutrition and Exercise Metabolism*. 2007;17(1):56–69.

Lanham-New SA, Stear S, Shirreffs S, Collins A, editors. *Sport and Exercise Nutrition*. John Wiley & Sons, Chichester, UK; 2011.

Lee JK, Lee JS, Park H, Cha YS, Yoon CS, Kim CK. Effect of L-carnitine supplementation and aerobic training on FABPc content and β-HAD activity in human skeletal muscle. *European Journal of Applied Physiology*. 2007;99(2):193–9.

Levers K, Dalton R, Galvan E, O'Connor A, Goodenough C, Simbo S, Mertens-Talcott SU, Rasmussen C, Greenwood M, Riechman S, Crouse S. Effects of powdered Montmorency tart cherry supplementation on acute endurance exercise performance in aerobically trained individuals. *Journal of the International Society of Sports Nutrition*. 2016;13(1):22.

Liang MT, Podolka TD, Chuang WJ. Panax notoginseng supplementation enhances physical performance during endurance exercise. *Journal of Strength and Conditioning Research*. 2005;19(1):108–14.

Lim K, Ryu S, Ohishi Y, Watanabe I, Tomi H, Suh H, Lee WK, Kwon T. Short-term (-)-hydroxycitrate ingestion increases fat oxidation during exercise in athletes. *Journal of Nutritional Science and Vitaminology*. 2002;48(2):128–33.

Lindh AM, Peyrebrune MC, Ingham SA, Bailey DM, Folland JP. Sodium bicarbonate improves swimming performance. *International Journal of Sports Medicine*. 2008;29(6):519–23.

Liu BL, Zhang X, Zhang W, Zhen HN. New enlightenment of French Paradox: Resveratrol's potential for cancer chemoprevention and anti-cancer therapy. *Cancer Biology and Therapy*. 2007;6(12):1833–6.

Lu TM, Chiu HF, Shen YC, Chung CC, Venkatakrishnan K, Wang CK. Hypocholesterolemic efficacy of quercetin rich onion juice in healthy mild hypercholesterolemic adults: A pilot study. *Plant Foods for Human Nutrition*. 2015;70(4):395–400.

Luden ND, Saunders MJ, Todd MK. Post-exercise carbohydrate-protein-antioxidant ingestion decreases plasma creatine kinase and muscle soreness. *International Journal of Sport Nutrition and Exercise Metabolism*. 2007;17(1):109–23.

Lukaski HC. Vitamin and mineral status: Effects on physical performance. *Nutrition*. 2004;20(7):632–44.

Lundy B. Nutrition for synchronized swimming: A review. *International Journal of Sport Nutrition and Exercise Metabolism*. 2011;21(5):436–45.

Ma G, Bavadekar SA, Davis YM, Lalchandani SG, Nagmani R, Schaneberg BT, Khan IA, Feller DR. Pharmacological effects of ephedrine alkaloids on human α1-and α2-adrenergic receptor subtypes. *Journal of Pharmacology and Experimental Therapeutics*. 2007;322(1):214–21.

Ma GD, Chiu CH, Hsu YJ, Hou CW, Chen YM, Huang CC. Changbai Mountain ginseng (panax ginseng CA Mey) extract supplementation improves exercise performance and energy utilization and decreases fatigue-associated parameters in mice. *Molecules*. 2017;22(2):237.

Malaguti M, Angeloni C, Hrelia S. Polyphenols in exercise performance and prevention of exercise-induced muscle damage. *Oxidative Medicine and Cellular Longevity.* 2013; 2013:825928.

Mandel H, Levy N, Izkovitch S, Korman SH. Elevated plasma citrulline and arginine due to consumption of Citrullus vulgaris (watermelon). *Journal of Inherited Metabolic Disease.* 2005;28(4):467–72.

Mao GX, Deng HB, Yuan LG, Li D, Yvonne Li Y, Wang Z. Protective role of salidroside against aging in a mouse model induced by D-galactose. *Biomedical and Environmental Sciences.* 2010;23(2):161–6.

Martínez-Sánchez A, Alacid F, Rubio-Arias JA, Fernández-Lobato B, Ramos-Campo DJ, Aguayo E. Consumption of watermelon juice enriched in L-citrulline and pomegranate ellagitannins enhanced metabolism during physical exercise. *Journal of Agricultural and Food Chemistry.* 2017a;65(22):4395–404.

Martínez-Sánchez A, Ramos-Campo DJ, Fernández-Lobato B, Rubio-Arias JA, Alacid F, Aguayo E. Biochemical, physiological, and performance response of a functional watermelon juice enriched in L-citrulline during a half-marathon race. *Food and Nutrition Research.* 2017b;61(1):1330098.

Matter M, Stittfall T, Graves J, Myburgh K, Adams B, Jacobs P, Noakes TD. The effect of iron and folate therapy on maximal exercise performance in female marathon runners with iron and folate deficiency. *Clinical Science (London).* 1987;72(4):415–22.

McLellan TM, Pasiakos SM, Lieberman HR. Effects of protein in combination with carbohydrate supplements on acute or repeat endurance exercise performance: A systematic review. *Sports Medicine.* 2014;44(4):535–50.

McNaughton LR, Siegler J, Midgley A. Ergogenic effects of sodium bicarbonate. *Current Sports Medicine Reports.* 2008;7(4):230–6.

Menzies KJ, Singh K, Saleem A, Hood DA. Sirtuin 1-mediated effects of exercise and resveratrol on mitochondrial biogenesis. *Journal of Biological Chemistry.* 2013;288(10):6968–79.

Molinos Domene Á. Effects of adaptogen supplementation on sport performance. A recent review of published studies. *Journal of Human Sport and Exercise.* 2013;8(4): 1054–66.

Moore DR, Phillips SM, Babraj JA, Smith K, Rennie MJ. Myofibrillar and collagen protein synthesis in human skeletal muscle in young men after maximal shortening and lengthening contractions. *American Journal of Physiology. Endocrinology and Metabolism.* 2005;288:E1153–9.

Moore DR. Nutrition to support recovery from endurance exercise: Optimal carbohydrate and protein replacement. *Current Sports Medicine Reports.* 2015;14(4):294–300.

Morihara N, Ushijima M, Kashimoto N, Sumioka I, Nishihama T, Hayama M, Takeda H. Aged garlic extract ameliorates physical fatigue. *Biological and Pharmaceutical Bulletin.* 2006;29(5):962–6.

Morris DM, Beloni RK, Wheeler HE. Effects of garlic consumption on physiological variables and performance during exercise in hypoxia. *Applied Physiology, Nutrition, and Metabolism.* 2013;38(4):363–7.

Muggeridge DJ, Howe CC, Spendiff O, Pedlar C, James PE, Easton C. A single dose of beetroot juice enhances cycling performance in simulated altitude. *Medicine and Science in Sports and Exercise.* 2014;46(1):143–50.

Muhamad AS, Keong CC, Kiew OF, Abdullah MR, Lam CK. Effects of Eurycoma longifolia Jack supplementation on recreational athletes' endurance running capacity and physiological responses in the heat. *International Journal of Applied Sports Sciences.* 2010;22(2):1–9.

Muoio DM, Leddy JJ, Horvath PJ, Awad AB, Pendergast DR. Effect of dietary fat on metabolic adjustments to maximal VO$_2$ and endurance in runners. *Medicine and Science in Sports and Exercise.* 1994;26:81–8.

Murray R, Bartoli WP, Eddy DE, Horn MK. Physiological and performance responses to nicotinic-acid ingestion during exercise. *Medicine and Science in Sports and Exercise.* 1995;27(7):1057–62.

Nielsen OB, Paoli F, Overgaard K. Protective effects of lactic acid on force production in rat skeletal muscle. *The Journal of Physiology.* 2001;536(1):161–6.

Nieman DC, Henson DA, Maxwell KR, Williams AS, Mcanulty SR, Jin F, Shanely RA, Lines TC. Effects of quercetin and EGCG on mitochondrial biogenesis and immunity. *Medicine and Science in Sports and Exercise.* 2009;41(7):1467–75.

Nieman DC, Williams AS, Shanely RA, Jin F, McAnulty SR, Triplett NT, Austin MD, Henson DA. Quercetin's influence on exercise performance and muscle mitochondrial biogenesis. *Medicine and Science in Sports and Exercise.* 2010;42(2):338-45.

Noakes TD, Sharwood K, Speedy D, Hew T, Reid S, Dugas J, Almond C, Wharam P, Weschler L. Three independent biological mechanisms cause exercise-associated hyponatremia: Evidence from 2,135 weighed competitive athletic performances. *Proceedings of the National Academy of Sciences of the United States of America.* 2005;102(51):18550–5.

Noreen EE, Buckley JG, Lewis SL, Brandauer J, Stuempfle KJ. The effects of an acute dose of Rhodiola rosea on endurance exercise performance. *The Journal of Strength and Conditioning Research.* 2013;27(3):839–47.

Nuri TH, Yee JC, Gupta M, Khan MA, Ming LC. A review of panax ginseng as an herbal medicine. *Archives of Pharmacy Practice.* 2016;7(5):61.

Oh TW, Ohta F. Capsaicin increases endurance capacity and spares tissue glycogen through lipolytic function in swimming rats. *Journal of Nutritional Science and Vitaminology.* 2003;49(2):107–11.

Oi Y, Imafuku M, Shishido C, Kominato Y, Nishimura S, Iwai K. Garlic supplementation increases testicular testosterone and decreases plasma corticosterone in rats fed a high protein diet. *The Journal of Nutrition.* 2001;131(8):2150–6.

Orer GE, Guzel NA. The effects of acute L-carnitine supplementation on endurance performance of athletes. *The Journal of Strength and Conditioning Research.* 2014;28(2):514–9.

Ota N, Soga S, Shimotoyodome A, Haramizu S, Inaba M, Murase T, Tokimitsu I. Effects of combination of regular exercise and tea catechins intake on energy expenditure in humans. *Journal of Health Science.* 2005;51(2):233–6.

Panda AK, Swain KC. Traditional uses and medicinal potential of Cordyceps sinensis of Sikkim. *Journal of Ayurveda and Integrative Medicine.* 2011;2(1):9.

Pandareesh MD, Anand T. Ergogenic effect of dietary L-carnitine and fat supplementation against exercise induced physical fatigue in Wistar rats. *Journal of Physiology and Biochemistry.* 2013;69(4):799–809.

Panjwani U, Thakur L, Anand JP, Singh SN, Singh SB, Banerjee PK, Banerjee PK. Effect of L-carnitine supplementation on endurance exercise in normobaric/normoxic and hypo-baric/hypoxic conditions. *Wilderness and Environmental Medicine.* 2007;18(3):169–76.

Panossian A, Wikman G. Evidence-based efficacy of adaptogens in fatigue, and molecular mechanisms related to their stress-protective activity. *Current Clinical Pharmacology.* 2009;4(3):198–219.

Parisi A, Tranchita E, Duranti G, Ciminelli E, Quaranta F, Ceci R, Cerulli C, Borrione P, Sabatini S. Effects of chronic Rhodiola rosea supplementation on sport performance and antioxidant capacity in trained male: Preliminary results. *Journal of Sports Medicine and Physical Fitness.* 2010;50(1):57–63.

Park SK, Jung IC, Lee WK, Lee YS, Park HK, Go HJ, Kim K, Lim NK, Hong JT, Ly SY, Rho SS. A combination of green tea extract and l-theanine improves memory and attention in subjects with mild cognitive impairment: A double-blind placebo-controlled study. *Journal of Medicinal Food.* 2011;14(4):334–43.

Pendergast DR, Horvath PJ, Leddy JJ, Venkatraman JT. The role of dietary fat on performance, metabolism, and health. *The American Journal of Sports Medicine.* 1996;24(6_suppl):S53–8.

Peters EM, Goetzsche JM, Grobbelaar B, Noakes TD. Vitamin C supplementation reduces the incidence of postrace symptoms of upper-respiratory-tract infection in ultramarathon runners. *The American Journal of Clinical Nutrition.* 1993;57(2):170–4.

Phillips SM, Van Loon LJ. Dietary protein for athletes: From requirements to optimum adaptation. *Journal of Sports Sciences.* 2011;29(sup1):S29–38.

Phung OJ, Baker WL, Matthews LJ, Lanosa M, Thorne A, Coleman CI. Effect of green tea catechins with or without caffeine on anthropometric measures: A systematic review and meta-analysis. *The American Journal of Clinical Nutrition.* 2010;91(1):73–81.

Price MJ, Simons C. The effect of sodium bicarbonate ingestion on high-intensity intermittent running and subsequent performance. *The Journal of Strength and Conditioning Research.* 2010;24(7):1834–42.

Rai D, Bhatia G, Sen T, Palit G. Anti-stress effects of Ginkgo biloba and panax ginseng: A comparative study. *Journal of Pharmacological Sciences.* 2003;93(4):458–64.

Rasmussen CJ. Nutrition before, during, and after exercise for the strength/power athlete. In Antonio j, Kalman DS, Stout JR, Greenwood M, Willoughby D, Haff GG, editors, *Essentials of Sports Nutrition and Supplements* (pp. 647–65). Humana Press, Totowa, NJ; 2008.

Richards JC, Lonac MC, Johnson TK, Schweder MM, Bell C. Epigallocatechin-3-gallate increases maximal oxygen uptake in adult humans. *Medicine and Science in Sports and Exercise.* 2010;42(4):739–44.

Rodriguez NR, DiMarco NM, Langley S. Position of the American Dietetic Association, Dietitians of Canada, and the American College of Sports Medicine: Nutrition and athletic performance. *Journal of the American Dietetic Association.* 2009;109(3):509–27.

Rutherford JA, Spriet LL, Stellingwerff T. The effect of acute taurine ingestion on endurance performance and metabolism in well-trained cyclists. *International Journal of Sport Nutrition and Exercise Metabolism.* 2010;20(4):322–9.

Ryan M. *Sports Nutrition for Endurance Athletes.* Velo Press, Boulder, CO; 2007.

Sale C, Harris RC, Delves S, Corbett J. Metabolic and physiological effects of ingesting extracts of bitter orange, green tea and guarana at rest and during treadmill walking in overweight males. *International Journal of Obesity.* 2006;30(5):764–73.

Sandhu JS, Shah B, Shenoy S, Chauhan S, Lavekar GS, Padhi MM. Effects of Withania somnifera (Ashwagandha) and Terminalia Arjuna (Arjuna) on physical performance and cardiorespiratory endurance in healthy young adults. *International Journal of Ayurveda Research.* 2010;1(3):144–49.

Saunders MJ, Kane MD, Todd MK. Effects of a carbohydrate-protein beverage on cycling endurance and muscle damage. *Medicine and Science in Sports and Exercise.* 2004;36(7):1233–8.

Schneiker KT, Bishop D, Dawson B, Hackett LP. Effects of caffeine on prolonged intermittent-sprint ability in team-sport athletes. *Medicine and Science in Sports and Exercise.* 2006;38(3):578–85.

Scholey A, Bauer I, Neale C, Savage K, Camfield D, White D, Maggini S, Pipingas A, Stough C, Hughes M. Acute effects of different multivitamin mineral preparations with and without guaraná on mood, cognitive performance and functional brain activation. *Nutrients.* 2013;5(9):3589–604.

Schumacher HR, Pullman-Mooar S, Gupta SR, Dinnella JE, Kim R, McHugh MP. Randomized double-blind crossover study of the efficacy of a tart cherry juice blend in treatment of osteoarthritis (OA) of the knee. *Osteoarthritis and Cartilage.* 2013;21(8):1035–41.

Semwal RB, Semwal DK, Vermaak I, Viljoen A. A comprehensive scientific overview of Garcinia Cambogia. *Fitoterapia.* 2015;102:134–48.

Seo DY, Kwak HB, Lee SR, Cho YS, Song IS, Kim N, Bang HS, Rhee BD, Ko KS, Park BJ, Han J. Effects of aged garlic extract and endurance exercise on skeletal muscle FNDC-5 and circulating irisin in high-fat-diet rat models. *Nutrition Research and Practice*. 2014;8(2):177–82.

Shanely RA, Nieman DC, Zwetsloot KA, Knab AM, Imagita H, Luo B, Davis B, Zubeldia JM. Evaluation of Rhodiola rosea supplementation on skeletal muscle damage and inflammation in runners following a competitive marathon. *Brain, Behavior, and Immunity*. 2014;39:204–10.

Shekelle P, Hardy ML, Morton SC, Maglione M, Suttorp M, Roth E, Jungvig L, Mojica WA, Gagne J, Rhodes S, McKinnon E. Ephedra and ephedrine for weight loss and athletic performance enhancement: Clinical efficacy and side effects. *Evidence Report/ Technology Assessment (Summary)*. 2003;76:1.

Shenoy S, Bhaskaran UC, Sandhu JS, Paadhi MM. The effect of Ashwagandha (Withania Somnifera) on anaerobic performance on elite Indian cyclist. *Medicina Sportiva: Journal of Romanian Sports Medicine Society*. 2012;8(3):1909.

Shergis JL, Zhang AL, Zhou W, Xue CC. Panax ginseng in randomised controlled trials: A systematic review. *Phytotherapy Research*. 2013;27(7):949–65.

Shimomura Y, Inaguma A, Watanabe S, Yamamoto Y, Muramatsu Y, Bajotto G, Sato J, Shimomura N, Kobayashi H, Mawatari K. Branched-chain amino acid supplementation before squat exercise and delayed-onset muscle soreness. *International Journal of Sport Nutrition and Exercise Metabolism*. 2010;20(3):236–44.

Simopoulos AP. Omega-3 fatty acids and athletics. *Current Sports Medicine Reports*. 2007;6(4):230–6.

Smith AE, Walter AA, Graef JL, Kendall KL, Moon JR, Lockwood CM, Fukuda DH, Beck TW, Cramer JT, Stout JR. Effects of β-alanine supplementation and high-intensity interval training on endurance performance and body composition in men; a double-blind trial. *Journal of the International Society of Sports Nutrition*. 2009;6(1):5.

Snell PG, Ward R, Kandaswami C, Stohs SJ. Comparative effects of selected non-caffeinated rehydration sports drinks on short-term performance following moderate dehydration. *Journal of the International Society of Sports Nutrition*. 2010;7(1):28–36.

Srinivasan K. Ginger rhizomes (Zingiber officinale): A spice with multiple health beneficial potentials. *PharmaNutrition*. 2017;5(1):18–28.

Srinivas-Shankar U, Roberts SA, Connolly MJ, O'Connell MD, Adams JE, Oldham JA, Wu FC. Effects of testosterone on muscle strength, physical function, body composition, and quality of life in intermediate-frail and frail elderly men: A randomized, double-blind, placebo-controlled study. *The Journal of Clinical Endocrinology and Metabolism*. 2010;95(2):639–50.

Stellingwerff T. Contemporary nutrition approaches to optimize elite marathon performance. *International Journal of Sports Physiology and Performance*. 2013;8(5):573–8.

Stout JR, Cramer JT, Zoeller RF, Torok D, Costa P, Hoffman JR, Harris RC, O'Kroy J. Effects of beta-alanine supplementation on the onset of neuromuscular fatigue and ventilatory threshold in women. *Amino Acids*. 2007;32(3):381–6.

Stuessi C, Hofer P, Meier C, Boutellier U. L-carnitine and the recovery from exhaustive endurance exercise: A randomised, double-blind, placebo-controlled trial. *European Journal of Applied Physiology*. 2005;95(5–6):431–5.

Sumiyoshi M, Kimura Y. Effects of Eleutherococcus senticosus Cortex on recovery from the forced swimming test and fatty acid β-oxidation in the liver and skeletal muscle of mice. *The Natural Products Journal*. 2016;6(1):49–55.

Sung DJ, Kim S, Kim J, An HS, So WY. Role of l-carnitine in sports performance: Focus on ergogenic aid and antioxidant. *Science and Sports*. 2016;31(4):177–88.

Sureda A, Córdova A, Ferrer MD, Tauler P, Pérez G, Tur JA, Pons A. Effects of L-citrulline oral supplementation on polymorphonuclear neutrophils oxidative burst and nitric oxide production after exercise. *Free Radical Research.* 2009;43(9):828–35.

Suzuki M, Itokawa Y. Effects of thiaminee supplementation on exerciseinduced fatigue. *Metabolic Brain Disease.* 1996;11(1):95–106.

Suzuki T, Morita M, Kobayashi Y, Kamimura A. Oral L-citrulline supplementation enhances cycling time trial performance in healthy trained men: Double-blind randomized placebo-controlled 2-way crossover study. *Journal of the International Society of Sports Nutrition.* 2016;13(1):1–8.

Tarazona-Díaz MP, Alacid F, Carrasco M, Martínez I, Aguayo E. Watermelon juice: Potential functional drink for sore muscle relief in athletes. *Journal of Agricultural and Food Chemistry.* 2013;61(31):7522–8.

Tesch PA, Colliander EB, Kaiser P. Muscle metabolism during intense, heavy-resistance exercise. *European Journal of Applied Physiology and Occupational Physiology.* 1986;55(4):362–6.

Theodorou AS, Paradisis G, Smpokos E, Chatzinikolaou A, Fatouros I, King RF, Cooke CB. The effect of combined supplementation of carbohydrates and creatine on anaerobic performance. *Biology of Sport.* 2017;34(2):169–75.

Thibault G. Ahead of the pack. *Training Conditional.* 2006;16:25–31.

Thivel D, Isacco L, Rousset S, Boirie Y, Morio B, Duché P. Intensive exercise: A remedy for childhood obesity? *Physiology and Behavior.* 2011;102(2):132–6.

Thompson D, inventor. Endurance sports drink utilizing tapioca starch. United States patent application US. 2015 Mar 5;14/476,727.

Thompson JL, Manore MM. Predicted and measured resting metabolic rate of male and female endurance athletes. *The Journal Am Diet Associação.* 1996;96(1):30–4.

Tomita K, Okuhara Y, Shigematsu N, Suh H, Lim K. (−)-Hydroxycitrate ingestion increases fat oxidation during moderate intensity exercise in untrained men. *Bioscience, Biotechnology, and Biochemistry.* 2003;67(9):1999–2001.

Trumbo P, Schlicker S, Yates AA, Poos M. Dietary reference intakes for energy, carbohydrate, fiber, fat, fatty acids, cholesterol, protein and amino acids. *Journal of the American Dietetic Association.* 2002;102(11):1621–30.

Veasey RC, Haskell-Ramsay CF, Kennedy DO, Wishart K, Maggini S, Fuchs CJ, Stevenson EJ. The effects of supplementation with a vitamin and mineral complex with Guaraná prior to fasted exercise on affect, exertion, cognitive performance, and substrate metabolism: A randomized controlled trial. *Nutrients.* 2015;7(8):6109–27.

Venkatakrishnan K, Chiu HF, Cheng JC, Chang YH, Lu YY, Han YC, Shen YC, Tsai KS, Wang CK. Comparative studies on the hypolipidemic, antioxidant and hepatoprotective activities of catechins enriched Green and Oolong tea in a double-blind clinical trial. *Food and Function.* 2018;9(2):1205–13. doi:10.1039/C7FO01449J.

Volek JS, Noakes T, Phinney SD. Rethinking fat as a fuel for endurance exercise. *European Journal of Sport Science.* 2015;15(1):13–20.

Volkov NI. Bioenergetics of sports activities. In *Theory and Practice of Physical Culture and Sports.* Moscow, Russia; 2010 [in Russian].

Von Dullivard SP, Braun WR, Markofski M, Beneke R, Leithauser R. Fluids and hydration in prolonged endurance performance. *Nutrition.* 2004;20(65):1–656.

Vukovich Matthew D, Adams GD. Effect of β-hydroxy β-methylbutyrate (HMB) on vo2peak and maximal lactate in endurance trained cyclists. *Medicine and Science in Sports and Exercise.* 1997;29(5):252.

Vukovich MD, Dreifort GD. Effect of β-hydroxy β-Methylbutyrate on the onset of blood lactate accumulation and O_2 peak in endurance-trained cyclists. *The Journal of Strength and Conditioning Research.* 2001;15(4):491–7.

Walker TB, Robergs RA. Does Rhodiola rosea possess ergogenic properties? *International Journal of Sport Nutrition and Exercise Metabolism.* 2006;16(3):305–15.

Wall BT, Stephens FB, Constantin-Teodosiu D, Marimuthu K, Macdonald IA, Greenhaff PL. Chronic oral ingestion of l-carnitine and carbohydrate increases muscle carnitine content and alters muscle fuel metabolism during exercise in humans. *The Journal of Physiology.* 2011;589(4):963–73.

Wang H, Wen Y, Du Y, Yan X, Guo H, Rycroft JA, Boon N, Kovacs EMR, Mela DJ. Effect of catechin enriched green tea on body composition. *Obesity.* 2010;18(4):773–9.

Wankhede S, Langade D, Joshi K, Sinha SR, Bhattacharyya S. Examining the effect of Withania somnifera supplementation on muscle strength and recovery: A randomized controlled trial. *Journal of the International Society of Sports Nutrition.* 2015;12(1):43.

Weckerle CS, Stutz MA, Baumann TW. Purine alkaloids in Paullinia. *Phytochemistry.* 2003;64(3):735–42.

Westerterp-Plantenga MS, Kovacs EM. The effect of (–)-hydroxycitrate on energy intake and satiety in overweight humans. *International Journal of Obesity.* 2002;26(6):870–2.

Wilkinson DJ, Hossain T, Hill DS, Phillips BE, Crossland H, Williams J, Loughna P, Churchward-Venne TA, Breen L, Phillips SM, Etheridge T. Effects of leucine and its metabolite β-hydroxy-β-methylbutyrate on human skeletal muscle protein metabolism. *The Journal of Physiology.* 2013;591(11):2911–23.

Williams MH. Dietary supplements and sports performance. *Minerals.* 2005;2:43–9.

Williams MH. Dietary supplements for endurance athletes. In Rawson S, Volpe SL, editors, *Nutrition for Elite Athletes* (p. 45). CRC Press, Boca Raton, FL; 2015.

Wilson GJ, Wilson JM, Manninen AH. Effects of beta-hydroxy-beta-methylbutyrate (HMB) on exercise performance and body composition across varying levels of age, sex, and training experience: A review. *Nutrition and Metabolism.* 2008;5(1):1.

Wilson JM, Fitschen PJ, Campbell B, Wilson GJ, Zanchi N, Taylor L, Wilborn C, Kalman DS, Stout JR, Hoffman JR, Ziegenfuss TN. International society of sports nutrition position stand: Beta-hydroxy-beta-methylbutyrate (HMB). *Journal of the International Society of Sports Nutrition.* 2013;10(1):6.

Wilson PB. Ginger (Zingiber officinale) as an analgesic and ergogenic aid in sport: A systemic review. *The Journal of Strength and Conditioning Research.* 2015;29(10):2980–95.

Wilson PB, Fitzgerald JS, Rhodes GS, Lundstrom CJ, Ingraham SJ, Ambegaonkar JP. Effectiveness of ginger root (Zingiber officinale) on running-induced muscle soreness and function: A pilot study. *International Journal of Athletic Therapy Training.* 2015;20(6):44–50.

Wong CP, Bandyopadhyay A, Chen CK. Effects of panax ginseng supplementation on physiology responses during endurance performance. *Journal of Men's Health.* 2011;8(S1):S78–80.

Wu RE, Huang WC, Liao CC, Chang YK, Kan NW, Huang CC. Resveratrol protects against physical fatigue and improves exercise performance in mice. *Molecules.* 2013;18(4):4689–702.

Wu YL, Lian LH, Jiang YZ, Nan JX. Hepatoprotective effects of salidroside on fulminant hepatic failure induced by D-galactosamine and lipopolysaccharide in mice. *Journal of Pharmacy and Pharmacology.* 2009;61(10):1375–82.

Xu J, Li Y. Effects of salidroside on exhaustive exercise-induced oxidative stress in rats. *Molecular Medicine Reports.* 2012;6(5):1195–8.

Yan F, Wang B, Zhang Y. Polysaccharides from Cordyceps sinensis mycelium ameliorate exhaustive swimming exercise-induced oxidative stress. *Pharmaceutical Biology.* 2014;52(2):157–61.

Yan F, Zhang Y, Wang B. Effects of polysaccharides from Cordyceps sinensis mycelium on physical fatigue in mice. *Bangladesh Journal of Pharmacology.* 2012;7(3):217–21.

Yeh TS, Chan KH, Hsu MC, Liu JF. Supplementation with soybean peptides, taurine, Pueraria isoflavone, and ginseng saponin complex improves endurance exercise capacity in humans. *Journal of Medicinal Food.* 2011;14(3):219–25.

Zafeiridis A. The effects of dietary nitrate (beetroot juice) supplementation on exercise performance: A review. *American Journal of Sports Science.* 2014;2(4):97–110.

Zanchi NE, Gerlinger-Romero F, Guimaraes-Ferreira L, de Siqueira Filho MA, Felitti V, Lira FS, Seelaender M, Lancha AH. HMB supplementation: Clinical and athletic performance-related effects and mechanisms of action. *Amino Acids.* 2011;40(4):1015–25.

Zehsaz F, Farhangi N, Mirheidari L. The effect of Zingiber officinale R. rhizomes (ginger) on plasma pro-inflammatory cytokine levels in well-trained male endurance runners. *Central European Journal of Immunology.* 2014;39:174–80.

Zhang M, Izumi I, Kagamimori S, Sokejima S, Yamagami T, Liu Z, Qi B. Role of taurine supplementation to prevent exercise-induced oxidative stress in healthy young men. *Amino Acids.* 2004;26(2):203–7.

Zhang XL, Ren F, Huang W, Ding RT, Zhou QS, Liu XW. Anti-fatigue activity of extracts of stem bark from Acanthopanax senticosus. *Molecules.* 2010;16(1):28–37.

Zhang Z, Xu S. Study of the effects of Schisandra chinensis (Turcz.) baill polysaccharides on anti-fatigue and anti-hypoxia in mice. In *World Automation Congress*, Puerto Vallarta, Mexico, (pp. 1–4). IEEE; 2012.

Zhang ZJ, Tong Y, Zou J, Chen PJ, Yu DH. Dietary supplement with a combination of Rhodiola crenulata and Ginkgo biloba enhances the endurance performance in healthy volunteers. *Chinese Journal of Integrative Medicine.* 2009;15(3):177–83.

6 Prosthetics and Limb Health in Extreme Sports

Sashwati Roy, Shomita S. Mathew-Steiner, and Chandan K. Sen

CONTENTS

6.1   Introduction 115
6.2   Types of Prosthetics, Design, and Materials 118
6.3   Socket Systems 118
6.4   Prosthetics and Extreme Sports 120
    6.4.1   Blades 120
    6.4.2   Moto Knee and Versa Foot 120
    6.4.3   Upper-Limb Prosthetics 120
6.5   Prosthetic Device Function 120
6.6   Prosthesis-Related Injuries 121
    6.6.1   Common Injuries for All Levels of Amputation 121
    6.6.2   Injuries to the Residual Limb 121
6.7   Measuring Residual Limb Health Outcomes 121
6.8   Summary and Conclusions 123
Bibliography 124

6.1   INTRODUCTION

Prosthetics are artificial replacements for portions of the body that have been removed or lost due to traumatic injury or illness. Typically, limbs or joints are targeted areas for prosthetic replacements which are sometimes used for cosmetic or functional purposes or both. Prosthetics are not to be confused with orthotics. Prosthetics replace a component of the musculo-skeletal system, while orthotics support or correct a weak or misaligned limbic structure.

The origin of the word prosthesis is from the Greek word "prostitheni" meaning addition, application or attachment. Prosthetics have been adapted for human use since the time of the early Egyptians (circa 950 BCE). Most of the earliest prosthetics were simple adaptations such as a peg leg or hand hook, made from wood or metal, and used mostly for form rather than function. In recent times, given the collision of the worlds of dynamic performance (hiking, biking, extreme adventure sports) and prosthetics, a burgeoning realm of advanced prosthetics has opened the door to unlimited possibilities for amputees. This chapter will focus primarily on lower-limb prosthetics.

A coalition of scientific disciplines such as biomechanical and structural engineering, kinesiology, and material fabrication are traditionally considered essential for the development of effective prosthetic devices for use in sport or regular living. Following fitting of the prosthetic, experts in sports medicine, physical therapy, orthopedic medicine, and athletic training add support for competitive amputees. A critical determinant in training for active performance with a prosthetic limb is the health of the residual limb. To this end, quantitative, non-invasive measurement of limb health outcomes including tissue perfusion, oxygenation, hydration, and skin barrier function can aid in the design and testing of advanced prosthetics and other therapeutic interventions while preserving residual limb health (Figure 6.1).

Several reports highlight the importance of the socket/limb interface. Almost 20 years ago, it was reported that ~98% of patients with lower limb loss ($N = 92$) identified prosthesis fit as their primary concern (Legro et al. 1999). It was later found that nearly one-third of respondents expressed dissatisfaction with prosthesis comfort (Pezzin et al. 2004). Following this, similar dissatisfaction was identified with the socket interface after a multi-stakeholder focus group study of the needs of lower-extremity amputees (Klute et al. 2009). That study reported that the current socket fitting process was too prolonged and assiduous, resulting in stress and strain on the residual limb that created problems with skin and tissue health. The authors concluded that there was a strong need for an objective in-socket fit measurement

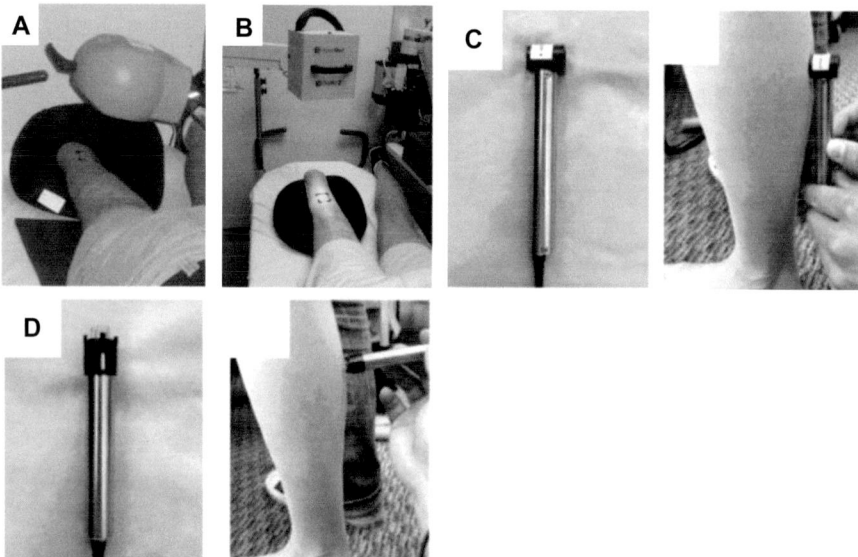

FIGURE 6.1   (See color insert.) Non-invasive imaging to monitor residual skin health. **A.** Laser speckle imaging (LSI) for skin perfusion. **B.** Hyperspectral imaging for skin oxygen saturation. **C.** Transepidermal water loss (TEWL) for skin barrier function. **D.** Surface electrical capacitance for skin hydration. (Reprinted with permission from Rink CL, et al. Standardized approach to quantitatively measure residual limb skin health in individuals with lower-limb amputation. (New York, Mary Ann Liebert, 2017), 225–232).

that was independent of user verbal feedback. Since this study, there have been multiple attempts to quantify prosthetic socket fit, but these studies employed technologies with limited clinical applications such as radiological (Commean, Smith, and Vannier 1997; Lilja, Johansson, and Oberg 1993; Papaioannou et al. 2010), acoustic (Convery and Murray 2000), and optical (Sanders et al. 2006). There were several issues with these studies, including the need for bulky equipment, limited range of measurement and limited time periods of measurement. The Ohio Willow Wood Company developed and commercialized a LimbLogic Communicator™ (also called In-Socket Digital Data Recorder (ISDDR)) supported by long-term research collaboration with our group (Figure 6.2) (Rink et al. 2016, 2017).

This technology enabled real-time, in-socket recording of patient-centric data. The device consisted of two components: a controller and a communicator. The controller consists of a distal or side-mounted housing that contains a six-axis accelerometer along

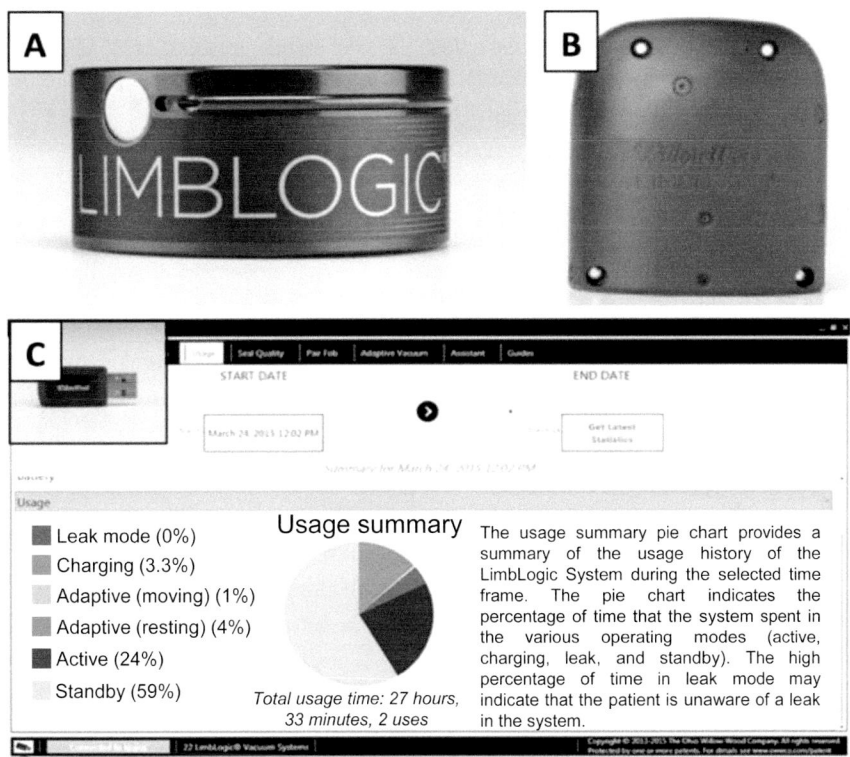

FIGURE 6.2 **(See color insert.)** The ISDDR Platform. ISDDR is a commercially available Willow Wood technology enabling real-time, in-socket recording of patient- centric data. The device consists of two components: **A.** and **B.** a controller, and **C.** a communicator. The controller consists of a **A.** distal or **B.** side-mounted housing that contains a six-axis accelerometer along with a vacuum pressure sensor capable of resolving global changes in the socket pressure waveform that correlate with in-socket motion and prosthesis fit. Using the communicator **C.** quantitative data related to socket motion and prosthesis usage can be transferred to a workstation in order to provide relevant patient-centric data to both the user and clinician about prosthesis performance.

with a vacuum pressure sensor capable of resolving global changes in the socket pressure waveform that correlate with in-socket motion and prosthesis fit. Using the communicator, the quantitative data related to socket motion and prosthesis usage can be transferred to a workstation in order to provide relevant patient-centric data to both the user and clinician about prosthesis performance. This data is not only useful for quantifying the quality of the initial fit, but also for tracking changes in fit quality over time (Rink et al. 2016, 2017). This simply means that by minimizing the in-socket movement of the residual limb due to an ideal fit, the health of the residual limb is conserved.

6.2 TYPES OF PROSTHETICS, DESIGN, AND MATERIALS

Essential considerations for prosthetic design include overall form (size, shape, and suspension used), fit (comfort and usability), and function (level of performance: balance, basic mobility, high-end performance, range of use, and device control).

Lower limb: Above knee amputation (AKA) or transfemoral (TF) amputation. At the end of the residual limb is where the prosthetic replacement is fitted. Key components include a socket combined with a supportive frame, an artificial knee, a pylon, and an artificial foot.

Below knee amputation (BKA) or transtibial amputation. Prosthetics for this type typically consist of a socket, pylon, and a foot. Sometimes a suspension sleeve or harness may be used in both cases.

The use of lighter and more resilient materials such as carbon fiber composites, titanium, and aluminum for prosthetic construction have changed the range of functionality for amputees, particularly those with a passion for extreme sports. Together with the Paralympic movement, the technological advances for high-end performance prosthetic applications have been outstanding. For example, advances such as the gait-adaptive knee, an artificial limb that can be adapted to the specific needs of the user, have been a game-changer for athletes with limb loss. With such adaptations, Paralympic athletes and those involved in extreme activities such as competitive snowboarding, snowmobiling, and mountain biking are not only able to participate in such high-impact activities but also to be successful in them. In many cases, such athletes can achieve results similar or close to their able-bodied competitors.

At present, while big advances are occurring in the physical structure and composition of prosthetics, enabling adaptation to high-performance activities, there are also significant advances being made to connect the user with the machine via the mechanism of neural linkage. The degree of connectivity is directly correlated with the degree of loss of the biological component, i.e., the more intact the limb, the better the integration of the artificial component. Much work is being done to integrate muscle and/or bone to the machine, but both are still a work in progress. Neural linkage has been most successful with prosthetic hands, which require simpler muscle connections to be functional.

6.3 SOCKET SYSTEMS

The critical component of the prosthesis is the socket. The fit of this component determines the functionality of the limb. Prosthetic sockets for lower limbs could be pin locking, suction/passive vacuum, and vacuum suspension. The vacuum suspension (VAS) or elevated vacuum suspension (EVS) system is a type of socket system that may have advantages for high-performance activities. This is different from the passive suction or valve systems. Unlike all other modes of suspension, the EVS system prevents loss of limb volume during use and provides better control over the prosthesis. An active vacuum system removes air between the liner and socket, creating a negative pressure environment that secures the limb within the socket. EVS sockets are better adapted to everyday and active living due to their improved fit and function (Board, Street, and Caspers 2001; Ferraro 2011; Samitier et al. 2016; Traballesi et al. 2012), decrease in pistoning (Board, Street, and Caspers 2001; Darter, Sinitski, and Wilken 2016; Gerschutz et al. 2010, 2015), and better residual limb volume management (Board, Street, and Caspers 2001; Goswami et al. 2003; Sanders and Fatone 2011). Quantitative studies performed using in- and out-of-socket measurements provided evidence that long-term use of EVS was significantly better at preserving the skin-barrier function of residual limbs compared to other types of sockets (Figure 6.3).

In fact, EVS use was found to provide physiological benefits to residual limb health in people with lower limb amputations (Rink et al. 2016).

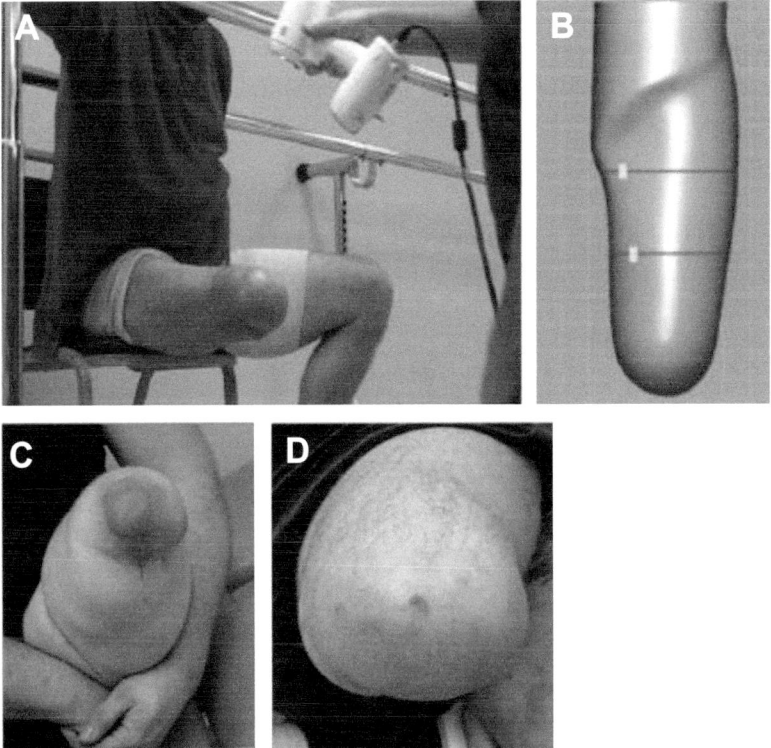

FIGURE 6.3 **(See color insert.) A.** Prosthetists use a scanning device to digitize limb shape. **B.** Digital model is modified to create a positive mold for socket fabrication tailored to the residual limb. **C.** Tissue injury as a result of using a pink-locking suspension system. **D.** Injury healed once the amputee was fit and began wearing an elevated vacuum suspension socket (EVS).

6.4   PROSTHETICS AND EXTREME SPORTS

The availability of advanced technology combined with cutting-edge material is not only enabling amputees to engage in their favorite sport or extreme activity (skiing, snowboarding, surfing, etc.) but also breaking the boundaries of their experience. Amputees like Oscar Pistorius (athletics) and Mike Schultz (X-Games) along with others in areas such as rock climbing, surfing, and snowboarding have been trailblazers in their sport of choice. Therefore, the disability is no longer a limiting factor and the choice of sport activity is limitless. However, the bigger debate is if these artificial limbs give advantages over people without prosthetics. Currently, the following types of prosthetics are in use by sports athletes today:

6.4.1   BLADES

The double-leg amputee Oscar Pistorius was the poster-child for this type of running prosthetic and labelled the "Blade Runner" due to the distinctly shaped curved lower-extremity prosthetics that he used in his London Olympics appearances. This type of prosthetic is made of carbon fiber and specially fabricated to match the runner's weight and impact level while providing the appropriate amount of traction.

6.4.2   MOTO KNEE AND VERSA FOOT

Following an accident that resulted in amputation, X Games snowmobile and motocross racer Mike Schultz invented his own prosthetic to customize the range of motion needed to race. This design was a combination of rugged but lightweight materials with shock absorbers and spring actions to withstand participation in extreme sports. His company BioDapt now manufactures this type of prosthetic for other athletes.

6.4.3   UPPER-LIMB PROSTHETICS

Specially modified prosthetics for upper-limb amputees include the Viau system for swimming, the Eagle for golfing, the Pinch Hitter for baseball, the Power Play for hockey, or hooks for bicycling. These artificial appendages mimic the functions of fingers, arms, and elbows.

6.5   PROSTHETIC DEVICE FUNCTION

Achieving a comfortable and functional connection between an amputee and their prosthetic limb is critical to the success of the prosthesis. The socket system, therefore, is the most significant component for overall success of the prosthesis (Lake 2008; Schultz, Baade, and Kuiken 2007). In an effort to maximize socket performance and comfort without adversely affecting residual limb health, a prosthetist custom fits a socket for every patient using plaster wraps or computer-aided design.

This process, however, is limited by the fact that there is no quantitative feedback to determine appropriate socket fit and it relies on anecdotal visual cues along with subjective verbal feedback from the patient. The mature residual limb (>18 months post-amputation (Berke 2004)) is subject to daily (Zachariah et al. 2004) and chronic (Fernie and Holliday 1982; Sanders et al. 2011) changes in volume that are likely to compromise socket fit and performance. In the context of extreme sports and other high-performance activities, these volume changes are very likely to be much more dynamic, adversely affecting fit, performance, and residual limb health (Sanders et al. 2011) – including skin breakdown and ulceration (Bui et al. 2009), which can impact the performance of these activities.

6.6 PROSTHESIS-RELATED INJURIES

6.6.1 COMMON INJURIES FOR ALL LEVELS OF AMPUTATION

High-performance activity on a prosthetic is not always as natural as that with two normal limbs and involves a lot of training. In addition to mental resilience, amputees have to strengthen their physical body, especially the residual limb and core, and obtain a great-fitting socket to enable high-level activity. With increasing levels of activity, there are increasing problems such as pain and injuries/sores due to loss of limb volume, pressure points, and movement in the socket. While socket fit is essential, monitoring the health of the skin on the residual limb in real time is a factor that is not always addressed.

6.6.2 INJURIES TO THE RESIDUAL LIMB

Common injuries that develop at the interface of the residual limb and prosthetic include skin abrasions, pressure sores, blisters, and rashes (Figure 6.3).

These could be caused by (a) an improper fit of the prosthesis causing pistoning of the residual limb in the socket which results in increased shear forces, or rubbing, of the skin causing an increased susceptibility for skin breakdown, (b) inadequate rest for the residual limb and (c) milking–distal stretch.

Sometimes more severe complications can occur including osteoarthritis, muscle strains on the prosthetic side, hamstring strains/tears (more common in below knee amputations), and lower back pain. In people with unilateral amputations, common injuries include overuse injuries such as plantar fasciitis, Achilles tendonosis, and stress fractures.

6.7 MEASURING RESIDUAL LIMB HEALTH OUTCOMES

Residual limb health is a key determinant of quality of life for individuals with lower-limb amputations. Skin-health problems, caused by shear forces and stress to the residual limb, are known to affect the ability of individuals with lower-limb loss to perform household tasks, use their prosthesis, engage in social functions, and participate in sports (Meulenbelt et al. 2011). To address the need for longitudinal evaluation of the residual limb in the socket, an objective, non-invasive measure of residual limb health in the form of an adaptive elevated vacuum socket (EVS) system with in-built detection systems for residual limb movement was developed. This system dynamically responds to optimize the fit and performance of the prosthetic device. Specifically, adaptive EVS measures and controls for movement between the liner and socket, limiting separation between the two. Innovative technologies that were included in this system included socket-integrated monitoring of movement relative to the residual limb and a 'smart' elevated vacuum suspension (EVS) system that adjusts vacuum level to limit motion and improve fit. The work, done in collaboration with Ohio Willow Wood Company, included state-of-the-art in-socket (probe-based) and out-of-socket (imaging) modalities to assess residual limb circulation and skin health in response to prosthetic socket use (Figure 6.4) (Rink et al. 2016, 2017).

Using a standardized approach including non-invasive imaging (hyperspectral and laser speckle imaging) and probe-based measures of oxygenation (transcutaneous oxygen measurement [TCOM]), perfusion (Laser Doppler flowmetry [LDF]), skin barrier function (transepidermal water loss [TEWL]), and skin hydration (surface electrical capacitance [SEC]) (Figures 6.1 and 6.5) on able-limbed and individuals with unilateral lower-limb amputation (transtibial and transfemoral), our group reported two important findings (Rink et al. 2017). First, that the residual limb transcutaneous oxygen tension was significantly lower in participants with lower-limb loss compared to able-limbed individuals. Second, in amputees, the TEWL and SEC

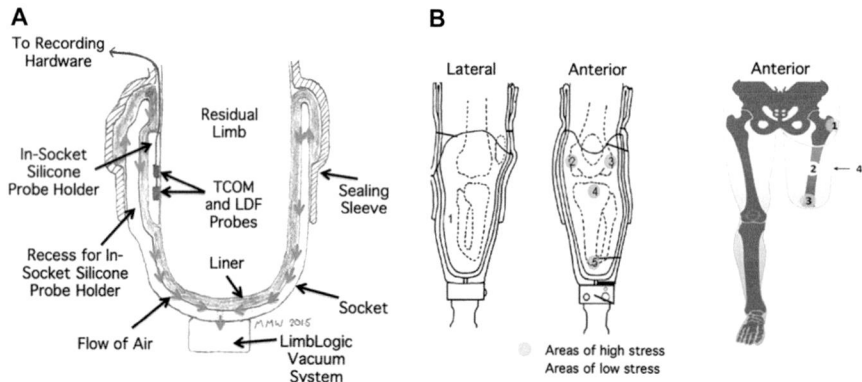

FIGURE 6.4   (See color insert.) Elevated vacuum suspension schematic and probe measurement points. **A.** Illustration of test socket with recess for in-socket silicone probe holder. **B.** Residual-limb measurement sites. Green and yellow indicate measurement sites of high and low stress, respectively. LDF = laser Doppler flowmetry, TCOM = transcutaneous oxygen measurement. (Reprinted with permission from *Rink C, et al. Elevated vacuum suspension preserves residual-limb skin health in people with lower-limb amputation: Randomized clinical trial.* (California, PLOS, 2016), 1121–32) *JRRD is now PLOS Veterans Disability & Rehabilitation Research Channel.*

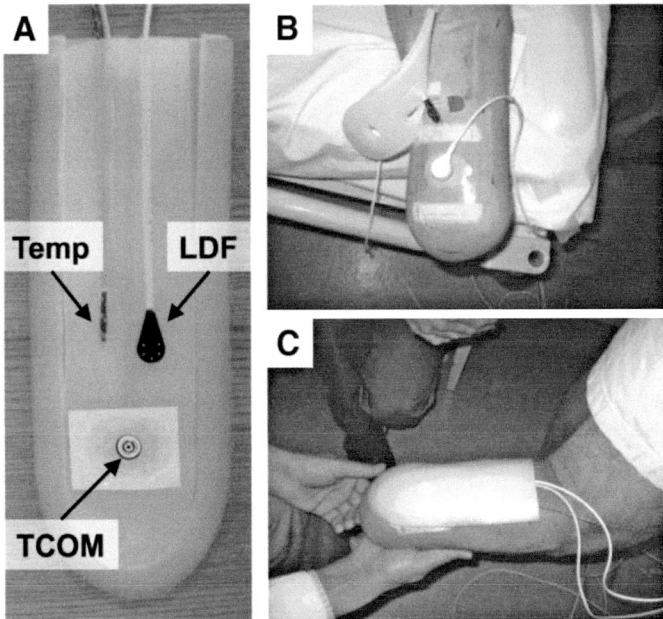

FIGURE 6.5   (See color insert.) Silicone gel probe holder for in-liner measurement. **A.** Temperature, transcutaneous oxygen measurement (TCOM) and laser Doppler flowmetry (LDF) probes were embedded in a silicone gel insert to enable real-time measurement of limb temperature, oxygenation, and perfusion respectively. **B.** Placement of probes on residual limb of trans- tibial participant. Oxygen permeable Tegaderm™ was used to adhere the TCOM probe to the limb. **C.** The silicone gel insert enabled reproducible placement and spacing of probes and buffered against the liner from pressing probes tightly against skin. (Reprinted with permission from Rink CL, et al. Standardized approach to quantitatively measure residual limb skin health in individuals with lower limb amputation. (New York, Mary Ann Liebert, 2017), 225–32).

were significantly more indicative of skin barrier disruption (Figure 6.6) (Rink et al. 2017). These findings corroborate the high incidence (36%) of active skin problems in the residual limb of people with lower-limb loss (Meulenbelt et al. 2011).

6.8   SUMMARY AND CONCLUSIONS

In conclusion, achieving a comfortable and functional connection between an amputee and their prosthetic limb is critical for all individuals, particularly those participating in high-performance activities. The socket system is the most important component for overall rehabilitative success of the prosthesis. The residual limb health within that socket determines sustained functional outcomes for the active person with an artificial limb. Several variations of the socket and prosthetics have dramatically altered the range of activities that amputees can engage in. Real-time monitoring and quantitative measurement of in-socket fitting related to movement

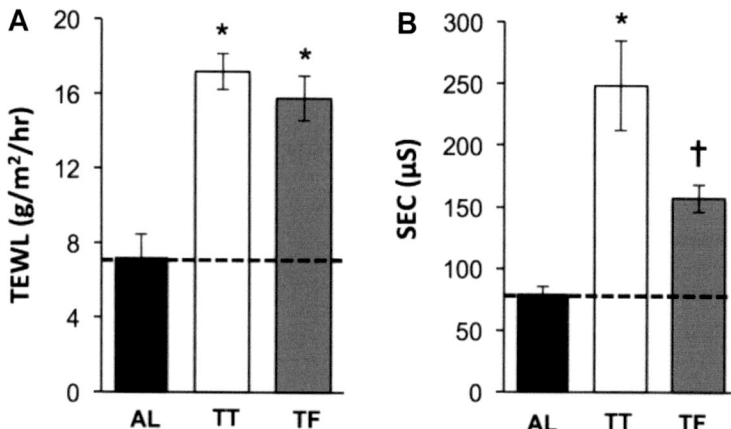

FIGURE 6.6   **A.** Loss of water through the skin epidermal layer was measured by TEWL probe in able-limb (AL, $n = 4$), transtibial (TT, $n = 5$), and transfemoral (TF, $n = 5$) participants while resting without a liner. AL measurements were matched to TT sites. **B.** Mean ± SE TEWL for all sites across groups. *Dashed line* represents mean value of AL without liner. *$p < 0.05$ versus AL. (Reprinted with permission from Rink CL, et al. Standardized approach to quantitatively measure residual limb skin health in individuals with lower limb amputation. (New York, Mary Ann Liebert, 2017), 225–32).

will promote comfort, function, and limb/soft tissue health. This, in turn, will translate to fewer complications related to skin injury caused by socket forces and motion, promoting a healthy limb environment and therefore sustained limb function for any kind of low- or high-performance activity.

BIBLIOGRAPHY

Berke, G. 2004. "Post-operative management of the lower extremity amputee: Standards of care. Official findings of the state-of-the-science conferences #2". *J Prosthet Orthot* 16:6–12.

Board, W. J., G. M. Street, and C. Caspers. 2001. "A comparison of trans-tibial amputee suction and vacuum socket conditions". *Prosthet Orthot Int* 25 (3):202–9.

Bui, K. M., G. J. Raugi, V. Q. Nguyen, and G. E. Reiber. 2009. "Skin problems in individuals with lower-limb loss: Literature review and proposed classification system". *J Rehabil Res Dev* 46 (9):1085–90.

Commean, P. K., K. E. Smith, and M. W. Vannier. 1997. "Lower extremity residual limb slippage within the prosthesis". *Arch Phys Med Rehabil* 78 (5):476–85.

Convery, P., and K. D. Murray. 2000. "Ultrasound study of the motion of the residual femur within a trans-femoral socket during gait". *Prosthet Orthot Int* 24 (3):226–32.

Darter, B. J., K. Sinitski, and J. M. Wilken. 2016. "Axial bone-socket displacement for persons with a traumatic transtibial amputation: The effect of elevated vacuum suspension at progressive body-weight loads". *Prosthet Orthot Int* 40 (5):552–7.

Fernie, G. R., and P. J. Holliday. 1982. "Volume fluctuations in the residual limbs of lower limb amputees". *Arch Phys Med Rehabil* 63 (4):162–5.

Ferraro, C. 2011. "Outcomes study of transtibial amputees using elevated vacuum suspension in comparison With pin suspension". *J Prosthet Orthot* 23 (2):78–81.

Gerschutz, M. J., J. A. Denune, J. M. Colvin, and G. Schober. 2010. "Elevated vacuum suspension influence on lower limb amputee's residual limb volume at different vacuum pressure settings.". *J Prosthet Orthot* 22 (4):252–6.

Gerschutz, M. J., M. L. Hayne, J. M. Colvin, and J. A. Denune. 2015. "Dynamic effectiveness evaluation of elevated vacuum suspension". *J Prosthet Orthot* 27 (4):161–5.

Goswami, J., R. Lynn, G. Street, and M. Harlander. 2003. "Walking in a vacuum-assisted socket shifts the stump fluid balance". *Prosthet Orthot Int* 27 (2):107–13.

Klute, G. K., C. Kantor, C. Darrouzet, H. Wild, S. Wilkinson, S. Iveljic, and G. Creasey. 2009. "Lower-limb amputee needs assessment using multistakeholder focus-group approach". *J Rehabil Res Dev* 46 (3):293–304.

Lake, C. 2008. "The evolution of upper limb prosthetic socket design". *J Prosthet Orthot* 20 (3):85–92.

Legro, M. W., G. Reiber, M. del Aguila, M. J. Ajax, D. A. Boone, J. A. Larsen, D. G. Smith, and B. Sangeorzan. 1999. "Issues of importance reported by persons with lower limb amputations and prostheses". *J Rehabil Res Dev* 36 (3):155–63.

Lilja, M., T. Johansson, and T. Oberg. 1993. "Movement of the tibial end in a PTB prosthesis socket: A sagittal X-ray study of the PTB prosthesis". *Prosthet Orthot Int* 17 (1):21–6.

Meulenbelt, H. E., J. H. Geertzen, M. F. Jonkman, and P. U. Dijkstra. 2011. "Skin problems of the stump in lower limb amputees: 1. A clinical study". *Acta Derm Venereol* 91 (2):173–7.

Papaioannou, G., C. Mitrogiannis, G. Nianios, and G. Fiedler. 2010. "Assessment of amputee socket-stump-residual bone kinematics during strenuous activities using Dynamic Roentgen Stereogrammetric Analysis". *J Biomech* 43 (5):871–8.

Pezzin, L. E., T. R. Dillingham, E. J. Mackenzie, P. Ephraim, and P. Rossbach. 2004. "Use and satisfaction with prosthetic limb devices and related services.". *Arch Phys Med Rehabil* 85 (5):723–9.

Rink, C., M. M. Wernke, H. M. Powell, S. Gynawali, R. M. Schroeder, J. Y. Kim, J. A. Denune, G. M. Gordillo, J. M. Colvin, and C. K. Sen. 2016. "Elevated vacuum suspension preserves residual-limb skin health in people with lower-limb amputation: Randomized clinical trial". *J Rehabil Res Dev* 53 (6):1121–32.

Rink, C. L., M. M. Wernke, H. M. Powell, M. Tornero, S. C. Gnyawali, R. M. Schroeder, J. Y. Kim, J. A. Denune, A. W. Albury, G. M. Gordillo, J. M. Colvin, and C. K. Sen. 2017. "Standardized approach to quantitatively measure residual limb skin health in individuals with lower limb amputation". *Adv Wound Care (New Rochelle)* 6 (7):225–32.

Samitier, C. B., L. Guirao, M. Costea, J. M. Camos, and E. Pleguezuelos. 2016. "The benefits of using a vacuum-assisted socket system to improve balance and gait in elderly transtibial amputees". *Prosthet Orthot Int* 40 (1):83–8.

Sanders, J. E., and S. Fatone. 2011. "Residual limb volume change: Systematic review of measurement and management". *J Rehabil Res Dev* 48 (8):949–86.

Sanders, J. E., D. S. Harrison, T. R. Myers, and K. J. Allyn. 2011. "Effects of elevated vacuum on in-socket residual limb fluid volume: Case study results using bioimpedance analysis". *J Rehabil Res Dev* 48 (10):1231–48.

Sanders, J. E., A. Karchin, J. R. Fergason, and E. A. Sorenson. 2006. "A noncontact sensor for measurement of distal residual-limb position during walking". *J Rehabil Res Dev* 43 (4):509–16.

Schultz, A. E., S. P. Baade, and T. A. Kuiken. 2007. "Expert opinions on success factors for upper-limb prostheses". *J Rehabil Res Dev* 44 (4):483–9.

Traballesi, M., A. S. Delussu, A. Fusco, M. Iosa, T. Averna, R. Pellegrini, and S. Brunelli. 2012. "Residual limb wounds or ulcers heal in transtibial amputees using an active suction socket system. A randomized controlled study". *Eur J Phys Rehabil Med* 48 (4):613–23.

Zachariah, S. G., R. Saxena, J. R. Fergason, and J. E. Sanders. 2004. "Shape and volume change in the transtibial residuum over the short term: Preliminary investigation of six subjects". *J Rehabil Res Dev* 41 (5):683–94.

7 Nutritional Requirements in Extreme Sports

Matthew Butawan, Jade L. Caldwell, and Richard J. Bloomer

CONTENTS

7.1   Introduction 127
7.2   General Nutritional Overview 128
    7.2.1   Macronutrients/Micronutrients.. 128
    7.2.2   Metabolic State 128
    7.2.3   General Health.. 129
    7.2.4   Chrono-Nutrition 130
7.3   Sport Nutrition.. 130
    7.3.1   Intensity/Duration/Volume.. 130
    7.3.2   Macronutrient Adjustments 131
    7.3.3   Goals.. 132
7.4   Nutritional Considerations for Extreme Sports 134
    7.4.1   Travel and Food Availability 134
    7.4.2   Cortisol 135
    7.4.3   Epinephrine/Norepinephrine.. 135
    7.4.4   Environment 136
    7.4.5   Hydration 137
7.5   Conclusion 138
References.. 138

7.1   INTRODUCTION

The human body has an incredible capacity to adapt to different types of stress. In 1936, Hans Selye proposed a model of the progression of any type of stressor, the General Adaptation Syndrome (GAS) (Selye 1936). In short, sympathoadrenal responses (alarm phase) to a stressor elicit metabolic and physiologic adaptations (resistance phase) until resolved or exhausted (exhaustion phase). Selye suggested the model could be applied to any type of stressor; for example, physical activity, exposure to toxins (illness), or enduring extreme temperatures.

It is currently well accepted that nutritional modifications can be a tool to enhance mental (Gómez-Pinilla 2008) and physical performance (Beck et al. 2015). With proper nourishment by foods, beverages, and even oxygen, an individual can support these adaptive processes. In contrast, failure to provide the appropriate quantities and qualities of nutritional components can result in metabolic derangements and reduced capacities (Selye 1938). Extreme sport athletes represent special cases in which stressors may compound simultaneously. While the nutritional recommendations for general health, as well as for traditional athletes, are becoming more commonplace and congruent (Auestad et al. 2015; Skuland and Ånestad 2012), research surrounding the nutritional demands of extreme sport athletes is still in its infancy—with a better understanding forthcoming. By adapting what is currently known about sport nutrition and added stressors, this chapter will aim to provide special considerations for extreme sport athletes, while first covering general nutritional overviews and recommendations for traditional athletes.

7.2 GENERAL NUTRITIONAL OVERVIEW

Nutrition is the ever-evolving scientific field of study focused on the use of foods and beverages to optimize human health and performance. Because the human body is such a dynamic organism, metabolic requirements and nutritional inputs are never fixed. That said, the most beneficial nutritional recommendations are individualized and centered on fact-based approaches. Though the field is moving toward individualized nutrition, it has not yet arrived and, therefore, may still require trial-and-error tweaks to well-established themes of healthy eating. This section will cover the current premise of healthy eating.

7.2.1 MACRONUTRIENTS/MICRONUTRIENTS

Macronutrients—carbohydrates, fats, and proteins—are the foundation of all diets, providing energy and substrates for metabolism. In order to facilitate some of these biochemical reactions, micronutrients, in the form of vitamins and minerals, are necessary to conformationally stabilize substrates and/or enzymes. Typical macronutrient recommendations are approximately 45–65%, 20–35%, and 10–35% of total energy for carbohydrates, fats, and protein, respectively. For a better understanding of the reference range differences based on health agencies around the world, compiled data can be viewed thanks to work done by Senekal, Naude, and Wentzel-Viljoen (2014). Though a consensus has not been made regarding macronutrient reference ranges, the differences are small and thus these recommendations represent the underlying themes of healthy eating to prevent chronic diseases (Shikany and White 2000). By adjusting macronutrients and ensuring adequate intake of micronutrients, individuals can theoretically make nutritional modifications to improve their overall health.

Certainly, each of these macronutrients can be explored in much greater detail by delving into the different forms, functions, and metabolic uses of each macronutrient subtype; however, that would be beyond the scope of this section and chapter. Instead, the reader should focus on the broad importance of using nutrition to address metabolic adaptations to stressors.

7.2.2 METABOLIC STATE

Metabolism is the summation of competing pathways of anabolism—the synthesis of energy-storing complex molecules—and catabolism—the breakdown of complex molecules yielding energy. Though different tissues have preferred fuel sources to meet their specific functions, the metabolic state of any tissue is determined by the predominant pathway at any given time. For a much more detailed explanation of metabolism of various tissues, the reader is referred to Chapter 30 of Berg, Tymoczko, and Stryer (2002). It is also important to mention that all tissues do not need to be in the same metabolic state. In fact, the metabolic state of a tissue will vary based on function and state of the whole body. In this way, the body can compartmentalize systems and distribute energy based on demand in order to adapt and overcome a variety of stressors.

These external stressors may come in the form of exercise, environmental conditions, or dietary choices (Oken, Chamine, and Wakeland 2015). During the alarm and resistance phases of Selye's GAS, external stressors modulate the cellular and tissue metabolism of the body, forcing it to adapt. For example, activation of the sympathoadrenal system (hypothalamic–pituitary–adrenal axis) triggers the release of epinephrine (EPI) and norepinephrine (NE) from the adrenal medulla. Adrenergic receptors are ubiquitously expressed throughout the body whereby they exert mostly catabolic effects such as mobilizing fat and glucose (Pernet et al. 1984). Furthermore, these catecholamines are also able to induce immune cell activation, proliferation, or apoptosis (Barnes, Carson, and Nair 2015; Brown et al. 2003) which could be attributed to altered immune cell metabolism and possibly even fuel-switching (van der Windt and Pearce 2012).

7.2.3 GENERAL HEALTH

Deviances from these recommended macronutrient reference ranges may be detrimental to health and promote the development of chronic diseases (Shikany and White 2000). Most notably, the "Western diet", which contains an abundance of highly processed and refined carbohydrates and oils, has been implicated in the development of chronic diseases such as heart disease (Hou et al. 2015), high blood pressure (Geleijnse, Grobbee, and Kok 2005), type 2 diabetes (Qi et al. 2009), and some cancers (Haggar and Boushey 2009). When combined with the reduced energy expenditure of a sedentary lifestyle, overconsumption is easily accomplished. Following excessive Calorie intake, such as after consuming a high-fat and high-carbohydrate meal, metabolic dysregulation sets in the form of postprandial oxidative stress which can potentially alter intracellular signaling (Bloomer et al. 2010). Chronic overconsumption may lead to obesity and the development of associated chronic co-morbidities such as insulin resistance (Cordain et al. 2005), which is a metabolic dysregulation in the form of cell-to-cell signaling (Pessin and Saltiel 2000). Repeated bouts with these metabolic abnormalities can make it more difficult to return to a healthy homeostasis, as successive deviations distance the new metabolic state from the initial metabolic state (Oken, Chamine, and Wakeland 2015).

In an effort to prevent chronic disease development, additional recommendations have been made to certain macronutrient subtypes. Overconsumption of refined sugars is one of the leading causes of obesity and insulin resistance (MacDonald 2016); thus, current recommendations suggest limiting consumption to below 10% of total daily energy intake (EI) (Johnson et al. 2009; Nishida et al. 2004). Increasing evidence suggests the microbiome can greatly influence host metabolism (Musso, Gambino, and Cassader 2011). To promote the growth of beneficial gut microbes, dietary fiber recommendations suggest >38 g/day and >25 g/day for males and females, respectively (Makki et al. 2018). Essential fatty acids such as omega-6 (ω-6) and omega-3 (ω-3) are responsible for many signaling pathways and inflammation (Glick and Fischer 2013). Currently the "Western diet" contains an abundance of ω-6 but a lack of ω-3, with a ω-6:ω-3 ratio close to 15:1. Studies suggest that reducing the ω-6:ω-3 ratio as much as possible (preferably <5:1) greatly prevents the development of chronic diseases (Simopoulos 2008).

7.2.4 CHRONO-NUTRITION

Chrono-nutrition is an emerging field within nutrition dealing with eating patterns in terms of timing. The expression of many genes involved in anabolic and catabolic pathways is regulated by circadian oscillations of the central and/or peripheral clocks (Asher and Schibler 2011). The central clock is located in the suprachiasmatic nucleus (SCN) and entrained primarily by photoperiods whereas the peripheral clocks are in many different peripheral tissues and entrained primarily by food but also by exercise (Tahara, Aoyama, and Shibata 2017). These peripheral clocks can be found in the liver, pancreas, adipose tissue, and skeletal muscle. Uncoupling of the peripheral and circadian clocks can result in metabolic dysfunction (Potter et al. 2016). For more information on the impacts of chrono-nutrition and metabolic disturbances, the reader is directed to a review by Almoosawi et al. (2016) (Almoosawi et al. 2016).

7.3 SPORT NUTRITION

It is well established that proper nutrition can improve mental (Gómez-Pinilla 2008) and physical performance (Beck et al. 2015). Because of the spectrum-like nature of athletic abilities and training routines, clearly defined sport nutrition recommendations are more difficult to individualize. Nevertheless, athletes use nutrition to reach their target goals by adjusting their macronutrient quantities and relative distribution based on their training intensity and volume. In an attempt to provide more personalized sport nutrition recommendations, various organizations make recommendations in units of grams/kilogram of body weight rather than percent of total EI. This section will provide a broad overview of exercise routines, macronutrient adjustments, and nutritional strategies for common goals. For a more comprehensive evaluation of traditional sports nutrition, the reader is directed to a review by Potgieter (2013), which summarizes the recommendations from the International Olympic Committee (IOC) (Maughan, Burke, and Coyle 2004), International Society for Sport Nutrition (ISSN) (Kerksick et al. 2008; Kreider et al. 2010), and American College of Sports Medicine (ACSM) (Rodriguez, DiMarco and Langley 2009).

7.3.1 INTENSITY/DURATION/VOLUME

Differences in training status and programs make it more complicated to provide nutritional recommendations for athletes than for non-athletes. Each training session can vary based on intensity and duration while the duration and sessions per unit time constitute the volume. Moreover, competitive athletes plan their training programs around competitions in an attempt to achieve peak performance during an event (i.e. periodization). Nutritional planning during the different periodization phases has recently been reviewed by Jeukendrup (2017). That said, there are many considerations when attempting to individualize nutrition for athletes.

To simplify this process as recommendations start moving toward individualization, athletes can be categorized into groups based on training volume (Kreider et al. 2010): 1) General Fitness/Low Volume (e.g. 30–40 minutes/day, 3 times per week); 2) Moderate Volume (e.g. 2–3 hours/day; 5–6 times per week); 3) High Volume (e.g. 3–6 hours/day as 1–2 sessions per day, 5–6 times per week). For novice athletes or even moderate-volume athletes, regular training will induce both cardiovascular and metabolic adaptations which allow the athlete to sustain energy production for longer durations. Thus, nutritional recommendations may also need to be modified as the athlete progresses.

Gender must also be considered, as cardiovascular and hormonal responses to exercise differ between men and women (Tarnopolsky 2000; Wheatley et al. 2014). For example, there appear to be gender differences in response to exercise-induced EPI and NE in terms of substrate metabolism (Horton et al. 1998; Tarnopolsky et al. 1990). At low to moderate intensity exercise, women appear to utilize fat more than men, despite having lower plasma EPI levels, suggesting women may be more sensitive to the lipolytic effects of EPI (Horton et al. 2009). This can also be observed with reduced muscle glycogen depletion and possibly increased intramuscular triglyceride oxidation (Roepstorff et al. 2006).

Following intense exercise bouts, an increase in metabolism above resting levels can be observed for up to several hours after exercise has ceased. This phenomenon is termed excess post-exercise oxygen consumption (EPOC) and while the exact cause is unknown, contributing factors have been suggested to include lactic acid accumulation, catecholamines, glucocorticoids, fatty acids, temperature, and other factors (Gaesser and Brooks 1984). Women appear to have a shorter duration of EPOC following different exercise intensities (Smith and Mc Naughton 1993). This phenomenon would contribute to the daily energy expenditure.

7.3.2 MACRONUTRIENT ADJUSTMENTS

For generally active individuals participating in a low volume of exercise, nutritional modifications may not be necessary, as general daily recommendations of 1800–2200 Calories would likely suffice (Kreider et al. 2010). Macronutrient adjustments may only be of benefit for athletes partaking in moderate to high volumes of intense exercise. Overall daily energy requirements vary primarily based on the current training status, relative training volume, and size of athlete. Larger athletes require more Calories to maintain their size due to the large amount of fat-free mass, which is directly proportional to resting metabolic rate (Sparti et al. 1997). As one would expect, with an increase in training volume, an increase in overall quantity of Calories is required.

Using indirect calorimetry, volume of oxygen consumption (VO_2) and volume of carbon dioxide production (VCO_2) can be measured to determine peak/max VO_2, energy expenditure (EE), and respiratory exchange ratio (RER). RER is an index of carbohydrate and/or fat utilization based on the VCO_2 per VO_2. A low RER value indicates that fats are primarily being oxidized for energy whereas a high RER indicates that carbohydrates are primarily being utilized. Examination of studies employing indirect calorimetry provides a basis for macronutrient recommendations. In general, as exercise intensity increases, carbohydrate utilization increases, whereas when exercise duration is prolonged and performed at low relative intensity, fat utilization increases (Gimenez et al. 2013). These may be partly attributed to catabolic effects of exercise-induced EPI and NE secretion (Ball 2014), as well as the activation of different muscle fiber types and their corresponding oxidative potential (Egan and Zierath 2013). At any given point, the body and these muscle fibers are only efficient enough to use a maximum volume of oxygen (VO_{2max}) for energy production. As exercise intensities approach an individual's VO_{2max}, the body is forced to rely on carbohydrates for energy production because carbohydrate oxidation requires less oxygen to produce ATP. That said, carbohydrate fueling is the most complex macronutrient adjustment. For more information, see Table 7.1.

7.3.3 Goals

Tailoring nutritional intake to achieve goals can be very effective if done properly. In general, goals and strategies are often sport specific but common themes can be observed across most sports. For instance, many athletes desire to increase their power-to-weight ratio for purposes of maximizing force production/efficiency or use nutrient timing to augment performance/recovery.

Whether attempting to lose fat, gain muscle, or a combination, the underlying theme to consider deals with EI versus EE. In order to induce any sort of weight loss including that of fat mass, a hypocaloric diet is almost always consumed. It should be mentioned that males tend to have more lean mass whereas females display more fat mass as an energetic depot to support gestation (Geer and Shen 2009). Thus, females appear to be more susceptible to metabolic dysregulations as a consequence of hypocaloric diets (Manore, Kam and Loucks 2007). This can be psychologically troublesome for female athletes, who may attempt to achieve an even more negative energy balance if not seeing the desired results. Weight loss in females may also be hindered based on the menstrual cycle, as estrogen acts as an anabolic hormone on adipose tissue (Brown and Clegg 2010). Rapid weight loss can be harmful; therefore, it is recommended athletes only lose less than 1.5% of body weight per week (Turocy et al. 2011). Furthermore, weight loss attempts should be made during the off season in order to avoid any detriments to competition. While consuming a hypocaloric diet, it is important to remember that the weight lost will likely be a combination of fat and muscle. To counteract the loss of muscle, it is recommended not to exceed a 500 Calorie deficit and to increase protein consumption to between 1.8–2.0 grams/kilogram of body weight/day (g/kg/d) (Phillips 2011). High-quality protein which is rich in leucine can be of great benefit, as leucine displays anti-catabolic effects (Xia et al. 2016).

While fat loss can be desirable for a number of reasons, athletes often also want to increase their overall lean mass. Maintenance of muscle mass is a dynamic process involving the balance of muscle breakdown and muscle protein synthesis. Weight/

TABLE 7.1

Sport Nutrition Recommendations

	Young, Generally Active	Moderate Volume High Intensity	High Volume High Intensity	
Before CHO	Not necessary	200–300 g 3–4 hr prior		ACSM
		8–10 g/kg/d for 1–3 day prior *OR*		ISSN
		1–2 g/kg for 3–4 hr prior to event		
		7–12 g/kg/24 hr *OR*		IOC
		36–48 hr 10–12 g/kg *OR*		
		1–4 g/kg 1–4 hr prior to exercise		
During CHO >60 min	Not necessary	0.7 g/kg/hr *OR*		ACSM
		30–60 g/hr		
		30–60 g/hr		ISSN
		45–75 min: small amounts		IOC
		stop/start exercise between 1–2.5 hr: 30–60 g/hr		
		ultra-endurance exercise between 2.5–3 hr: up to 90 g/hr		
After CHO	Not necessary	1.0–1.5 g/kg 30 min *AND* again every 2 hr for 4–6 hr		ACSM
		1.5 g/kg *OR*		ISSN
		0.6–1.0 g/kg first 30 min and again every 2 hours for next 4–6 hr		
		1–1.2 g/kg/hr for 1st 4 hours		IOC
Daily CHO	General recommendations	6–10 g/kg/d		ACSM
		5–8 g/kg/d	8–10 g/kg/d	ISSN
		5–7 g/kg/d	4–12* g/kg/d	IOC
Daily PRO	General recommendations	1.2–1.7 g/kg		ACSM
		1.0–1.5 g/kg/d	1.5–2.0 g/kg/d	ISSN
		1.3–1.8 g/kg and 1.6–1.7 g/kg/d strength training		IOC
Daily FAT	General recommendations	20–35%; never below 20%;		ACSM
		30%	30–50%	ISSN
		minimum 15–20%		IOC

Abbreviations: ACSM – American College of Sports Medicine; ISSN – International Society of Sports Nutrition; IOC – International Olympic Committee.

*4–7 g/kg/d for high volume strength training athletes; 8–12 g/kg/d for high volume aerobic competitors

resistance training appears to be the best stimulus for the muscle protein synthesis when combined with proper fueling to facilitate muscle hypertrophy. In order to accumulate muscle mass, a hypercaloric diet containing 1.3–1.8 g/kg/d of high-quality protein is often recommended (Potgieter 2013). Larger athletes are advised to consume the higher end of this reference range. A portion of these Calories should be consumed immediately after resistance exercise or within 30 minutes of completion, with co-ingestion of carbohydrates (Potgieter 2013). High-quality protein such as whey, milk, egg, and soy isolate provide easily digestible sources of amino acids which are rich in leucine and can stimulate muscle protein synthesis through activation of mammalian target of rapamycin (mTOR) (Xia et al. 2016).

Nutrient administration relative to an event can improve performance, reduce injury, and increase recovery (Kerksick et al. 2008). Not surprisingly, carbohydrates appear to be the most important macronutrient to plan consumption around an event in order to maximize muscle and liver glycogen stores. These energy stores can be readily accessed during exercise, and with longer duration exercise, they can be depleted and must be replenished during the recovery period. The recommendations for carbohydrate timing vary slightly based on agency but apply mainly to endurance athletes competing in a moderate to high volume of intense exercise. Consuming carbohydrates before an event in an attempt to increase glycogen stores or increase the amount of circulating glucose is generally beneficial (Kerksick et al. 2008). Carbohydrate recommendations before an event vary based on organization. For instance, current recommendations are listed as either 200–300 g 3–4 hours prior to an event (Rodriguez, DiMarco, and Langley 2009); 1–4 g/kg/hr 1–4 hours prior to event (Maughan, Burke, and Coyle 2004); or 1–2 g/kg/hr 3–4 hours prior to an event (Kreider et al. 2010). Sport nutrition committees agree that recreationally active individuals or athletes exercising for less than 60 minutes do not need to consume additional carbohydrates during an event (Potgieter 2013). The methods to replenish glycogen stores following an event are not clearly defined. For more detailed information and specific recommendations based on organization, see Table 7.1.

In addition to consuming carbohydrates post-exercise, high-quality protein is also recommended, especially for resistance-trained athletes as mentioned above. Currently, there are no recommendations regarding fat consumption in relation to a training event, but these Calorie-dense foods provide a viable means to adjust macronutrient quantities.

7.4 NUTRITIONAL CONSIDERATIONS FOR EXTREME SPORTS

Extreme sport athletes participate in activities that add further stressors to the human body on top of the stress of exercise. The duration and intensity of these events vary wildly and could last anywhere between a few minutes (e.g. bungee jumping) or up to a few days/weeks (e.g. high-altitude expedition). These added stressors can come in the form of environmental influences that need to be overcome or psychological factors that result in hormonal secretions that alter metabolism. Though hormonal secretions of EPI and NE are certainly expected with any exercise, these may even be exaggerated in extreme sport athletes. Because direct evidence within extreme sport athletes is scant and the activities undergone by these athletes vary greatly, this section will attempt to introduce the reader to special considerations for extreme sport athletes.

7.4.1 Travel and Food Availability

Considering the unique environments that some extreme sports are conducted in, traveling may be an important consideration for extreme athletes. Frequent long-distance traveling induces circadian misalignment of the central clock (Weingarten and Collop 2013) and consequently desynchronizes peripheral oscillators. This could have major implications for chrono-nutrition as the body attempts to readjust to the newly localized light–dark cycle. The process of central clock entrainment takes time but resynchronization can be aided by re-entrainment of peripheral clocks through nutrition and exercise (Tahara, Aoyama and Shibata 2017). For athletes with the means, early arrival at a destination competition or event may allow for re-entrainment of the central clock and synchronization of peripheral clocks, thereby allowing for usual expression of anabolic/catabolic processes throughout the day.

Another chief concern for extreme sport athletes is the availability of food and dietary options. In circumstances where food is not available for an extended period of time, the concern should obviously shift from adjusting macronutrient contributions toward ensuring adequate energy and water intake. Through proper planning, nutrient-dense meal-replacement bars or shakes can serve as portable meals.

7.4.2 Cortisol

Cortisol is a catabolic hormone and circadian rhythm marker. Cortisol reaches a peak in the morning hours usually just before waking up and acts to mobilize glucose and fatty acids. During intense exercise of 80% VO_{2max}, cortisol levels rise to stimulate energy-producing pathways, which may involve increased glycogenolysis or proteolysis (to produce amino acid precursors for gluconeogenesis in the liver) (Hill et al. 2008). Cortisol spikes are also known to occur with acute stress or fear exposure. Extreme athletes participating in ultra-endurance events (Kraemer et al. 2007), high-altitude expeditions (Hackney et al. 1995), bungee jumping (van Westerloo et al. 2011), potholing (spelunking) (Stenner et al. 2007), and sky-diving (Thatcher et al. 2003) display elevated cortisol levels. Considering the biological half-life of cortisol is approximately 66 minutes (Weitzman et al. 1971), it is possible that at least 25% of the cortisol spike may still affect metabolism two hours post-exercise. Of course, being a circadian marker, the time of day the exercise is performed would affect this greatly. This is supported by a study demonstrating intense exercise performed during the trough of the cortisol cycle results in a quicker return to the basal cortisol cycle than exercise performed at the peak of the cortisol cycle (Erdemir and Bozdogan 2013). Extreme athletes performing exceptionally long events or competitions such as marathons or climbing expeditions may benefit from following the sport nutrition recommendations for high-volume athletes (Table 7.2).

7.4.3 Epinephrine/Norepinephrine

As mentioned previously, EPI and NE secretion is dependent on exercise intensity following stress activation of the sympathoadrenal system. During exercise, EPI and NE plasma concentrations are known to increase (Ball 2014). The plasma concentrations increase to greater levels for anaerobic exercises than aerobic (Zouhal et al. 2008). As intensity of aerobic exercise increases, plasma EPI and NE concentrations increase. However, these levels quickly reach a steady state minutes after the initiation of exercise. For longer duration exercises (e.g. >60 minutes), plasma EPI levels start to rise even further, presumably as fatigue starts to set in (Perrault et al. 1991). Once plasma NE reaches a "pseudo-steady state," minutes after starting an exercise, the plasma NE concentration will slowly rise with prolonged exercise (Perrault et al. 1991).

TABLE 7.2

Special Considerations Associated with Extreme Sport Athletes

| | Extreme Sport Nutritional Considerations | | | | | |
| | Environmental | | | Psychological | | |
	Cold Exposure	Heat Exposure	Hypoxia	Epinephrine	Norepinephrine	Cortisol
Gluconeogenesis				↑	↑	↑
Glycogenesis	↓	↓	↓	↓	↓	↓
Glycogenolysis	↑↑	↑↑	↑	↑	↑	↑
Lipogenesis	↓	↑	↓	↓	↓	↑
Lipolysis	↑	↓	↑	↑	↑	↓
Ketone production				↓	↓	↓
Protein synthesis		↓		↑	↑	↓
Proteolysis		↑		↑	↑	↑

At low exercise intensities, increases to plasma EPI and NE concentrations display lipolytic effects and strong glucoregulatory effects by stimulating glucose production, but as intensity increases (from 25% to 45% VO_{2max}), the lipolytic effects decreases (Mora-Rodriguez and Coyle 2000). The biological half-life of both of these catecholamines is incredibly short (~2–3 minutes). That said, for longer-duration intense exercise to exhaustion, increases to overall consumption of carbohydrates should likely increase slightly or the athlete should aim to consume toward the higher end of the suggested athlete reference ranges. For short-duration events or exercises, modifications are likely not required.

7.4.4 Environment

Environmental conditions can prompt thermoregulatory processes that can alter substrate metabolism as an individual attempts to maintain an appropriate body temperature. These environmental conditions can occur in the form of heat exposure, cold exposure, or hypoxic conditions such as hypobaric hypoxia or recurrent underwater apneic events.

When exposed to heat stress without exercise, individuals experience increases in plasma EPI, NE, and cortisol (McMorris et al. 2006). EPI and NE can affect cardiac output and cause vasodilation in order to maximize the distribution of blood and heat as heat gets expelled through sweat loss and/or respiration. The ability of athletes to accomplish this goal depends on the individual's acclimation to heat, cardiopulmonary fitness, and hydration status (Sawka et al. 1993). Exercise with heat stress increases the overall metabolic rate and energy expenditure with a shift from fat utilization to carbohydrate use (Febbraio 2001). This could be attributed to the exacerbation of EPI and NE release of exercise under heat stress in comparison to exercise alone. Because catabolic processes are activated when exposed to hot environments, increases to overall daily Caloric consumption should increase based on exercise duration and intensity with a larger proportion of macronutrients coming from carbohydrates.

When exposed to cold environments, opposite cardiovascular thermoregulatory mechanisms occur whereby vasoconstriction attempts to limit the blood supply to extremities to reduce heat loss and preserve body temperature. Moreover, metabolic rate and energy expenditure increase to fulfill thermoregulatory and basal metabolic processes (Carlson and Marriott 1996). For instance, shivering occurs to promote heat production which causes a dramatic increase in carbohydrate oxidation and fatty acid oxidation to a lesser degree (Vallerand and Jacobs 1989). Interestingly, chronic exposure to heat may also promote the transition of white adipose tissue to thermogenic brown adipose tissue (Lee et al. 2014). When participating in an extreme sport in a cold environment, the athlete should consider the duration spent in the cold environment. If a lengthy expedition in the cold is planned, a hypercaloric diet in the weeks leading up to the event may be beneficial in order to increase fat mass for heat insulation. During such an expedition, careful planning of food supplies will be important to limit carrying load while ensuring adequate nutrition. For athletes spending a brief time in a cold environment, modifications are likely unnecessary.

Exposure to hypoxic conditions, like those experienced at high altitudes or prolonged free diving sessions, limit the amount of available oxygen for substrate metabolism. Under hypobaric hypoxic conditions, carbohydrate utilization and energy expenditure become elevated and remain elevated after exercise (Katayama et al. 2010), possibly for similar reasons to EPOC. Following hypobaric hypoxia, mitochondrial function is diminished, which suggests a large majority of energy comes from glycolytic metabolism (Murray 2016). Alternatively, during repeat apneic bouts, as seen during free diving, metabolic alterations occur in order to buffer elevated blood lactate concentrations (Joulia et al. 2003). For extreme athletes exposed to hypobaric hypoxic conditions, an increase in carbohydrate consumption may be beneficial, whereas standard sport nutritional recommendations are probably acceptable for divers.

7.4.5 Hydration

Hydration status is difficult to assess, thus making recommendations problematic. Fluids and electrolytes comprise the medium through which all cells communicate. At the cellular level, fluids can control anabolic and catabolic pathways by regulating cell size (Häussinger 1996). Failure to maintain proper hydration status of tissues has been linked to a number of cardiopulmonary disorders (El-Sharkawy, Sahota, and Lobo 2015). Furthermore, exercising in a hypohydrated state can result in sport performance impairments (Sawka, Cheuvront, and Kenefick 2015). Interestingly, resistance exercise while in a hypohydrated state increased exercise-induced plasma NE and cortisol spike and reduced clearance rate as well as altering substrate metabolism (Judelson et al. 2008). Ensuring adequate fluid and electrolyte intake is important for all athletes, especially those competing in hot environments or high-altitude, dry climates where sweat loss is high.

7.5 CONCLUSION

Nutritional recommendations have come a long way toward a better understanding of personalized nutrition. That said, there is still significant work needed before individualized plans are ready to be implemented for general health purposes. Despite the fact that nutritional recommendations are still developing, sport nutrition plans have advanced with guidelines available for many athletic endeavors. Unfortunately, these have not yet reached the extreme sport athletes who often have varied nutritional requirements dependent on the duration and intensity of their activity, as well as other factors such as environmental and psychological stressors. Our current understanding is limited to the few studies that have investigated these factors individually, but rarely together. Taken with the nutritional recommendations for traditional athletes based on gender, exercise intensity/duration, and overall volume, extreme sport athletes should consider the effects of the added stressors (e.g. environment and psychological stress). While the recommendations for traditional athletes are suitable for most extreme athletes, ultra-endurance athletes and extreme environment expeditioners should plan dietary choices for all phases of their events (pre, during, and post) and understand that trial and error will likely be necessary to determine what works best for their condition and their particular body.

REFERENCES

Almoosawi, S, S Vingeliene, LG Karagounis, and GK Pot. 2016. Chrono-nutrition: A review of current evidence from observational studies on global trends in time-of-day of energy intake and its association with obesity. *Proceedings of the Nutrition Society* 75 (4):487–500.

Asher, Gad, and Ueli Schibler. 2011. Crosstalk between components of circadian and metabolic cycles in mammals. *Cell Metabolism* 13 (2):125–137.

Auestad, Nancy, Judith S Hurley, Victor L Fulgoni, and Cindy M Schweitzer. 2015. Contribution of food groups to energy and nutrient intakes in five developed countries. *Nutrients* 7 (6):4593–4618.

Ball, Derek. 2014. Metabolic and endocrine response to exercise: Sympathoadrenal integration with skeletal muscle. *Journal of Endocrinology* 224 (2). doi:10.1530/JOE-14-JOE-0408.

Barnes, Mark A, Monica J Carson, and Meera G Nair. 2015. Non-traditional cytokines: How catecholamines and adipokines influence macrophages in immunity, metabolism and the central nervous system. *Cytokine* 72 (2):210–219.

Beck, Kathryn L, Jasmine S Thomson, Richard J Swift, and Pamela R Von Hurst. 2015. Role of nutrition in performance enhancement and postexercise recovery. *Open Access Journal of Sports Medicine* 6:259.

Berg, JM, JL Tymoczko, and L Stryer. 2002. The integration of metabolism. In *Biochemistry*, edited by S. Moran. New York: W H Freeman.

Bloomer, Richard J, Mohammad M Kabir, Kate E Marshall, Robert E Canale, and Tyler M Farney. 2010. Postprandial oxidative stress in response to dextrose and lipid meals of differing size. *Lipids in Health and Disease* 9 (1):79.

Brown, LM, and D J Clegg. 2010. Central effects of estradiol in the regulation of food intake, body weight, and adiposity. *The Journal of Steroid Biochemistry and Molecular Biology* 122 (1–3):65–73.

Brown, Scott W, Randall T Meyers, Karen M Brennan, et al. 2003. Catecholamines in a macrophage cell line. *Journal of Neuroimmunology* 135 (1–2):47–55.

Carlson, Sydne J, and Bernadette M Marriott. 1996. *Nutritional Needs in Cold and High-Altitude Environments: Applications for Military Personnel in Field Operations*: National Academies Press, Washington, D.C.

Cordain, Loren, S Boyd Eaton, Anthony Sebastian, et al. 2005. Origins and evolution of the Western diet: Health implications for the 21st century. *The American Journal of Clinical Nutrition* 81 (2):341–354.

Egan, Brendan, and Juleen R Zierath. 2013. Exercise metabolism and the molecular regulation of skeletal muscle adaptation. *Cell Metabolism* 17 (2):162–184.

El-Sharkawy, Ahmed M, Opinder Sahota, and Dileep N Lobo. 2015. Acute and chronic effects of hydration status on health. *Nutrition Reviews* 73 (suppl_2):97–109.

Erdemir, Ibrahim, and Tuba Kizilet Bozdogan. 2013. Effects of exercise on circadian rhythms of cortisol. *International Journal of Sports Science* 3 (3):68–73.

Febbraio, Mark A. 2001. Alterations in energy metabolism during exercise and heat stress. *Sports Medicine* 31 (1):47–59.

Gaesser, Glenn A, and George A Brooks. 1984. Metabolic bases of excess post-exercise oxygen consumption: a review. *Medicine and Science in Sports and Exercise* 16 (1):29–43.

Geer, Eliza B, and Wei Shen. 2009. Gender differences in insulin resistance, body composition, and energy balance. *Gender Medicine* 6:60–75.

Geleijnse, J M, D E Grobbee, and F J Kok. 2005. Impact of dietary and lifestyle factors on the prevalence of hypertension in Western populations. *Journal of Human Hypertension* 19 (S3):S1–S4.

Gimenez, Philippe, Hugo Kerhervé, Laurent A Messonnier, Léonard Féasson, and Guillaume Y Millet. 2013. Changes in the energy cost of running during a 24-h treadmill exercise. *Medicine and Science in Sports and Exercise* 45 (9):1807–1813.

Glick, Norris R, and Milton H Fischer. 2013. The role of essential fatty acids in human health. *Journal of Evidence-Based Complementary and Alternative Medicine* 18 (4):268–289.

Gómez-Pinilla, Fernando. 2008. Brain foods: The effects of nutrients on brain function. *Nature Reviews. Neuroscience* 9 (7):568–578.

Hackney, AC, S Feith, R Pozos, and J Seale. 1995. Effects of high altitude and cold exposure on resting thyroid hormone concentrations. *Aviation, Space, and Environmental Medicine* 66 (4):325–329.

Haggar, Fatima A, and Robin P Boushey. 2009. Colorectal cancer epidemiology: Incidence, mortality, survival, and risk factors. *Clinics in Colon and Rectal Surgery* 22 (4):191–197.

Häussinger, Dieter. 1996. The role of cellular hydration in the regulation of cell function. *Biochemical Journal* 313 (3):697–710.

Hill, EE, E Zack, C Battaglini, M Viru, A Viru, and A C Hackney. 2008. Exercise and circulating cortisol levels: The intensity threshold effect. *Journal of Endocrinological Investigation* 31 (7):587–591.

Horton, Tracy J, Suzanne Dow, Michael Armstrong, and W Troy Donahoo. 2009. Greater systemic lipolysis in women compared with men during moderate-dose infusion of epinephrine and/or norepinephrine. *Journal of Applied Physiology* 107 (1):200–210.

Horton, Tracy J, Michael J Pagliassotti, Karen Hobbs, and James O Hill. 1998. Fuel metabolism in men and women during and after long-duration exercise. *Journal of Applied Physiology* 85 (5):1823–1832.

Hou, Lina, Fei Li, Yuanyuan Wang, et al. 2015. Association between dietary patterns and coronary heart disease: A meta-analysis of prospective cohort studies. *International Journal of Clinical and Experimental Medicine* 8 (1):781.

Jeukendrup, Asker E. 2017. Periodized nutrition for athletes. *Sports Medicine* 47 (1):51–63.

Johnson, Rachel K, Lawrence J Appel, Michael Brands, et al. 2009. Dietary sugars intake and cardiovascular health: A scientific statement from the American Heart Association. *Circulation* 120 (11):1011–1020.

Joulia, Fabrice, Jean Guillaume Steinberg, Marion Faucher, et al. 2003. Breath-hold training of humans reduces oxidative stress and blood acidosis after static and dynamic apnea. *Respiratory Physiology and Neurobiology* 137 (1):19–27.

Judelson, Daniel A, Carl M Maresh, Linda M Yamamoto, et al. 2008. Effect of hydration state on resistance exercise-induced endocrine markers of anabolism, catabolism, and metabolism. *Journal of Applied Physiology* 105 (3):816–824.

Katayama, Keisho, Kazushige Goto, Koji Ishida, and Futoshi Ogita. 2010. Substrate utilization during exercise and recovery at moderate altitude. *Metabolism* 59 (7):959–966.

Kerksick, Chad, Travis Harvey, Jeff Stout, et al. 2008. International Society of Sports Nutrition position stand: Nutrient timing. *Journal of the International Society of Sports Nutrition* 5 (1):17.

Kraemer, William J, Maren S Fragala, Jeff S Volek, et al. 2007. Hormonal responses to a 160 Km race across frozen Alaska. *British Journal of Sports Medicine* 42 (2): 116–120.

Kreider, Richard B, Colin D Wilborn, Lem Taylor, et al. 2010. ISSN exercise & sport nutrition review: Research & recommendations. *Journal of the International Society of Sports Nutrition* 7 (1):1–43.

Lee, Paul, Sheila Smith, Joyce Linderman, et al. 2014. Temperature-acclimated brown adipose tissue modulates insulin sensitivity in humans. *Diabetes* 63 (11):3686–3698.

MacDonald, Ian A. 2016. A review of recent evidence relating to sugars, insulin resistance and diabetes. *European Journal of Nutrition* 55 (2):17–23.

Makki, Kassem, Edward C Deehan, Jens Walter, and Fredrik Bäckhed. 2018. The impact of dietary fiber on gut microbiota in host health and disease. *Cell Host and Microbe* 23 (6):705–715.

Manore, Melinda M, Kam Lynn Ciadella, and Anne B Loucks. 2007. The female athlete triad: Components, nutrition issues, and health consequences. *Journal of Sports Sciences* 25 (S1):S61–S71.

Maughan, Ron, Louise M Burke, and Edward F Coyle. 2004. *Food, Nutrition and Sports Performance II: The International Olympic Committee Consensus on Sports Nutrition*: Routledge New York.

McMorris, Terry, Jon Swain, Marcus Smith, et al. 2006. Heat stress, plasma concentrations of adrenaline, noradrenaline, 5-hydroxytryptamine and cortisol, mood state and cognitive performance. *International Journal of Psychophysiology* 61 (2):204–215.

Mora-Rodriguez, Ricardo, and Edward F Coyle. 2000. Effects of plasma epinephrine on fat metabolism during exercise: Interactions with exercise intensity. *American Journal of Physiology-Endocrinology and Metabolism* 278 (4):E669–E676.

Murray, Andrew J. 2016. Energy metabolism and the high-altitude environment. *Experimental Physiology* 101 (1):23–27.

Musso, Giovanni, Roberto Gambino, and Maurizio Cassader. 2011. Interactions between gut microbiota and host metabolism predisposing to obesity and diabetes. *Annual Review of Medicine* 62 (1):361–380.

Nishida, Chizuru, Ricardo Uauy, Shiriki Kumanyika, and Prakash Shetty. 2004. The joint WHO/FAO expert consultation on diet, nutrition and the prevention of chronic diseases: Process, product and policy implications. *Public Health Nutrition* 7 (1a):245–250.

Oken, Barry S, Irina Chamine, and Wayne Wakeland. 2015. A systems approach to stress, stressors and resilience in humans. *Behavioural Brain Research* 282:144–154.

Pernet, A, M Walker, GV Gill, H Orskov, KG Alberti, and DG Johnston. 1984. Metabolic effects of adrenaline and noradrenaline in man: Studies with somatostatin. *Diabete et metabolisme* 10 (2):98–105.

Perrault, H, M Cantin, G Thibault, GR Brisson, G Brisson, and M Beland. 1991. Plasma atriopeptin response to prolonged cycling in humans. *Journal of Applied Physiology* 70 (3):979–987.

Pessin, Jeffrey E, and Alan R Saltiel. 2000. Signaling pathways in insulin action: Molecular targets of insulin resistance. *The Journal of Clinical Investigation* 106 (2):165–169.

Phillips, Stuart M. 2011. The science of muscle hypertrophy: Making dietary protein count. *Proceedings of the Nutrition Society* 70 (1):100–103.

Potgieter, Sunita. 2013. Sport nutrition: A review of the latest guidelines for exercise and sport nutrition from the American College of Sport Nutrition, the International Olympic Committee and the International Society for Sports Nutrition. *South African Journal of Clinical Nutrition* 26 (1):6–16.

Potter, Gregory DM, Debra J Skene, Josephine Arendt, Janet E Cade, Peter J Grant, and Laura J Hardie. 2016. Circadian rhythm and sleep disruption: Causes, metabolic consequences, and countermeasures. *Endocrine Reviews* 37 (6):584–608.

Qi, Lu, Marilyn C Cornelis, Cuilin Zhang, Rob M Van Dam, and Frank B Hu. 2009. Genetic predisposition, Western dietary pattern, and the risk of type 2 diabetes in men. *The American Journal of Clinical Nutrition* 89 (5):1453–1458.

Rodriguez, Nancy R, Nancy M DiMarco, and Susie Langley. 2009. Position of the American Dietetic Association, Dietitians of Canada, and the American College of Sports Medicine: Nutrition and athletic performance. *Journal of the American Dietetic Association* 109 (3):509–527.

Roepstorff, Carsten, Morten Donsmark, Maja Thiele, et al. 2006. Sex differences in hormone-sensitive lipase expression, activity, and phosphorylation in skeletal muscle at rest and during exercise. *American Journal of Physiology-Endocrinology and Metabolism* 291 (5):E1106–E1114.

Sawka, Michael N, Samuel N Cheuvront, and Robert W Kenefick. 2015. Hypohydration and human performance: Impact of environment and physiological mechanisms. *Sports Medicine* 45 (1):51–60.

Sawka, Michael N, C Bruce Wenger, Andrew J Young, and Kent B Pandolf. 1993. Physiological responses to exercise in the heat. In *Nutritional Needs in Hot Environments: Applications for Military Personnel in Field Operations* p. 55.

Selye, Hans. 1936. A syndrome produced by diverse nocuous agents. *Nature* 138 (3479):32.

Selye, Hans. 1938. Adaptation energy. *Nature* 141 (3577):926.

Senekal, M, C Naude, and E Wentzel-Viljoen. 2014. Dietary recommendations for health: Fact sheet. University of Cape Town, Cape Town, South Africa.

Shikany, James M, and GL White Jr. 2000. Dietary guidelines for chronic disease prevention. *Southern Medical Journal* 93 (12):1138–1151.

Simopoulos, Artemis P. 2008. The importance of the omega-6/omega-3 fatty acid ratio in cardiovascular disease and other chronic diseases. *Experimental Biology and Medicine* 233 (6):674–688.

Skuland, Silje Elisabeth, and Siv Elin Ånestad. 2012. The mainstreaming of sports nutrition consumption in the Norwegian food culture. *Anthropology of Food* S7.

Smith, Jo, and Lars Mc Naughton. 1993. The effects of intensity of exercise on excess postexercise oxygen consumption and energy expenditure in moderately trained men and women. *European Journal of Applied Physiology and Occupational Physiology* 67 (5):420–425.

Sparti, Andrea, James P DeLany, A Jacques, Gary E Sander, and George A Bray. 1997. Relationship between resting metabolic rate and the composition of the fat-free mass. *Metabolism* 46 (10):1225–1230.

Stenner, Elisabetta, Elisabetta Gianoli, Clara Piccinini, Bruno Biasioli, Andrea Bussani, and Giorgio Delbello. 2007. Hormonal responses to a long duration exploration in a cave of 700 m depth. *European Journal of Applied Physiology* 100 (1):71–78.

Tahara, Yu, Shinya Aoyama, and Shigenobu Shibata. 2017. The mammalian circadian clock and its entrainment by stress and exercise. *The Journal of Physiological Sciences* 67 (1):1–10.

Tarnopolsky, LJ, JD MacDougall, SA Atkinson, MA Tarnopolsky, and JR Sutton. 1990. Gender differences in substrate for endurance exercise. *Journal of Applied Physiology* 68 (1):302–308.

Tarnopolsky, Mark A. 2000. Gender differences in metabolism; nutrition and supplements. *Journal of Science and Medicine in Sport* 3 (3):287–298.

Thatcher, Joanne, Sue Reeves, Debbie Dorling, and Anna Palmer. 2003. Motivation, stress, and cortisol responses in skydiving. *Perceptual and Motor Skills* 97 (3):995–1002.

Turocy, Paula Sammarone, Bernard F DePalma, C A Horswill, et al. 2011. National Athletic Trainers' Association position statement: Safe weight loss and maintenance practices in sport and exercise. *Journal of Athletic Training* 46 (3):322–336.

Vallerand, André L, and Ira Jacobs. 1989. Rates of energy substrates utilization during human cold exposure. *European Journal of Applied Physiology and Occupational Physiology* 58 (8):873–878.

van der Windt, Gerritje J, and Erika L Pearce. 2012. Metabolic switching and fuel choice during T-cell differentiation and memory development. *Immunological Reviews* 249 (1):27–42.

van Westerloo, David J, Goda Choi, Ester C Löwenberg, et al. 2011. Acute stress elicited by bungee jumping suppresses human innate immunity. *Molecular Medicine* 17 (3–4):180.

Weingarten, Jeremy A, and Nancy A Collop. 2013. Air travel: Effects of sleep deprivation and jet lag. *Chest* 144 (4):1394–1401.

Weitzman, Elliot D, David Fukushima, Christopher Nogeire, Howard Roffwarg, TF Gallagher, and Leon Hellman. 1971. Twenty-four hour pattern of the episodic secretion of cortisol in normal subjects. *The Journal of Clinical Endocrinology and Metabolism* 33 (1):14–22.

Wheatley, Courtney M, Eric M Snyder, Bruce D Johnson, and Thomas P Olson. 2014. Sex differences in cardiovascular function during submaximal exercise in humans. *Springerplus* 3 (1):445.

Xia, Zhi, Jason Cholewa, Yan Zhao, et al. 2016. Hypertrophy-promoting effects of leucine supplementation and moderate intensity aerobic exercise in pre-senescent mice. *Nutrients* 8 (5):246.

Zouhal, Hassane, Christophe Jacob, Paul Delamarche, and Arlette Gratas-Delamarche. 2008. Catecholamines and the effects of exercise, training and gender. *Sports Medicine* 38 (5):401–423.

8 Dietary Supplements for Use in Extreme Sports

Nicholas J.G. Smith, Matthew Butawan, and Richard J. Bloomer

CONTENTS

8.1 Overview of Dietary Supplements..144
    8.1.1 Regulation of Dietary Supplements...144
    8.1.2 Safety of Dietary Supplements: Adulterants and Third-Party Supplement Testing..145
    8.1.3 Safety of Dietary Supplements: Additional Considerations 146
8.2 Dietary Supplements for Overall Health 146
    8.2.1 Multivitamin/Mineral Supplements 147
    8.2.2 Vitamin D3 147
    8.2.3 Fish Oil (Omega-3 Fatty Acids)..148
    8.2.4 Protein Supplements 148
8.3 Dietary Supplements to Aid Physical Performance 148
    8.3.1 Caffeine 149
        8.3.1.1 Main Takeaways 150
    8.3.2 Creatine...151
        8.3.2.1 Main Takeaways 152
    8.3.3 Beta-Alanine...152
        8.3.3.1 Main Takeaways 153
    8.3.4 Sodium Bicarbonate 153
        8.3.4.1 Main Takeaways 154
    8.3.5 Nitrate (Beetroot Juice)...155
        8.3.5.1 Main Takeaways 156
8.4 Supplements to Aid Cognitive Performance 156
    8.4.1 Caffeine 156
    8.4.2 Rhodiola Rosea...157
    8.4.3 Ginseng...157
    8.4.4 L-Theanine..158
    8.4.5 Creatine...158
    8.4.6 Theacrine 158
8.5 Dietary Supplements to Aid Exercise Recovery 159
    8.5.1 Protein...159
        8.5.1.1 Main Takeaways 160

8.5.2   Creatine.. 160
         8.5.2.1   Main Takeaways 160
8.5.3   Beta-Hydroxy-Beta-Methylbutyrate (HMB) 160
         8.5.3.1   Main Takeaways 161
8.5.4   Carbohydrates.. 161
         8.5.4.1   Main Takeaways 161
8.5.5   Specific Amino Acid Mixtures.. 161
         8.5.5.1   Main Takeaways 162
8.6   Conclusions... 162
References... 163

8.1   OVERVIEW OF DIETARY SUPPLEMENTS

Over the past three decades, a multitude of dietary supplements has flooded the market, many of which are marketed specifically to athletes. Such supplements often claim to boost athletic performance or to enhance the recovery process. However, with thousands of these products on the market today, athletes may find themselves asking questions, including which products actually work; which products are safe; which products are backed by science and can yield the type of improvements that are alluded to in the advertising materials; or which products are best suited for a particular sport? For athletes interested in dietary supplements, the answers to these questions can be the difference between money well spent and money wasted. It can also be the difference between achieving their athletic goals and falling just short. Thus, the aim of this chapter is to provide an overview of the current landscape with regards to dietary supplements and ergogenic aids. Specifically, we include a brief overview of the regulation of dietary supplements, followed by sections that describe the efficacy of popular dietary supplements—with a specific focus on supplements designed to enhance overall health, physical performance, cognitive performance, and exercise recovery.

When reading this chapter, it is important to keep in mind the following key points:

1. Dietary supplements are intended to *supplement* the diet. They cannot replace a healthy diet. For more information regarding nutritional advice, please see Chapter 7: Nutritional requirements in extreme sports.
2. Many of the supplements described in this chapter can induce improvements in some facet of overall health, physical performance, cognitive performance, and/or exercise recovery. However, these improvements are likely to be small in magnitude relative to the changes experienced when significant alterations in exercise training and/or dietary intake are made. The focus of any athlete should be the use of sound exercise training and nutritional approaches to enhance performance and recovery.

8.1.1   REGULATION OF DIETARY SUPPLEMENTS

Before considering the use of dietary supplements, individuals should be familiar with the regulation of the dietary supplement industry and its impacts on the safety and purity of dietary supplements. In 1994, the U.S. Congress approved the Dietary Supplement Health and Education Act (DSHEA), a piece of legislation that has had profound impacts on the supplement industry. Under DSHEA, a dietary supplement is "a product (other than tobacco) intended to supplement the diet that bears or contains one or more of the following dietary ingredients: (A) a vitamin; (B) a mineral; (C) an herb or other botanical; (D) an amino acid; (E) a dietary substance for use by man to supplement the diet by increasing the total dietary intake; or (F) a concentrate, metabolite, constituent, extract, or combination of any ingredient described in clause (A), (B), (C), (D), or (E)."[1] Dietary supplements must be designed specifically for oral consumption and display labels on packaging designating them as dietary supplements. Additionally, they must not be marketed "for use as a conventional food or as a sole item of a meal or the diet."

In accordance with this definition of dietary supplement, DSHEA enacted a number of new regulations to govern the supplement industry, charging the Food and Drug Administration (FDA) with enforcing these regulations. These regulations are still in effect today and have been met with mixed approval by companies and consumers. To better protect consumers, DSHEA requires dietary supplement manufacturers to validate the safety of the individual dietary ingredients contained within their products and appropriately label their products in accordance with DSHEA and FDA labeling regulations. DSHEA also prohibits companies from producing or marketing adulterated products. That said, there is no requirement for companies to demonstrate the efficacy of their products, and they are permitted to manufacture and sell dietary supplements without conducting extensive safety testing, as would be the requirement for pharmaceuticals. These latter policies have allowed companies to flood the market with dietary supplements that boast dubious claims and sometimes questionable safety profiles. As a result, the FDA has been forced to adopt a reactionary regulation strategy in which supplements are monitored more carefully only after they become available on the market; the FDA does not test most supplements for contaminants or purity, unless the product produces severe negative health outcomes (i.e. liver damage) in unsuspecting consumers. It should be noted that an announcement made in February 2019 indicated that the FDA is planning to strengthen the regulation of dietary supplements.

8.1.2 Safety of Dietary Supplements: Adulterants and Third-Party Supplement Testing

Because the production and sale of dietary supplements is somewhat loosely regulated under DSHEA, dietary supplements have the potential to be contaminated by adulterants, a safety concern for athletes and non-athletes alike. Supplements may be contaminated via one or two methods. Contamination can occur via the intentional addition of an adulterant (i.e. anabolic agent), a relatively uncommon practice that can occur primarily with non-reputable sports supplement companies. Alternatively, substance impurity can occur when adulterants are added via cross-contamination (being exposed to adulterated substances). In this scenario, a potentially well-intentioned company can unwittingly contaminate an otherwise good product during production.

Adulterated supplements can pose a risk to all individuals. For example, consumption of certain contaminants (i.e. heavy metals) can cause harm with repeated or high-dose exposure. Additionally, consumption (even unknown consumption) of dietary ingredients that are banned by the World Anti-Doping Association (WADA) can result in disqualification for athletes that are drug tested for banned substances. Therefore, all individuals need guarantees that the dietary supplements they consume are not adulterated. Athletes can best assure purity by purchasing products tested by third-party organizations (e.g. US Pharmacopeia (USP), InformedChoice.org, etc.).

In response to questions of supplement safety, a number of third-party organizations – independent of the government and of supplement companies – have been founded to test the quality of dietary supplements. Examples of reputable supplement-testing organizations include the USP, NSF International, ConsumerLab.com, and InformedChoice.org. All of these organizations test supplements using the latest technology to ensure product purity, with NSF International and InformedChoice. org specifically testing for substances banned by WADA and other athletic agencies. Supplements certified by these agencies will bear some form of mark on their packaging. To help avoid contamination, individuals should seek to consume supplements approved by one of these organizations. This is especially important for athletes, who may be drug tested. Products consumed by these individuals should be evaluated through organizations such as NSF International and InformedChoice.org. While the above is important to keep in mind, it should be noted that the enforcement of current Good Manufacturing Practices (cGMPs) should help to minimize the number of problems related to adulterated dietary supplements.

8.1.3 SAFETY OF DIETARY SUPPLEMENTS: ADDITIONAL CONSIDERATIONS

Though third-party approved dietary supplements are generally considered safe for consumption by healthy adults, some supplements may not be appropriate for certain individuals or populations. This includes those who may be using prescription medications, with which the dietary supplement may adversely react. Moreover, some individuals are sensitive to certain ingredients (e.g. caffeine) and should use caution prior to ingesting certain dietary supplements. To prevent negative health outcomes, individuals should consult with their healthcare professionals (i.e. pharmacist, physician) before consuming any dietary supplement.

8.2 DIETARY SUPPLEMENTS FOR OVERALL HEALTH

Many of the dietary supplements found on the market today are purported to improve various parameters of health. Popular options include vitamins, minerals, or herbals/botanicals, which account for 56% of all supplement sales.[2] Most of these products will likely not lead to any significant improvement in overall health for otherwise healthy individuals consuming a balanced diet, but some (i.e. vitamin D3 and fish oil) may actually help to improve various markers of health.

Before discussing these supplements, it is important to note that it is particularly difficult to evaluate the efficacy of dietary supplements on "overall health" using only clinical trials (often considered the gold standard of supplementation research). Clinical trials that evaluate these dietary supplements often use outcome measures such as the development of chronic disease or mortality following chronic supplementation. Because it can take many years or even decades for these supplements to display positive effects on overall health, clinical trials examining these supplements are particularly susceptible to confounding factors – such as genetics, diet, physical activity, disease state, and supplementation protocol. Thus, though peer-reviewed literature regarding these supplements will be discussed, the basis for the recommendation of many of these supplements is based largely on shorter-term trials that use surrogate measures of health as outcome variables, as opposed to long-term studies using hard endpoints (e.g. death).

8.2.1 MULTIVITAMIN/MINERAL SUPPLEMENTS

Multivitamin/mineral supplements (MVMs) are one of the most popular dietary supplements on the market today.[3,4] As the name implies, MVMs are dietary supplements that contain a combination of vitamins and minerals. A variety of MVM exists, but the most common form is a once-daily tablet or capsule containing a cocktail of the recommended daily intake (RDI) of the common vitamins and minerals.[5]

The efficacy of MVMs is a polarizing topic. Only a limited number of clinical studies have linked regular MVM supplementation with reductions in chronic disease,[6] while a majority of studies reports no significant benefit of MVM supplementation. However, as discussed above, it is difficult to assess the effect of a dietary supplement on chronic disease development given the multitude of confounding factors. Thus, because MVMs are both safe[7] and inexpensive, it may be prudent for individuals to invest in MVMs as a means to "fill nutritional gaps," theoretically augmenting physiological function while potentially attenuating the risk of illness or disease by ensuring that RDIs are met.

8.2.2 VITAMIN D3

Vitamin D (cholecalciferol) performs many vital physiological functions, and an individual's Vitamin D status (defined using concentration of serum 25-hydroxyvitamin D [25(OH)D]) is an important marker for overall health.[8] Research indicates that a large portion of the population is vitamin D insufficient (serum 25(OH)D 30–50 nmol/L) or deficient (serum 25(OH)D <30 nmol/L).[9,10] Under normal circumstances, vitamin D is absorbed from the diet or synthesized following sun exposure. Vitamin D insufficiency and deficiency is more common in obese individuals, individuals with limited sun exposure, and individuals with dark skin.[9] Additionally, the risk of developing vitamin D insufficiency and deficiency increases during the winter and spring months.

Vitamin D status appears to be a meaningful marker of overall health. Vitamin D adequate men have been shown to have higher testosterone levels, relative to vitamin D insufficient/deficient men.[11] Adequate vitamin D levels may protect individuals from a variety of acute and chronic illnesses, including infectious disease, cancer, cardiovascular disease, and diabetes mellitus.[12] Moreover, vitamin D insufficient and deficient individuals may be at a higher risk of all-cause mortality. Thus, vitamin D insufficient and deficient individuals should attempt to increase 25(OH)D levels which can be achieved through regular vitamin D3 supplementation, as vitamin D3 supplementation has been reported to effectively increase 25(OH)D, particularly in both vitamin D deficient and insufficient individuals.[13]

8.2.3 Fish Oil (Omega-3 Fatty Acids)

Omega-3 fatty acids are fatty acid chains with double bonds located three carbons from the methyl end of the fatty acid chain. Though a variety of omega-3s exists, alpha-linolenic acid (ALA), eicosapentaenoic acid (EPA), and docosahexaenoic acid (DHA) are the most well researched omega-3s. ALA is found in plant oils (i.e. flax seeds), and DHA and EPA are found primarily in fish and krill oils. These omega-3s perform a variety of important physiological functions. Notably, studies have shown that ALA, DHA, and EPA reduce systemic inflammation via competitive inhibition of omega-6 fatty acids.[14,15] Increased consumption of DHA and EPA has been linked to decreased incidence of various negative health outcomes, such as cardiovascular disease, cancer, and cognitive decline.[16] Thus, it would seem prudent for individuals not meeting the recommended daily consumption of omega-3 fatty acids (1.6 g/d for men; 1.1 g/day for women) to consider the use of fish oil supplements to benefit overall long-term health.

8.2.4 Protein Supplements

As described in Chapter 7 protein is a chief component of a well-balanced diet. Normal, healthy individuals should aim to consume at least 0.8 grams of protein per kilogram of body weight per day to optimize health, though this recommendation changes based on physical activity level and athletic goals (i.e. lean mass gain). For most individuals, it will be easy to meet this recommendation by consuming a normal diet. However, some individuals such as vegans or those attempting to lose weight may struggle to meet their protein needs, in particular "complete" sources of protein containing all essential amino acids. A protein supplement may help these individuals meet their daily protein needs, thus maintaining optimal health.

8.3 DIETARY SUPPLEMENTS TO AID PHYSICAL PERFORMANCE

Physical performance is an important component of athletic performance. Broadly, physical performance is classified using various exercise tests, including cardiovascular endurance, power, strength, and muscular endurance exercise testing. Cardiovascular endurance exercise testing involves prolonged aerobic-type exercise (i.e. running or cycling). Types of endurance exercise tests include time-to-exhaustion (endurance exercise until volitional failure), time trial (either time-based or distance-based), or graded exercise tests. High-intensity "power" exercise tests include short sprint, longer sprint (<8 min; i.e. 1600 m sprint), and repeated sprint (short >10 s bouts of maximal-effort sprinting, separated by relatively short rest intervals) exercise tests. Strength tests are typically administered as one-repetition maximum tests (max amount of weight lifted on a given exercise during one repetition). Muscular endurance tests are typically administered as maximum-repetitions-to-failure exercise tests (max number of repetitions completed during a given exercise at a set intensity). These types of exercise tests will be used to define physical performance within this section of the chapter. It is important to note that not all exercise tests are equal in terms of application value. Time-to-exhaustion tests are generally considered less ecologically valid than time trial tests.[17–20] Repeated sprint tests are considered highly applicable to sport performance because many sports involve similar repeated bouts of high-intensity exercise.[21] In general, adequate training and a balanced diet is the best way to improve performance on these types of tests, but in recent years, a variety of dietary supplements have been explored as a means to augment physical performance.

Many of the products sold today are multi-ingredient dietary supplements that contain a proprietary blend of purported ergogenic agents. Many of these products contain ingredients that may be either potentially harmful (e.g. those with high levels of stimulants) or lack efficacy. Clearly, only a small percentage of multi-ingredient products currently being sold have actually been evaluated using clinical trials or laboratory tests. Thus, this section will focus primarily on single-ingredient dietary supplements (with the exception of beetroot juice) that are supported by peer-reviewed scientific research. Aside from carbohydrate, which is well-known to aid exercise performance, a selected few of these single ingredient supplements such as caffeine, creatine, beta-alanine, sodium bicarbonate, and dietary nitrate appear to have efficacy as ergogenic supplements. In general, these supplements may generate small-to-moderate improvements in physical performance in many individuals. However, it is important to understand that these supplements will not replace an appropriate training regimen or a well-balanced diet. Additionally, the individual response to these supplements varies widely based on a litany of genetic and non-genetic factors.

8.3.1 Caffeine

Caffeine, a naturally occurring psychoactive compound, is one of the most popular ergogenic aids and has been studied extensively with regard to physical performance. When consumed prior to exercise, caffeine can stimulate the central nervous system via the inhibition of adenosine receptors. This may cause reductions in perceptions of fatigue and pain, improving exercise performance across a number of exercise modalities.

A number of factors must be considered when using caffeine as an ergogenic aid. Moderate doses (3–6 mg/kg) of caffeine administered approximately 60 minutes prior to exercise are often reported to elicit the best improvements in physical performance,[22–24] with no benefits (and often performance decrements) reported when high (>9 mg/kg) doses are used.[22] Low (<3 mg/kg) doses are often not considered ergogenic, with the exception of continuous caffeine ingestion during prolonged (>120 minute) endurance exercise.[25] Further, it should be noted that a number of genetic and non-genetic factors (including chronic caffeine usage) affect caffeine absorption and metabolism, and individual response to caffeine varies widely (see Pickering, 2018 for a review).[26] For instance, some individuals require significantly more time to metabolize caffeine than others, potentially related to genetic predispositions. Nevertheless, studies have shown that moderate doses of caffeine administered approximately 60 minutes prior to exercise consistently aid physical performance in a number of populations.

In recent years, scientific reviews have indicated that acute, moderate-dose caffeine supplementation can be ergogenic in most performance settings.[22,25,27–29] The greatest performance improvements are often reported during exercise lasting longer than 5 minutes, particularly during aerobic/endurance-type protocols. A meta-analysis conducted by Doherty et al. indicated caffeine supplementation improved endurance performance by 21.4% on testing ≤120 minutes and 17.7% on testing lasting >120 minutes.[27] Doherty et al. also noted that these ergogenic effects are seen most frequently on time-to-exhaustion testing. Other reviews have reported similar findings.[22,29] However, it is also evident that closed-ended protocols of varying durations can benefit from acute caffeine supplementation. A systematic review conducted by Ganio reported that caffeine has an ergogenic effect on time trial exercise testing (>5 min), with a mean improvement of 3.2% following caffeine supplementation.[28] Additionally, a recent meta-analysis indicated that caffeine significantly improves performance during short-duration (45 s–8 min), closed-ended exercise testing.[23]

Comparatively fewer studies have examined caffeine supplementation in conjunction with sprint-type performance. In general, it appears that caffeine can improve performance on repeated-sprint performance but does not enhance single sprint performance lasting less than 30 seconds. In their meta-analysis, Astorino et al. concluded that, in general, moderate caffeine consumption can improve sport-specific exercise testing (i.e. repeated sprints) in trained athletes.[24] Eleven of the 17 studies they reviewed reported an ergogenic effect of caffeine for at least one trial, leading to a mean improvement of 6.5% relative to placebo. Caffeine supplementation improved performance on activities such as 100-m sprint swimming and 4 s sprints on a cycle ergometer. However, as noted by Astorino et al., most studies that reported performance improvements following caffeine ingestion involved trained athletes (i.e. competitive swimmers), not recreationally active, healthy individuals. A subsequent review of caffeine's effects on power/sport-specific high-intensity exercise reported similar discrepant findings.[22] In this review, McLellan et al. indicated that moderate caffeine supplementation generally does not benefit all-out efforts lasting 60 s or less, as measured by peak power or fatigue. Moreover, caffeine supplementation can enhance performance on repeated sprinting when longer (90 s) rest intervals are used between sprints, though caffeine does not appear ergogenic in these settings when short (<20 s) rest intervals are used.

In relation to resistance exercise, moderate caffeine supplementation appears to improve muscular endurance but not muscular strength.[24,30] Polito et al. conducted a systematic review and meta-analysis to determine caffeine's effects on isotonic muscular strength and endurance.[30] Findings of this review indicated that moderate dose (4–6.2 mg/kg) caffeine supplementation 60 minutes prior to resistance exercise can improve the max number of repetitions performed on a given exercise at a given resistance. However, evidence indicated that caffeine supplementation did not improve maximal strength as measured by maximal weight lifted during one repetition of a given exercise.

8.3.1.1   Main Takeaways

Moderate (3–6 mg/kg) doses of caffeine administered approximately 60 minutes prior to exercise generally improves performance during exercise lasting longer than 60 seconds. Additionally, caffeine may improve performance during repeated sprint testing, as well as during muscular endurance testing.

8.3.2 Creatine

Creatine (Cr) is a naturally occurring organic compound that is synthesized endogenously and consumed in a standard diet. When activated (i.e. combined with a phosphate group to form phospho-creatine [PCr]), PCr is capable of rapidly producing energy by creating adenosine triphosphate (ATP; the energy "currency" of cellular reactions) through a process known as substrate level phosphorylation. This substrate-level phosphorylation is a vital component of energy production during short-duration, high-intensity activities (i.e. 8 s sprint). Research has established that creatine supplementation (CrS) increases muscle Cr concentrations,[31,32] thereby improving performance on high-intensity exercise (i.e. repeated sprinting and resistance training). Indeed, the International Society of Sports Nutrition has touted creatine monohydrate (the most widely used form of creatine supplementation) as "the most effective ergogenic nutritional supplement" for increasing performance in high-intensity exercise.[33] Creatine supplementation has also been shown to enhance performance in sport-specific settings.[34] In general, Cr appears to be an effective ergogenic aid capable of eliciting a number of performance enhancing effects.

Research has indicated that oral CrS, frequently administered as creatine monohydrate, is successful in increasing PCr levels in most humans. Typical supplementation guidelines recommend undergoing a loading phase of 20 g/day of Cr for 5–7 days to increase PCr levels by 20–40%.[33] Following the loading phase, individuals seeking to augment training gains frequently undergo a maintenance phase, consuming 3–5 g/day (larger individuals may need 5–10 g/day) to ensure that skeletal muscles remain saturated with PCr. It should be noted that studies have reported large intersubject variability with regards to Cr absorption. Scientific literature describes CrS "responders" and "non-responders," with responders and non-responders experiencing a >20 mmol/kg and <10 mmol/kg dry weight increase in total intramuscular creatine and phosphocreatine following creatine loading, respectively.[35,36] This is likely a product of various natural physiological components, including the prevalence of type II muscle fibers and physiological levels of Cr and PCr. Accordingly, responders should expect a greater increase in performance with CrS than non-responders.

As many reviews have discussed, it is well established that both Cr loading (~20 g/day for 5–7 days) and prolonged CrS (Cr loading followed by multiple weeks/ months of ~5 g/day) improve short-duration, high-intensity performance, notably during repeated-sprint testing.[32,33,37–39] Using a variety of rest intervals ranging from 10–120 s, studies have consistently demonstrated that CrS improves repeated-sprint performance on tests of varying durations, increasing power, work, and sprint velocity.[40–46] For example, Preen et al. reported that 5 days of CrS (20 g/day) increased total work and peak power during 10 sets of repeated cycling sprints, with sprints separated by 24, 54, or 84 s.[42] More recent studies have demonstrated the ergogenic effects of creatine loading on a number of other repeated-sprint tests, including the Running-based Anaerobic Sprint Test (six 35 m sprints separated by 10 s of rest).[44,45] It appears likely that CrS enhances performance in this type of testing through an increased rate of PCr resynthesis between sprints. Additionally, it appears likely that these performance-enhancing benefits translate well to training. Studies have reported that prolonged CrS combined with exercise training significantly enhances training adaptations, leading to greater improvements on repeated-sprint testing relative to exercise training alone.[47]

In addition to enhancing repeated-sprint performance, CrS may also augment performance during other modalities of short-duration, high-intensity exercise. Studies have shown that CrS enhances performance on resistance exercise, increasing muscular strength, power, and endurance. These effects are most profound when prolonged CrS (i.e. creatine loading followed by a maintenance phase) is combined with resistance exercise. Reviews have reported moderately large increases in muscular strength (3–8%) and muscular endurance (14%), relative to placebo, when prolonged CrS is combined with resistance training.[48–50] Additionally, CrS can improve performance on single sprint testing. Several studies have reported that CrS is capable of inducing small but meaningful improvements on single-sprint testing,[43,51–53] though these reports are contested by a number of studies reporting conflicting evidence.[54–57] Moreover, with regards to jump performance, CrS has been reported to increase max jump height during vertical jump testing and attenuate performance declines during repeated jump testing.[58–60] Creatine may also have a role in sport-specific activities, such as soccer agility drills performed while dribbling a soccer ball.[45]

It should also be noted that CrS has demonstrated the ability to affect parameters of exercise performance during prolonged exercise. For instance, studies have shown that CrS decreases lactate accumulation during submaximal exercise[61] and increases lactate threshold during graded exercise testing.[62] However, these reports are in direct contrast to a large body of studies that have reported that CrS does not affect lactate production or other markers or aerobic performance, such as VO_{2max}.[63,64] Thus, while it has shown promise in some areas of aerobic performance, CrS is not widely recommended for endurance athletes.

8.3.2.1 Main Takeaways

Evidence indicates creatine supplementation improves performance during short-duration, high-intensity exercise, particularly during repeated-sprints. Current guidelines recommend individuals follow a loading (~20 g/day for 7 days) and subsequent maintenance (~5 g/day) supplementation schedule to elicit maximum performance gains from creatine supplementation.

8.3.3 BETA-ALANINE

In recent years, beta-alanine has gained popularity as an ergogenic supplement. A non-proteogenic amino acid, humans produce beta-alanine naturally in the liver. Beta-alanine is relevant to exercise because it acts as the rate-limiting precursor to the formation of carnosine. A dipeptide found in large quantities in the brain and skeletal muscle, carnosine acts as a pH buffer in skeletal muscle during intense anaerobic exercise. Supplementing beta-alanine through a prolonged loading dose (~4–6 g/day for 28 days) significantly increases the concentration of muscle carnosine in most individuals.[65] This increase in muscle carnosine should be accompanied by a concomitant increase in the buffering capacity of skeletal muscle and result in an attenuation of metabolic acidosis during intense anaerobic exercise. Thus far, research has suggested that beta-alanine supplementation is ergogenic for intense, single-effort exercise lasting 0.5–10 min (i.e. 1500 m running), particularly in untrained individuals.[66] These performance-enhancing effects are more evident during open-ended testing (i.e. test to volitional exhaustion) than closed-ended testing (i.e. time trial). However, the literature indicates beta-alanine has little-to-no ergogenic effects on other types of exercise, such as resistance training, short sprinting (<30 s; i.e. 100 m sprint), repeated sprinting, or endurance exercise lasting longer than 10 minutes.

A number of publications have addressed beta-alanine in the context of physical performance.[23,66–68] These publications indicate beta-alanine may enhance endurance capacity during intense, single-effort exercise lasting 0.5–10 minutes.[66] Specifically, studies have reported that beta-alanine supplementation improves performance on anaerobic time-to-exhaustion protocols, with the greatest improvements reported during exercise lasting under 270 seconds.[67] For example, Danaher et al. recently reported that 4 weeks of beta-alanine loading improved exercise capacity during cycling at 110% maximal workload.[69] Other studies utilizing similar protocols have reported parallel results.[70] However, these ergogenic benefits do not appear to consistently translate to closed-ended testing, as a number of studies[71–75] and meta-analyses[23,66,68] have reported equivocal results utilizing closed-ended testing (i.e. time trials or simulated races with a predetermined endpoint) following beta-alanine loading. These reports call into question the efficacy of beta-alanine for sport performance, considering closed-ended testing is often considered more valid than open-ended testing.[17–20]

To date, beta-alanine supplementation has not consistently demonstrated ergogenic effects on all types of exercise. Studies have reported that beta-alanine does not improve performance during short sprints (i.e. <30 s)[76] or repeated sprints.[77,78] Additionally, although beta-alanine has been reported to increase total training volume and reduce fatigue during resistance training,[76,79,80] preliminary research has not consistently indicated that beta-alanine improves either muscular strength or muscular endurance.[79–82] It also does not appear to augment performance during longer-duration (>10 min) aerobic exercise, though more studies are needed to confirm this finding.[66] These findings are to be expected, as acidosis is not considered to be a major limiting factor in exercise that is extremely short (i.e. single-effort sprints or resistance exercise) or extending beyond 10 minutes in duration. Thus, it would appear that beta-alanine's ergogenic effects are limited primarily to short-duration, single-effort, open-ended exercise testing lasting 0.5–10 minutes. Further research may expand the implications for beta alanine in the future.

8.3.3.1 Main Takeaways

Beta alanine loading (~4–6 g/day for 28 days) may be ergogenic for sustained, single-effort, high-intensity exercise lasting 0.5–10 minutes, particularly for individuals who are not well-trained. However, current research indicates that beta-alanine supplementation does not enhance performance during short sprints (<30 s), repeated sprints, endurance exercise (>10 min), or certain aspects of resistance training.

8.3.4 Sodium Bicarbonate

Sodium bicarbonate ($NaHCO_3$) supplementation has been suggested to increase buffering capacity, enhancing performance during short-duration, high-intensity exercise. Produced endogenously via conversion of CO_2, bicarbonate (HCO_3^-) plays a large role in the natural buffering system of the blood. It helps to maintain physiological pH, including during high-intensity exercise. Acute (200–300 mg/kg) supplementation of $NaHCO_3$ has been reported to increase bicarbonate levels with acute administration of 300 mg/kg being the most studied dosage.[83] Peak bicarbonate concentrations are most frequently observed 60–180 min post-ingestion of 300 mg/kg.[84] However, because some individuals report experiencing significant gastrointestinal distress (i.e. nausea, vomiting, diarrhea, etc.) post-ingestion of a large bolus of sodium bicarbonate, current supplementation guidelines recommend either co-ingestion of 300 mg/kg with a meal or serial (~500 mg/kg/day for up to 5 days) bicarbonate supplementation.[83] Both methods have been reported to significantly increase plasma bicarbonate concentrations.[85] Regardless of supplementation protocol, increased plasma bicarbonate concentrations have been associated with improvements in short-duration, high-intensity performance, notably during sprint-type exercise testing.

Bicarbonate supplementation improves performance on high-intensity exercise, principally during sprint-type activities. Both individual investigations and pooled meta-analyses[83] have consistently indicated that bicarbonate supplementation meaningfully improves performance during sustained high-intensity exercise tests lasting 1–10 minutes. These improvements have been noted utilizing both open-ended (time-to-exhaustion) and closed-ended (i.e. time trial) exercise testing.[83] Meta-analyses have indicated individuals are more likely to experience meaningful improvements (~2%) on shorter high-intensity, single-effort exercise tests (~1 min) when compared to longer high-intensity, single-effort exercise tests (>10 minutes). Additionally, bicarbonate supplementation appears to benefit repeated sprint performance more than single-sprint performance, with studies reporting improvements as great as 8% on intermittent sprint testing.[86–89] Given the relevance of closed-ended and repeated-sprint exercise testing to sports, these reports indicate that bicarbonate supplementation should translate well to high-intensity sport performance involving components of sprinting or moving explosively. Early research into this field has shown promising results. Reports have demonstrated ergogenic effects of bicarbonate supplementation on exercise tests specific to tennis,[90] boxing,[91] judo,[87] and swimming.[91]

With reference to other modalities of high-intensity performance, more research is needed before recommendations can be made. Notably, future studies should examine bicarbonate's role with respect to muscular endurance and in combination with prolonged exercise training. Some evidence suggests that bicarbonate supplementation can positively influence muscular endurance during acute bouts of resistance training.[92] However, few studies have been published in this area, and more research is needed to draw meaningful conclusions. Similarly, prolonged bicarbonate ingestion during training has not been well studied. At least one study has reported greater gains following 8 weeks of bicarbonate supplementation combined with exercise training,[93] but again, more research in this area is needed before conclusions can be made.

8.3.4.1 Main Takeaways

Acute (~300 mg/kg, preferably co-ingested with a meal) and serial (1–5 mg/kg/day) sodium bicarbonate supplementation appears effective for increasing single-effort and repeated-effort sprints and, thus, is likely a relevant ergogenic supplement for sport performance. More research is needed to elucidate bicarbonate's effects on resistance training, as well as the safety and effectiveness of prolonged supplementation in combination with training. It is important for individuals considering bicarbonate supplementation to experiment with bicarbonate supplementation during training sessions prior to utilizing bicarbonate during competitions, as large boluses of bicarbonate are known to cause significant gastrointestinal distress.

8.3.5   Nitrate (Beetroot Juice)

Dietary nitrate (NO_3^-) supplementation has been proposed to improve exercise economy during endurance exercise by inducing vasodilation. Nitrate is a naturally occurring molecule found in many common foods, particularly green leafy vegetables and beetroot. Via the nitrate-nitrite-nitric oxide pathway, ingested nitrate can be converted to nitric oxide (NO), a potent signaling molecule that may stimulate vasodilation. Increased vasodilation may lead to improved blood flow to metabolic tissues (i.e. skeletal muscle) which can potentially have meaningful impacts on exercise via the improved delivery of oxygen and nutrients to skeletal muscle and a more efficient removal of metabolic wastes.

A number of reviews and meta-analyses have examined the relationship between nitrate supplementation and exercise performance. Generally, nitrate supplementation exhibits a small ergogenic effect on endurance exercise.[94] Nitrate's ergogenic effects are most commonly seen on protocols utilizing time-to-exhaustion exercise tests. This is possibly the result of improved muscle efficiency following nitrate supplementation, as nitrate supplementation has been shown to decrease steady state oxygen consumption (VO_2) at submaximal intensities.[95,96] Nitrate supplementation is less effective for time trial performance, for well-trained individuals (especially elite aerobic athletes).[94]

Nitrate supplementation is not well understood with respect to other types of exercise testing. Some studies indicate that nitrate supplementation can enhance sustained short-duration, high-intensity performance (i.e. 1500 m running),[97,98] while other studies suggest that nitrate does not improve this type of performance, including short-duration time trials (45 s–8 min).[23] Because of the equivocal evidence, more studies are needed to elucidate the true effect of nitrate supplementation on sprint-type performance. Performance during repeated effort sprints does not appear to be affected by nitrate supplementation.[99–101] Moreover, to our knowledge, only two studies have examined nitrate's effects on resistance exercise performance.[102,103] These studies reported equivocal results with respect to physical performance during resistance exercise (as measured by maximum repetitions to failure). It should be noted that the studies utilized differing exercise tests (bench press versus back squat), nitrate sources, and supplementation protocols. Thus, more research is needed before conclusions can be drawn regarding nitrate's effects on resistance exercise performance.

It should be noted that optimal nitrate dosing strategies have yet to be elucidated. Nitrate supplementation has been administered in the form of nitrate salts, nitrate water, pomegranate extract, or beetroot juice, with beetroot juice being by far the most common (and potentially most effective) form of administration because nitrate salts and waters are tightly regulated and/or banned in many countries.[94] In general, acute nitrate supplementation results in a dose-dependent increase in plasma nitrite concentrations. High doses of nitrate (i.e. >6.5 mmol) in the form of beetroot juice appear to confer the greatest performance benefits with respect to acute bouts of exercise. Moreover, nitrate loading (i.e. ~5.5 mmol of nitrate for 6 days) may be more effective than acute nitrate supplementation. However, given the potential safety concerns associated with the consumption of highly concentrated nitrates, individuals should exercise caution when consuming highly concentrated nitrate supplements.

8.3.5.1 Main Takeaways

Nitrate supplementation may improve endurance capacity (i.e. time-to-exhaustion) when supplemented in relatively high doses (i.e. >6.5 mmol), particularly in the form of beetroot juice. Nitrate supplementation may also improve performance in sustained high-intensity exercise.

8.4 SUPPLEMENTS TO AID COGNITIVE PERFORMANCE

In addition to physical performance, cognitive processes–such as memory, reaction speed, attention, decision-making, coordination, and motor control–can influence athletic performance to a large degree. To truly maximize athletic potential, athletes must strive to optimize cognitive performance as well as physical performance. Major factors that influence cognitive performance include age, sleep status, stress levels, and diet. With respect to diet, eating a healthy diet composed of appropriate amounts of fruits, vegetables, whole grains, proteins, healthy fats, and essential micronutrients can assist in optimizing cognitive performance. Additionally, supplementing a healthy diet with selected dietary supplements has been shown to enhance cognitive function in certain situations.

Many dietary supplements have been proposed to aid cognitive function. However, it is beyond the scope of this chapter to examine every proposed mental-performance enhancer. Instead, we focus on the supplements used by athletes to enhance cognitive function that appear most popular, such as caffeine, *Rhodiola rosea,* ginseng, L-theanine, Cr, and theacrine. Additionally, this section will focus on these supplements' ability to affect cognitive performance (including motor-control/skill-specific tasks) during and after exercise.

8.4.1 CAFFEINE

As described in the physical performance section, caffeine is a naturally-occurring psychoactive compound capable of stimulating the central nervous system, primarily through the inhibition of adenosine receptors. Caffeine has been well researched with respect to cognitive performance, and as detailed in a recent comprehensive review by McLellan et al., caffeine generally improves various cognitive functions.[22] Low order cognitive functions, such as vigilance, reaction time, and attention,[104–107] are most improved following acute caffeine ingestion, while high order functions (i.e. problem-solving) may or may not be improved with caffeine supplementation.

Additionally, learning and mood may also be enhanced with acute caffeine consumption. These cognition-enhancing effects are seen primarily with low-to-moderate doses of caffeine (32–300 mg), although increased doses (200–600 mg) may be more beneficial for sleep-deprived individuals.[108–111]

With regard to athletic-specific situations, increasing evidence suggests acute, moderate-dose caffeine supplementation enhances cognitive and motor-skill-specific performance during and after exercise. Multiple studies have indicated that caffeine supplementation improves performance on general cognitive tests during and/or following strenuous exercise.[112–114] For example, Hogervost et al. reported that athletes consuming 100 mg of caffeine (in a performance bar) demonstrated increased concentration, response times, and visual processing after prolonged endurance exercise, relative to two placebo groups (isocaloric non-caffeinated performance bar and 300 ml of placebo beverage).[113] More recent studies have examined caffeine's effects on skill-related tasks specific to sport (see Baker, 2014 for a review).[115] These studies have been conducted across multiple sport disciplines (i.e. soccer, field hockey, rugby) using a variety of tests.[116–119] Some studies reported increases in motor/skill performance (i.e. increased passing accuracy or better ball handling) during sport specific tests following bouts of exercise. It should be mentioned, though, that studies that do not implement exhaustive exercise or simulated game play prior to sport-specific skill tests are less likely to show ergogenic effects.[120–122] Thus, it appears that caffeine is most beneficial to sport-specific skills when fatigue levels are high.

8.4.2 RHODIOLA ROSEA

Rhodiola rosea (R. rosea) is a plant grown in mountainous regions of the northern hemisphere whose extract is used for medicinal purposes in various regions of Europe and Asia.[123] Though its effects on cognitive performance are not well researched in humans, proponents of *R. rosea* extract suggest it is capable of enhancing mental performance, particularly during stressful situations. At least three studies support this claim.[124,125] Recently, Jowko et al. reported that 26 healthy male students improved simple and choice reaction time during a battery of psychomotor tests following 4 weeks of *R. rosea* supplementation (600 mg/day), relative to placebo.[126] However, equivocal evidence exists with regard to *R. rosea*'s possible effects on cognitive performance. Of particular relevance to athletes, two studies have reported that *R. rosea* does not improve cognitive performance during or after exercise.[127,128] This equivocal evidence, in combination with the questionable quality of supporting research, has prompted several recent reviews to conclude that *R. rosea* is not efficacious for improving cognitive performance.[115,123,129] Thus, though future research is warranted, *R. rosea* is not currently recommended for athletes looking to improve mental performance.

8.4.3 GINSENG

Ginseng is another herb that has been used throughout history for medicinal purposes. Today, ginseng extract is commonly found in products such as energy drinks (i.e. Monster™). Though it has been reported to enhance various parameters of cognition (particularly functions related to memory), evidence regarding acute doses of ginseng in healthy humans remains equivocal, and chronic dosing regimens in healthy humans have not been studied.[130] Further, only one known study has reported testing sport-specific skill following ginseng supplementation. The study reported that ginseng supplementation improved shooting accuracy during a biathlon.[131] However, given that only one study has utilized ginseng in a sport-like setting, and other reports of ginseng supplementation are equivocal, more research is needed before ginseng can be recommended to athletes to improve cognitive performance.

8.4.4   L-Theanine

Found primarily in green tea, L-theanine is a non-proteogenic amino acid that is structurally similar to glutamine. L-theanine has not been studied extensively with respect to cognition, but some studies have reported performance enhancements following L-theanine ingestion. Alone, L-theanine appears to have limited effects on cognitive performance,[132] with only one known study reporting enhanced cognition (vigilance) in healthy adults following L-theanine ingestion.[133] Instead, L-theanine supplementation may have additive effects on cognitive performance when co-ingested with caffeine. Several studies have reported that L-theanine supplementation can synergistically improve various cognitive parameters, such as attention, reaction time, memory, and accuracy, when combined with caffeine, relative to caffeine alone.[132] However, given that no work has been conducted in an athletic setting, more research regarding L-theanine and caffeine is needed before it can be recommended to athletes.

8.4.5   Creatine

As discussed in review by Twycross-Lewis et al., there is some evidence to suggest that creatine supplementation can improve cognitive performance in individuals with impaired cognitive processing.[134] Specifically, creatine has been suggested to enhance cognitive performance in elderly individuals[135] and during hypoxia[136] and sleep-deprivation.[137] Because some individuals may face sleep deprivation and hypoxia during extreme sports, creatine supplementation may be of interest with regards to cognitive performance. However, research in these situations is preliminary and has not frequently been applied to athletic settings. Further research is needed before creatine can be recommended as a cognitive aid for athletes.

8.4.6   Theacrine

In recent years, theacrine, an agent similar in structure to caffeine, has gained popularity in the sports supplement world and is currently being used in multi-ingredient pre-workout supplements. Currently, research suggests that theacrine can improve subjective feelings related to cognition and arousal, including perceived energy, fatigue, concentration, and motivation to exercise.[138] However, to date, no study has demonstrated that theacrine has positive effects on any objective measure of cognition. Future research is warranted and may provide additional evidence for or against the use of theacrine as an agent to enhance cognitive performance during exercise.

8.5   DIETARY SUPPLEMENTS TO AID EXERCISE RECOVERY

Currently, many dietary supplements are being promoted as exercise recovery aids. Proposed recovery aids include protein supplements, creatine, beta-hydroxy-beta-methylbutyrate (HMB), carbohydrate supplements, and branched chain amino acids (BCAAs), amongst others. All such products claim to enhance the recovery process, generally via one or more of the following mechanisms: (1) limit skeletal muscle breakdown (2) reduce inflammation/oxidative stress (3) promote an anabolic state. If achieved, these aims should theoretically reduce the time needed for recovery between competitions and training sessions, augment exercise-induced adaptations (i.e. increase lean mass), and/or reduce the risk of overtraining. However, as is common with dietary supplements, only a selected few of these products can be recommended to athletes based on the available literature. Some, like protein supplements, have well-researched, practical uses. Others, like HMB, appear less effective for trained athletes. Still others have only demonstrated the ability to improve relatively impractical measures of the recovery process, such as blood metabolites (i.e. creatine kinase and lactate dehydrogenase), but not practical markers of recovery (i.e. muscle function or force production). This section will discuss the most well-researched recovery aids with a focus on practical uses for athletes.

8.5.1   PROTEIN

Protein supplements (i.e. protein powders or bars) are a commonly used, well-researched recovery aid. Because they have been suggested to improve the regenerative capacity of skeletal muscle, protein supplements are most often used by individuals seeking to augment lean mass gains. Common supplementation practice involves consuming anywhere from 20–50 g of protein (i.e. whey protein isolate) immediately following a bout of high-intensity training. A number of studies[139–142] and reviews[143–145] have reported increased lean mass gains when resistance training is combined with protein supplementation, as compared to resistance training alone. A recent report by Morton et al. indicated that protein supplementation combined with 6+ weeks of resistance training enhanced lean mass gains by 0.30 kg in healthy individuals, relative to resistance training alone.[146] Factors such as age and training status influenced the effects of protein supplementation, with young and resistance trained individuals generally benefiting from protein supplementation more than older and untrained individuals. However, the authors noted that gains in lean mass were most evident when optimal *total* protein intake (~1.6 g/kg/day distributed equally into 5–6 meals) was met, leading Morton et al. to conclude total daily protein intake is more important for lean mass gains than the specifics of protein supplementation (i.e. timing, dose, type). This conclusion generally supports the findings of other reviews[116] and meta-analyses[147] conducted in similar populations. Therefore, protein supplementation is most beneficial to individuals who are in a negative nitrogen balance in regards to lean mass gains. Such individuals may include certain clinical populations or those following specific diets (i.e. a vegan diet or hypocaloric diet).

With respect to other indirect measures of recovery, a recent systematic review by Pasiakos et al. indicated that some evidence exists to support the notion that protein supplementation reduces muscle soreness, attenuates muscle damage, and enhances recovery of muscle function following an acute bout of high intensity exercise.[148] These recovery-enhancing effects of protein supplementation are primarily seen when protein supplements are consumed after daily training sessions and in individuals that are in a nitrogen or caloric deficit. However, because research regarding these factors is largely conflicting, Pasiakos et al. concluded that supplementation cannot be recommended with 100% confidence to individuals seeking to improve these specific indirect measures of muscle recovery.

8.5.1.1 Main Takeaways

Protein supplementation may assist in maximizing lean mass gains via helping individuals meet the optimal protein intake (~1.6 g/kg/day) for lean mass gains.

8.5.2 CREATINE

With regards to recovery, creatine supplementation appears most useful for individuals attempting to gain muscle mass. Serial creatine supplementation (~20 g/kg/day for 7 days followed by ~5 g/kg/day) has consistently been associated with increased lean mass gains in both trained and untrained individuals when combined with resistance training.[142] The exact mechanisms by which lean mass gains are augmented remains to be elucidated, but in general, it appears that they are at least partially the result of a creatine-induced post-exercise anabolic state.[149]

Creatine has also been suggested to attenuate muscle damage, but research regarding creatine's effects on muscle damage is equivocal. Several studies have shown that creatine supplementation can diminish the development of muscle damage following intense exercise.[150-152] These studies primarily measure muscle damage using indirect markers of muscle damage, mainly in untrained individuals. For example, Cooke et al. indicated that 5 days of creatine loading (0.3 g/kg/day) prior to intense lower body exercise increased post-exercise isometric and isokinetic knee extension strength while decreasing serum creatine kinase levels in 14 healthy males.[152] However, conflicting research exists, and few studies have been conducted in well-trained individuals.[153] Moreover, a reduction in creatine kinase does not necessarily equate to a reduction in the degree of muscle damage. Therefore, creatine supplementation cannot be recommended for athletes specifically looking to reduce muscle damage.

8.5.2.1 Main Takeaways

Serial creatine supplementation (20 g/kg/day for 7 days followed by ~5 g/kg/day) in combination with resistance training may be effective for augmenting lean mass gains in both trained and untrained individuals. Additionally, creatine supplementation may attenuate the development of some indirect markers of exercise-induced muscle damage, but more research is needed in this area.

8.5.3 BETA-HYDROXY-BETA-METHYLBUTYRATE (HMB)

A leucine metabolite, HMB has been suggested as a potential recovery aid to limit muscle damage and speed up recovery, resulting in increased strength and lean mass gains.

Several recent reviews have highlighted the use of HMB in an athletic setting, and while research regarding HMB is still developing, it currently appears that HMB is mainly beneficial for untrained individuals.[154,155] HMB supplementation has been shown to reduce some indirect markers of skeletal muscle damage - such as creatine kinase, lactate dehydrogenase, and urea nitrogen - following high-intensity resistance training in untrained individuals.[156] HMB supplementation may also augment hypertrophy in untrained individuals. However, research in moderately trained,[157] and well-trained individuals[158] is equivocal in regards to skeletal muscle damage and recovery. Specifically, it does not appear as though HMB is useful for athletes undergoing strenuous training.

8.5.3.1 Main Takeaways

HMB supplementation can simultaneously improve the hypertrophic response and attenuate the accumulation of indirect markers of muscle damage following high-intensity resistance training in untrained individuals. Trained individuals do not appear to reap similar benefits from HMB.

8.5.4 CARBOHYDRATES

Post-exercise carbohydrate supplementation has been proposed as a method to enhance glycogen synthesis and improve exercise recovery. Research indicates that post-exercise carbohydrate supplementation (1–1.2 g/kg/hour for 4 hours post-exercise) does improve the rate of glycogen restoration. However, this is likely only beneficial for athletes that will complete a subsequent exercise bout within 8 hours of completing the initial exercise bout; standard consumption of a "normal" diet will likely result in similar glycogen restoration 24-hours post-exercise, compared to carbohydrate supplementation.[159] With regard to other aspects of recovery, post-exercise carbohydrate supplementation does not appear to attenuate markers of exercise-induced muscle damage,[160] but it may help with exercise-induced immunosuppression,[161,162] which may enhance cellular immunity and help to maintain the health of an athlete.

8.5.4.1 Main Takeaways

Post-exercise carbohydrate supplementation (1–1.2 g/kg/hour for 4 hours post-exercise) may augment glycogen restoration for athletes participating in multiple exercise sessions <8 hours apart and may enhance cellular immunity.

8.5.5 SPECIFIC AMINO ACID MIXTURES

In recent years, products containing some mixture of specific amino acids have gained popularity as sports supplements. Two types of amino acid mixtures in particular have been used as recovery aides: branched chain amino acid blends and essential amino acid blends. Branched chain amino acid (BCAA) supplements are typically composed of leucine, isoleucine, and valine in a 2:1:1 ratio. Today, BCAA mixtures are commonly used both alone or included within multi-ingredient dietary supplements. Research examining the effects of BCAAs on recovery is relatively scant, but early evidence suggests that BCAA supplementation may reduce the development of muscle damage following intense exercise. Studies conducted in both athletes and non-athletes alike have reported that BCAA supplementation reduces the accumulation of various indirect markers of muscle damage (i.e. serum creatine kinase and lactate dehydrogenase levels) in the blood following intense exercise (see Rahimi, 2017[163] for a meta-analysis). Additionally, a recent study in trained weight lifters indicated that BCAA supplementation (0.087 g/kg) attenuated reductions in isometric strength following exercise-induced muscle damage.[164] Collectively, these studies indicate that BCAA supplementation may be an effective recovery aid for athletes. However, more research is necessary to corroborate the efficacy of BCAA supplementation in an athletic population (especially in trained individuals) and to elucidate the most effective dosage for recovery.

Essential amino acid (EAA) mixtures commonly contain some mixture of the 9 metabolically essential amino acids: histidine, isoleucine, leucine, lysine, methionine, phenylalanine, threonine, tryptophan, and valine. EAA mixtures have been used as recovery aides in an attempt to favorably alter post-exercise protein turnover. When administered post-exercise in combination with a carbohydrate supplement, EAA supplements appear to attenuate protein degradation and increase protein synthesis in untrained individuals.[165–167] An increase in protein synthesis and decrease in protein degradation should, theoretically, be accompanied by an increase in lean mass gains and a decrease in skeletal muscle breakdown. However, this may not always be the case, as evidenced by studies that show that acute post-exercise protein synthesis may not be directly correlated with exercise-induced lean mass gains.[168] Certainly, more research into the role of EAAs and recovery is needed.

8.5.5.1 Main Takeaways

Though branched chain amino acid and essential amino acid mixtures display promise, more research is needed before these supplements can be strongly recommended for athletes seeking to augment recovery.

8.6 CONCLUSIONS

Dietary supplements are an evolving field within sports nutrition, and, thus, recommendations regarding dietary supplements for athletes are constantly being updated. Based on current research, extreme sports athletes should consider a number of dietary supplements to augment general health, physical performance, cognitive performance, and/or exercise recovery. In regards to overall health, multivitamin/minerals, vitamin D3, fish oil, and protein supplements may be useful to individuals for maintaining, or even improving, various markers of overall health. With respect to physical performance, caffeine is likely the most generally beneficial ergogenic aid, improving performance during exercise lasting longer than 60 seconds across many modalities. Other supplements may enhance performance during specific exercise types. Creatine, beta-alanine, and sodium bicarbonate supplementation may improve performance during short-duration, high-intensity exercise, and nitrate supplementation may enhance endurance performance during aerobic-type exercise. Athletes seeking to boost cognitive performance may consider caffeine supplementation, as it has consistently demonstrated the ability to improve measures of cognition. Protein and carbohydrate appear to be the most widely utilized and effective nutrients to augment various measures of exercise recovery.

Considering the above, it is important for all individuals to take certain precautionary measures when considering the use of dietary supplements. Athletes should ensure that all supplements they ingest are free of adulterants, which is best achieved by exclusively using products that are batch tested by third party organizations such as NSF International and InformedChoice.org. Additionally, athletes should experiment with products on themselves during training period prior to use in competition. This will help the athlete to determine tolerance to the supplement and to identify any negative side effects. Through these methods, athletes can ensure that they only utilize supplements that are appropriate for their use and will ultimate aid in exercise performance and recovery.

REFERENCES

1. Dietary supplement health and education act of 1994. https://ods.od.nih.gov/About/DSHEA_Wording.aspx. Accessed April 12, 2018.
2. Nutrition Business Journal. Supplement business report 2016. https://www.newhope.com/sites/newhope360.com/files/2016%20NBJ%20Supplement%20Business%20report_lowres_TOC.pdf. Accessed April 12, 2018.
3. Dickinson A, Blatman J, El-Dash N, Franco JC. Consumer usage and reasons for using dietary supplements: Report of a series of surveys. *Journal of the American College of Nutrition*. 2014;33(2):176–182. http://www.ncbi.nlm.nih.gov/pubmed/24724775. doi:10.1080/07315724.2013.875423.
4. Nutrition Business Journal. Supplements today: Why the future looks bright. http://www.newhope.com/sites/newhope360.com/files/Expo-West-2017-Supplements-Today-1.pdf. Accessed April 12, 2018.
5. National Institutes of Health: Office of Dietary Supplements. Multivitamin/mineral supplements. https://ods.od.nih.gov/factsheets/MVMS-Consumer/. Accessed Feb 17, 2017; Updated 2016.
6. Guallar E, Stranges S, Mulrow C, Appel LJ, Miller 3rd ER. Enough is enough: Stop wasting money on vitamin and mineral supplements. *Annals of Internal Medicine*. 2013;159(12):850–851. http://www.ncbi.nlm.nih.gov/pubmed/24490268.
7. Biesalski HK, Tinz J. Multivitamin/mineral supplements: Rationale and safety. *Nutrition*. 2016;36(60):60–66. https://search.proquest.com/docview/1884235677. doi:10.1016/j.nut.2016.06.003.
8. Bendik I, Friedel A, Roos FF, Weber P, Eggersdorfer M. Vitamin D: A critical and essential micronutrient for human health. *Frontiers in Physiology*. 2014;5(248). http://www.ncbi.nlm.nih.gov/pubmed/25071593. doi:10.3389/fphys.2014.00248.
9. Hilger J, Friedel A, Herr R, et al. A systematic review of vitamin D status in populations worldwide. *The British Journal of Nutrition*. 2014;111(1):23–45. http://www.ncbi.nlm.nih.gov/pubmed/23930771. doi:10.1017/S0007114513001840.
10. Farrokhyar F, Tabasinejad R, Dao D, Peterson D, Ayeni OR, Hadioonzadeh R, Bhandari M. Prevalence of vitamin D inadequacy in athletes: A systematic-review and meta-analysis. *Sports Med. Sports Medicine*. 2015;45(3):365–378. http://www.ncbi.nlm.nih.gov/pubmed/25277808. doi:10.1007/s40279-014-0267-6.
11. Wehr E, Pilz S, Boehm BO, Marz W, Obermayer-Pietsch B. Association of vitamin D status with serum androgen levels in men. *Clinical Endocrinology*. 2010;73(2):243–248. http://www.ingentaconnect.com/content/bsc/cend/2010/00000073/00000002/art00017. doi:10.1111/j.1365-2265.2009.03777.x.

12. Pludowski P, Holick MF, Pilz S, et al. Vitamin D effects on musculoskeletal health, immunity, autoimmunity, cardiovascular disease, cancer, fertility, pregnancy, dementia and mortality - A review of recent evidence. *Autoimmunity Reviews.* 2013;12(10):976–989. http://www.narcis.nl/publication/RecordID/oai:research.vu.nl:publications%2F46e51111-0338-451b-9892-ede820dd6163. doi:10.1016/j.autrev.2013.02.004.

13. Whiting SJ, Bonjour J, Payen FD, Rousseau B. Moderate amounts of vitamin D3 in supplements are effective in raising serum 25-hydroxyvitamin D from low baseline levels in adults: A systematic review. *Nutrients.* 2015;7(4):2311–2323. http://www.ncbi.nlm.nih.gov/pubmed/25835074. doi:10.3390/nu7042311.

14. Calder PC. Omega-3 polyunsaturated fatty acids and inflammatory processes: Nutrition or pharmacology? *British Journal of Clinical Pharmacology.* 2013;75(3):645–662. http://onlinelibrary.wiley.com/doi/10.1111/j.1365-2125.2012.04374.x/abstract. doi:10.1111/j.1365-2125.2012.04374.x.

15. Calder PC. Marine omega-3 fatty acids and inflammatory processes: Effects, mechanisms and clinical relevance. *Biochimica et Biophysica Acta (BBA) - Molecular and Cell Biology of Lipids.* 2015;4(4):469–484. doi:10.1016/j.bbalip.2014.08.010.

16. Wall R, Ross RP, Fitzgerald GF, Stanton C. Fatty acids from fish: The anti-inflammatory potential of long-chain omega-3 fatty acids. *Nutrition Reviews.* 2010;68(5):280–289. http://www.ncbi.nlm.nih.gov/pubmed/20500789.doi:10.1111/j.1753-4887.2010.00287.x.

17. Laursen P, Rhodes E, Langill R, McKenzie D, Taunton J. Relationship of exercise test variables to cycling performance in an ironman triathlon. *European Journal of Applied Physiology.* 2002;87(4):433–440. http://www.ncbi.nlm.nih.gov/pubmed/12172884. doi:10.1007/s00421-002-0659-4.

18. Laursen PB, Francis GT, Abbiss CR, Newton MJ, Nosaka K. Reliability of time-to-exhaustion versus time-trial running tests in runners. *Medicine and Science in Sports and Exercise.* 2007;39(8):1374–1379. http://www.ncbi.nlm.nih.gov/pubmed/17762371. doi:10.1249/mss.0b013e31806010f5.

19. Currell K, Jeukendrup AE. Validity, reliability and sensitivity of measures of sporting performance. *Sports Medicine.* 2008;38(4):297–316.

20. Stevens CJ, Dascombe BJ. The reliability and validity of protocols for the assessment of endurance sports performance: An updated review. *Measurement in Physical Education and Exercise Science.* 2015;19(4):177–185.doi:10.1080/1091367X.2015.1062381.

21. Bishop D, Girard O, Mendez-Villanueva A. Repeated-sprint ability – Part II. *Sports Medicine.* 2011;41(9):741–756. http://www.ncbi.nlm.nih.gov/pubmed/21846163. doi:10.2165/11590560-000000000-00000.

22. McLellan TM, Caldwell JA, Lieberman HR. A review of caffeine's effects on cognitive, physical and occupational performance. *Neuroscience and Biobehavioral Reviews.* 2016;71:294–312. doi:10.1016/j.neubiorev.2016.09.001.

23. Christensen PM, Shirai Y, Ritz C, Nordsborg NB. Caffeine and bicarbonate for speed. A meta-analysis of legal supplements potential for improving intense endurance exercise performance. *Frontiers in Physiology.* 2017;8:240. https://doaj.org/article/c293883cfce24564bbdc0501c3520dbb. doi:10.3389/fphys.2017.00240.

24. Astorino T, Roberson D. Efficacy of acute caffeine ingestion for short-term high-intensity exercise performance: A systematic review. *Journal of Strength and Conditioning Research.* 2010;24(1):257–265. http://www.ncbi.nlm.nih.gov/pubmed/19924012. doi:10.1519/JSC.0b013e3181c1f88a.

25. Spriet L. Exercise and sport performance with low doses of caffeine. *Sports Medicine.* 2014;44(S2):175–184. http://www.ncbi.nlm.nih.gov/pubmed/25355191. doi:10.1007/s40279-014-0257-8.

26. Pickering C, Kiely J. Are the current guidelines on caffeine use in sport optimal for everyone? Inter-individual variation in caffeine ergogenicity, and a move towards personalised sports nutrition. *Sports Med. Sports Medicine.* 2018;48(1):7–16. doi:10.1007/s40279-017-0776-1.

27. Doherty M, Smith PM. Effects of caffeine ingestion on exercise testing: A meta-analysis. *International Journal of Sport Nutrition and Exercise Metabolism*. 2004;14(6): 626–646. http://www.ncbi.nlm.nih.gov/pubmed/15657469.

28. Ganio M, Klau J, Casa D, Armstrong L, Maresh C. Effect of caffeine on sport-specific endurance performance: A systematic review. *Journal of Strength and Conditioning Research*. 2009;23(1):315–324. http://www.ncbi.nlm.nih.gov/pubmed/19077738. doi:10.1519/JSC.0b0 13e31818b979a.

29. Goldstein ER, Ziegenfuss T, Kalman D, et al. International society of sports nutrition position stand: Caffeine and performance. *Journal of the International Society of Sports Nutrition*. 2010;7(1):5. http://www.ncbi.nlm.nih.gov/pubmed/20205813. doi:10.1186/1550-2783-7-5.

30. Polito MD, Souza DB, Casonatto J, Farinatti P. Acute effect of caffeine consumption on isotonic muscular strength and endurance: A systematic review and meta-analysis. *Science and Sports*. 2016;31(3):119–128. https://www.sciencedirect.com/science/article/pii/S0765159716000563. doi:10.1016/j.scispo.2016.01.006.

31. Hultman E, Soderlund K, Timmons JA, Cederblad G, Greenhaff PL. Muscle creatine loading in men. *Journal of Applied Physiology*. 1996;81(1):232–237. http://jap.physiology.org/content/81/1/232.

32. Kreider RB. Creatine supplementation: Analysis of ergogenic value, medical safety, and concerns. *Journal of Exercise Physiology*. 1998;1(1):1–16.

33. Kreider RB, Kalman DS, Antonio J, et al. International society of sports nutrition position stand: Safety and efficacy of creatine supplementation in exercise, sport, and medicine. *Journal of the International Society of Sports Nutrition*. 2017;14(1):1–8. https://search.proquest.com/docview/1915806253. doi:10.1186/s12970-017-0173-z.

34. Bishop D. Dietary supplements and team-sport performance. *Sports Medicine*. 2010;40(12):995–1017. http://vuir.vu.edu.au/7128/.

35. Demant TW, Rhodes EC. Effects of creatine supplementation on exercise performance. *Sports Medicine*. 1999;28(1):49–60.

36. Syrotuik DG, Bell GJ. Acute creatine monohydrate supplementation: A descriptive physiological profile of responders vs. nonresponders. *Journal of Strength and Conditioning Research*. 2004;18(3):610–617. http://www.ncbi.nlm.nih.gov/pubmed/15320650. doi:10.1519/12392.1.

37. Williams MH, Branch JD. Creatine supplementation and exercise performance: An update. *Journal of the American College of Nutrition*. 1998;17(3):216–234. http://www.jacn.org/cgi/content/abstract/17/3/216.

38. Cooper R, Naclerio F, Allgrove J, Jimenez A. Creatine supplementation with specific view to exercise/sports performance: An update. *Journal of the International Society of Sports Nutrition*. 2012;9(1):33. http://www.ncbi.nlm.nih.gov/pubmed/22817979. doi:10.1186/1550-2783-9-33.

39. Dorrell HF, Gee TI, Middleton G. An update on effects of creatine supplementation on performance: A review. *Sports Nutrition and Therapy*. 2016;1:107. doi:10.4172/2473-6449.1000107.

40. Wiroth J, Bermon S, Andreï S, Dalloz E, Hébuterne X, Dolisi C. Effects of oral creatine supplementation on maximal pedalling performance in older adults. *European Journal of Applied Physiology*. 2001;84(6):533–539. http://www.ncbi.nlm.nih.gov/pubmed/11482548. doi:10.1007/s004210000370.

41. van Loon LJC, Oosterlaar AM, Hartgens F, Hesselink MKC, Snow RJ, Wagenmakers AJM. Effects of creatine loading and prolonged creatine supplementation on body composition, fuel selection, sprint and endurance performance in humans. *Clinical Science*. 2003;104(2):153–162. http://www.narcis.nl/publication/RecordID/oai:cris.maastrichtuniversity.nl:publications%2F3ff03f98-e3d5-403e-9f5e-2b29f406990b. doi:10.1042/CS20020159.

42. Preen D, Dawson B, Goodman C, Lawrence S, Beilby J, Ching S. Effect of creatine loading on long-term sprint exercise performance and metabolism. *Medicine and Science in Sports and Exercise.* 2001;33(5):814–821. http://www.ncbi.nlm.nih.gov/pubmed/11323554. doi:10.1097/00005768-200105000-00022.

43. Skare OC, Skadberg Ø Wisnes AR. Creatine supplementation improves sprint performance in male sprinters. *Scandinavian Journal of Medicine and Science in Sports.* 2001;11(2):96–102. http://onlinelibrary.wiley.com/doi/10.1034/j.1600-0838.2001.011002096.x/abstract. doi:10.1034/j.1600-0838.2001.011002096.x.

44. Deminice R, Rosa FT, Franco GS, Jordao AA, de Freitas EC. Effects of creatine supplementation on oxidative stress and inflammatory markers after repeated-sprint exercise in humans. *Nutrition (Burbank, Los Angeles County, California).* 2013;29(9):1127–1132. http://www.ncbi.nlm.nih.gov/pubmed/23800565. doi:10.1016/j.nut.2013.03.003.

45. Mohebbi H, Rahnama N, Moghadassi M, Ranjbar K. Effect of creatine supplementation on sprint and skill performance in young soccer players. *Middle-East Journal of Scientific Research.* 2012;12(3):397–401.

46. Dabidi Roshan V, Babaei H, Hosseinzadeh M, Arendt-Nielsen L. The effect of creatine supplementation on muscle fatigue and physiological indices following intermittent swimming bouts. *The Journal of Sports Medicine and Physical Fitness.* 2013;53(3):232. http://www.ncbi.nlm.nih.gov/pubmed/23715246.

47. Ramírez-Campillo R, González-Jurado JA, Martínez C, et al. Effects of plyometric training and creatine supplementation on maximal-intensity exercise and endurance in female soccer players. *Journal of Science and Medicine in Sport/Sports Medicine Australia.* 2016;19(8):682–687. http://www.ncbi.nlm.nih.gov/pubmed/26778661. doi:10.1016/j.jsams.2015.10.005.

48. Rawson ES, Volek JS. Effects of creatine supplementation and resistance training on muscle strength and weightlifting performance. *Journal of Strength and Conditioning Research.* 2003;17(4):822–831. http://www.ncbi.nlm.nih.gov/pubmed/14636102. doi:10.1519/00124278-200311000-00031.

49. Lanhers C, Pereira B, Naughton G, Trousselard M, Lesage F, Dutheil F. Creatine supplementation and lower limb strength performance: A systematic review and meta-analyses. *Sports Medicine.* 2015;45(9):1285–1294. http://www.ncbi.nlm.nih.gov/pubmed/25946994. doi:10.1007/s40279-015-0337-4.

50. Lanhers C, Pereira B, Naughton G, Trousselard M, Lesage F, Dutheil F. Creatine supplementation and upper limb strength performance: A systematic review and meta-analysis. *Sports Medicine.* 2017;47(1):163–173. https://search.proquest.com/docview/1924204573. doi:10.1007/s40279-016-0571-4.

51. Rossiter HB, Cannell ER, Jakeman PM. The effect of oral creatine supplementation on the 1000-m performance of competitive rowers. *Journal of Sports Sciences.* 1996;14(2):175–179. http://www.ncbi.nlm.nih.gov/pubmed/8737325. doi:10.1080/02640419608727699.

52. Dawson B, Cutler M, Moody A, Lawrence S, Goodman C, Randall N. Effects of oral creatine loading on single and repeated maximal short sprints. *Australian Journal of Science and Medicine in Sport.* 1995;27(3):56. http://www.ncbi.nlm.nih.gov/pubmed/8599745.

53. Faraji H, Arazi H, Vatani D, Hakimi M. The effects of creatine supplementation on sprint running performance and selected hormonal responses. *South African Journal for Research in Sport, Physical Education and Recreation.* 2010;32(2). doi:10.4314/sajrs.v32i2.59293.

54. Burke LM, Pyne DB, Telford RD. Effect of oral creatine supplementation on single-effort sprint performance in elite swimmers. *International Journal of Sport Nutrition.* 1996;6(3):222–233. http://www.ncbi.nlm.nih.gov/pubmed/8876342.

55. Peyrebrune MC, Nevill ME, Donaldson FJ, Cosford DJ. The effects of oral creatine supplementation on performance in single and repeated sprint swimming. *Journal of Sports Sciences.* 1998;16(3):271–279. http://www.tandfonline.com/doi/abs/10.1080/026404198366803. doi:10.1080/026404198366803.

56. Mujika I, Chatard JC, Lacoste L, Barale F, Geyssant A. Creatine supplementation does not improve sprint performance in competitive swimmers. *Medicine and Science in Sports and Exercise.* 1996;28(11):1435–1441. http://www.ncbi.nlm.nih.gov/pubmed/8933496. doi:10.1097/00005768-199611000-00014.

57. Snow RJ, McKenna MJ, Selig SE, Kemp J, Stathis CG, Zhao S. Effect of creatine supplementation on sprint exercise performance and muscle metabolism. *Journal of Applied Physiology.* 1998;84(5):1667–1673. http://jap.physiology.org/content/84/5/1667.

58. Ostojic SM. Creatine supplementation in young soccer players. *International Journal of Sport Nutrition and Exercise Metabolism.* 2004;14(1):95–103. http://www.ncbi.nlm.nih.gov/pubmed/15129933.

59. Kirksey B, Stone MH, Warren BJ, et al. The effects of 6 weeks of creatine monohydrate supplementation on performance measures and body composition in collegiate track and field athletes. *Journal of Strength and Conditioning Research.* 1999;13(2):148–156. doi:10.1519/00124278-199905000-00009.

60. Stone MH, Sanborn K, Smith LL, et al. Effects of in-season (5 weeks) creatine and pyruvate supplementation on anaerobic performance and body composition in American football players. *International Journal of Sport Nutrition.* 1999;9(2):146–165. http://www.ncbi.nlm.nih.gov/pubmed/10362452.

61. Tang F, Chan C, Kuo P. Contribution of creatine to protein homeostasis in athletes after endurance and sprint running. *European Journal of Nutrition.* 2014;53(1):61–71. http://www.ncbi.nlm.nih.gov/pubmed/23392621. doi:10.1007/s00394-013-0498-6.

62. Chwalbińska-Moneta J. Effect of creatine supplementation on aerobic performance and anaerobic capacity in elite rowers in the course of endurance training. *International Journal of Sport Nutrition and Exercise Metabolism.* 2003;13(2):173–183. http://www.ncbi.nlm.nih.gov/pubmed/12945828.

63. Branch JD. Effect of creatine supplementation on body composition and performance: A meta-analysis. *International Journal of Sport Nutrition and Exercise Metabolism.* 2003;13(2):198–226. http://www.ncbi.nlm.nih.gov/pubmed/12945830.

64. Zoeller RF, Stout JR, O'Kroy JA, Torok DJ, Mielke M. Effects of 28 days of beta-alanine and creatine monohydrate supplementation on aerobic power, ventilatory and lactate thresholds, and time to exhaustion. *Amino Acids.* 2007;33(3):505–510. http://www.ncbi.nlm.nih.gov/pubmed/16953366. doi:10.1007/s00726-006-0399-6.

65. Blancquaert L, Everaert I, Derave W. Beta-alanine supplementation, muscle carnosine and exercise performance. *Current Opinion in Clinical Nutrition and Metabolic Care.* 2015;18(1):63–70. http://www.ncbi.nlm.nih.gov/pubmed/25474013. doi:10.1097/MCO.0000000000000127.

66. Saunders B, Elliott-Sale K, Artioli GG, et al. B-alanine supplementation to improve exercise capacity and performance: A systematic review and meta-analysis. *British Journal of Sports Medicine.* 2017;51(8):658–669. http://dx.doi.org/10.1136/bjsports-2016-096396. doi:10.1136/bjsports-2016-096396.

67. Trexler ET, Smith-Ryan AE, Stout JR, et al. International society of sports nutrition position stand: Beta-alanine. *Journal of the International Society of Sports Nutrition.* 2015;12:30. http://www.ncbi.nlm.nih.gov/pubmed/26175657. doi:10.1186/s12970-015-0090-y.

68. Hobson RM, Saunders B, Ball G, Harris RC, Sale C. Effects of [beta]-alanine supplementation on exercise performance: A meta-analysis. *Amino Acids.* 2012;43(1):25–37. https://search.proquest.com/docview/1783901042. doi:10.1007/s00726-011-1200-z.

69. Danaher J, Gerber T, Wellard R, Stathis C. The effect of β-alanine and NaHCO3 co-ingestion on buffering capacity and exercise performance with high-intensity exercise in healthy males. *European Journal of Applied Physiology*. 2014;114(8):1715–1724. http://www.ncbi.nlm.nih.gov/pubmed/24832191. doi:10.1007/s00421-014-2895-9.

70. Hobson RM, Harris RC, Martin D, Smith P, Macklin B, Gualano B, Sale C. Effect of beta-alanine with and without sodium bicarbonate on 2,000-m rowing performance. *International Journal of Sport Nutrition and Exercise Metabolism*. 2013;23(5):480–487. http://www.ncbi.nlm.nih.gov/pubmed/24172994.

71. Howe ST, Bellinger PM, Driller MW, Shing CM, Fell JW. The effect of beta-alanine supplementation on isokinetic force and cycling performance in highly trained cyclists. *International Journal of Sport Nutrition and Exercise Metabolism*. 2013;23(6):562–570. http://www.ncbi.nlm.nih.gov/pubmed/23630052.

72. Painelli Vde S, Roschel H, Jesus Fd, et al. The ergogenic effect of beta-alanine combined with sodium bicarbonate on high-intensity swimming performance. *Applied Physiology, Nutrition, and Metabolism*. 2013;38(5):525. http://www.ncbi.nlm.nih.gov/pubmed/23668760. doi:10.1139/apnm-2012-0286.

73. Ducker KJ, Dawson B, Wallman KE. Effect of beta-alanine supplementation on 2,000-m rowing-ergometer performance. *International Journal of Sport Nutrition and Exercise Metabolism*. 2013;23(4):336–343. http://www.ncbi.nlm.nih.gov/pubmed/23994898.

74. Ducker KJ, Dawson B, Wallman KE. Effect of beta-alanine supplementation on 800-m running performance. *International Journal of Sport Nutrition and Exercise Metabolism*. 2013;23(6):554–561. http://www.ncbi.nlm.nih.gov/pubmed/23630039.

75. Bellinger PM, Minahan CL. The effect of β-alanine supplementation on cycling time trials of different length. *European Journal of Sport Science*. 2016;16(7):829–836. http://www.tandfonline.com/doi/abs/10.1080/17461391.2015.1120782. doi:10.1080/17461391.2015.1120782.

76. Derave W, Özdemir MS, Harris RC, et al. B-alanine supplementation augments muscle carnosine content and attenuates fatigue during repeated isokinetic contraction bouts in trained sprinters. *Journal of Applied Physiology*. 2007;103(5):1736–1743. http://jap.physiology.org/content/103/5/1736. doi:10.1152/japplphysiol.00397.2007.

77. Sweeney K, Wright G, Glenn Brice A, Doberstein S. The effect of β-alanine supplementation on power performance during repeated sprint activity. *Journal of Strength and Conditioning Research*. 2010;24(1):79–87. http://www.ncbi.nlm.nih.gov/pubmed/19935102. doi:10.1519/JSC.0b013e3181c63bd5.

78. Saunders B, Sale C, Harris RC, Sunderland C. Effect of beta-alanine supplementation on repeated sprint performance during the Loughborough intermittent shuttle test. *Amino Acids*. 2012;43(1):39–47. http://www.ncbi.nlm.nih.gov/pubmed/22434182. doi:10.1007/s00726-012-1268-0.

79. Hoffman J, Ratamess N, Ross R, et al. B-alanine and the hormonal response to exercise. *International Journal of Sports Medicine*. 2008;29(12):952–958. http://www.thieme-connect.de/DOI/DOI?10.1055/s-2008-1038678. doi:10.1055/s-2008-1038678.

80. Hoffman JR, Ratamess NA, Faigenbaum AD, Ross R, Kang J, Stout JR, Wise JA. Short-duration β-alanine supplementation increases training volume and reduces subjective feelings of fatigue in college football players. *Nutrition Research*. 2008;28(1):31–35. https://www.sciencedirect.com/science/article/pii/S0271531707002771. doi:10.1016/j.nutres.2007.11.004.

81. Kern B, Robinson T. Effects of β-alanine supplementation on performance and body composition in collegiate wrestlers and football players. *Journal of Strength and Conditioning Research*. 2011;25(7):1804–1815. http://ovidsp.ovid.com/ovidweb.cgi?T=JS&NEWS=n&CSC=Y&PAGE=fulltext&D=ovft&AN=00124278-201107000-00005. doi:10.1519/JSC.0b013e3181e741cf.

82. Kendrick I, Harris R, Kim H, et al. The effects of 10 weeks of resistance training combined with β-alanine supplementation on whole body strength, force production, muscular endurance and body composition. *Amino Acids*. 2008;34(4):547–554. http://www.ncbi.nlm.nih.gov/pubmed/18175046. doi:10.1007/s00726-007-0008-3.

83. Carr A, Hopkins W, Gore C. Effects of acute alkalosis and acidosis on performance. *Sports Medicine*. 2011;41(10):801–814. http://www.ncbi.nlm.nih.gov/pubmed/21923200. doi:10.2165/11591440-000000000-00000.

84. McNaughton LR, Gough L, Deb S, Bentley D, Sparks SA. Recent developments in the use of sodium bicarbonate as an ergogenic aid. *Current Sports Medicine Reports*. 2016;15(4):233. http://www.ncbi.nlm.nih.gov/pubmed/27399820.

85. Burke LM, Pyne DB. Bicarbonate loading to enhance training and competitive performance. *International Journal of Sports Physiology and Performance*. 2007;2(1):93–97. http://www.ncbi.nlm.nih.gov/pubmed/19255457.

86. Lancha Junior A, de Salles Painelli V, Saunders B, Artioli G. Nutritional strategies to modulate intracellular and extracellular buffering capacity during high-intensity exercise. *Sports Medicine*. 2015;45(S1):71–81. http://www.ncbi.nlm.nih.gov/pubmed/26553493. doi:10.1007/s40279-015-0397-5.

87. Tobias G, Benatti F, de Salles Painelli V, et al. Additive effects of beta-alanine and sodium bicarbonate on upper-body intermittent performance. *Amino Acids*. 2013;45(2):309–317. http://www.ncbi.nlm.nih.gov/pubmed/23595205. doi:10.1007/s00726-013-1495-z.

88. Price M, Moss P, Rance S. Effects of sodium bicarbonate ingestion on prolonged intermittent exercise. *Medicine and Science in Sports and Exercise*. 2003;35(8):1303–1308. http://www.ncbi.nlm.nih.gov/pubmed/12900682. doi:10.1249/01.MSS.0000079067.46555.3C.

89. Bishop D, Claudius B. Effects of induced metabolic alkalosis on prolonged intermittent-sprint performance. *Medicine and Science in Sports and Exercise*. 2005;37(5):759–767. http://www.ncbi.nlm.nih.gov/pubmed/15870629. doi:10.1249/01.MSS.0000161803.44656.3C.

90. Wu C, Shih M, Yang C, Huang M, Chang C. Sodium bicarbonate supplementation prevents skilled tennis performance decline after a simulated match. *Journal of the International Society of Sports Nutrition*. 2010;7(33):1–8. http://www.ncbi.nlm.nih.gov/pubmed/20977701. doi:10.1186/1550-2783-7-33.

91. Siegler J, Hirscher K. Sodium bicarbonate ingestion and boxing performance. *Journal of Strength and Conditioning Research*. 2010;24(1):103–108. http://www.ncbi.nlm.nih.gov/pubmed/19625976. doi:10.1519/JSC.0b013e3181a392b2.

92. Duncan M, Weldon A, Price M. The effect of sodium bicarbonate ingestion on back squat and bench press exercise to failure. *Journal of Strength and Conditioning Research*. 2014;28(5):1358–1366. http://www.ncbi.nlm.nih.gov/pubmed/24126895. doi:10.1519/JSC.0000000000000277.

93. Edge J, Bishop D, Goodman C. Effects of chronic NaHCO3 ingestion during interval training on changes to muscle buffer capacity, metabolism, and short-term endurance performance. *Journal of Applied Physiology*. 2006;101(3):918–925. http://jap.physiology.org/content/101/3/918. doi:10.1152/japplphysiol.01534.2005.

94. McMahon N, Leveritt M, Pavey T. The effect of dietary nitrate supplementation on endurance exercise performance in healthy adults: A systematic review and meta-analysis. *Sports Medicine*. 2017;47(4):735–756. https://search.proquest.com/docview/1924618342. doi:10.1007/s40279-016-0617-7.

95. Bailey SJ, Winyard P, Vanhatalo A, et al. Dietary nitrate supplementation reduces the O2 cost of low-intensity exercise and enhances tolerance to high-intensity exercise in humans. *Journal of Applied Physiology*. 2009;107(4):1144–1155. http://jap.physiology.org/content/107/4/1144. doi:10.1152/japplphysiol.00722.2009.

96. Larsen FJ, Weitzberg E, Lundberg JO, Ekblom B. Effects of dietary nitrate on oxygen cost during exercise. *Acta Physiologica.* 2007;191(1):59–66. http://www.ingentaconnect.com/content/bsc/aps/2007/00000191/00000001/art00008. doi:10.1111/j.1748-1716.2007.01713.x.

97. Thompson C, Vanhatalo A, Jell H, et al. Dietary nitrate supplementation improves sprint and high-intensity intermittent running performance. *Nitric Oxide.* 2016;61:55–61. doi:10.1016/j.niox.2016.10.006.

98. McQuillan JA, Dulson DK, Laursen PB, Kilding AE. The effect of dietary nitrate supplementation on physiology and performance in trained cyclists. *International Journal of Sports Physiology and Performance.* 2017;12:684–689. doi:10.1123/ijspp.2016-0202.

99. Christensen PM, Nyberg M, Bangsbo J. Influence of nitrate supplementation on VO$_2$ kinetics and endurance of elite cyclists. *Scandinavian Journal of Medicine and Science in Sports.* 2013;23(1):e31. http://onlinelibrary.wiley.com/doi/10.1111/sms.12005/abstract. doi:10.1111/sms.12005.

100. Martin K, Smee D, Thompson KG, Rattray B. No improvement of repeated-sprint performance with dietary nitrate. *International Journal of Sports Physiology and Performance.* 2014;9(5):845–850. http://www.ncbi.nlm.nih.gov/pubmed/24436354. doi:10.1123/ijspp.2013-0384.

101. Muggeridge DJ, Howe CCF, Spendiff O, Pedlar C, James PE, Easton C. The effects of a single dose of concentrated beetroot juice on performance in trained flatwater kayakers. *International Journal of Sport Nutrition and Exercise Metabolism.* 2013;23(5):498–506. http://www.ncbi.nlm.nih.gov/pubmed/23580456.

102. Flanagan SD, Looney DP, Miller MJS, et al. The effects of nitrate-rich supplementation on neuromuscular efficiency during heavy resistance exercise. *Journal of the American College of Nutrition.* 2016;35(2):100–107. http://www.tandfonline.com/doi/abs/10.1080/07315724.2015.1081572. doi:10.1080/07315724.2015.1081572.

103. Mosher S, Sparks S, Williams E, Bentley D, Mc Naughton L. Ingestion of a nitric oxide enhancing supplement improves resistance exercise performance. *Journal of Strength and Conditioning Research.* 2016;30(12):3520–3524. https://search.proquest.com/docview/1845707633. doi:10.1519/JSC.0000000000001437.

104. Nehlig A. Is caffeine a cognitive enhancer? *Journal of Alzheimer's Disease: JAD.* 2010;20(Suppl 1):S85–S94. http://www.ncbi.nlm.nih.gov/pubmed/20182035.

105. Snel J, Lorist MM, Tieges Z. Coffee, caffeine, and cognitive performance. In: Nehlig A, ed. *Coffe, Tea, Chocolate and the Brain.* Boca Raton, FL: CRC Press LLC; 2004:53–73.

106. Einöther S, Giesbrecht T. Caffeine as an attention enhancer: Reviewing existing assumptions. *Psychopharmacology.* 2013;225(2):251–274. http://www.ncbi.nlm.nih.gov/pubmed/23241646. doi:10.1007/s00213-012-2917-4.

107. Smith AP. Caffeine, practical implications. In: Kanarek RB, Lieberman HR, eds. *Diet, Brain, Behavior.* 1st ed. Boca Raton, FL: CRC Press; 2011:271–292. http://www.crcnetbase.com/isbn/9781439821572.

108. Lieberman H, Tharion W, Shukitt-Hale B, Speckman K, Tulley R. Effects of caffeine, sleep loss, and stress on cognitive performance and mood during U.S. navy SEAL training. *Psychopharmacology.* 2002;164(3):250–261. https://search.proquest.com/docview/218958967. doi:10.1007/s00213-002-1217-9.

109. Penetar D, McCann U, Thorne D, et al. Caffeine reversal of sleep deprivation effects on alertness and mood. *Psychopharmacology.* 1993;112(2–3):359–365. http://www.ncbi.nlm.nih.gov/pubmed/7871042. doi:10.1007/BF02244933.

110. Smith A, Sutherland D, Christopher G. Effects of repeated doses of caffeine on mood and performance of alert and fatigued volunteers. *Journal of Psychopharmacology.* 2005;19(6):620–626. http://journals.sagepub.com/doi/full/10.1177/0269881105056534. doi:10.1177/0269881105056534.

111. Wesensten N, Belenky G, Kautz M, Thorne D, Reichardt R, Balkin T. Maintaining alertness and performance during sleep deprivation: Modafinil versus caffeine. *Psychopharmacology.* 2002;159(3):238–247. http://www.ncbi.nlm.nih.gov/pubmed/ 11862356. doi:10.1007/s002130100916.

112. Hogervorst E, Riedel WJ, Kovacs EMR, Brouns FJPH, Jolles J. Caffeine improves cognitive performance after strenuous physical exercise. *International Journal of Sports Medicine.* 1999;20(6):354–361. http://www.narcis.nl/publication/RecordID/oai:cris. maastrichtuniversity.nl:publications%2F07c54583-0296-4e49-8b65-5aa3b5b388f5. doi:10.1055/s-2007-971144.

113. Hogervorst E, Bandelow S, Schmitt J, et al. Caffeine improves physical and cognitive performance during exhaustive exercise. *Medicine and Science in Sports and Exercise.* 2008;40(10):1841–1851. http://www.ncbi.nlm.nih.gov/pubmed/18799996. doi:10.1249/ MSS.0b013e31817bb8b7.

114. Kruk B, Chmura J, Krzeminski K, Ziemba A, Nazar K, Pekkarinen H, Kaciuba-Uscilko H. Influence of caffeine, cold and exercise on multiple choice reaction time. *Psychopharmacology.* 2001;157(2):197–201. http://www.ncbi.nlm.nih.gov/pubmed/ 11594446. doi:10.1007/s002130100787.

115. Baker LB, Nuccio RP, Jeukendrup AE. Acute effects of dietary constituents on motor skill and cognitive performance in athletes. *Nutrition Reviews.* 2014;72(12):790–802. http://onlinelibrary.wiley.com/doi/10.1111/nure.12157/abstract. doi:10.1111/nure.12157.

116. Phillips S. A brief review of critical processes in exercise-induced muscular hypertrophy. *Sports Medicine.* 2014;44(S1):71–77. http://www.ncbi.nlm.nih.gov/pubmed/24791918. doi:10.1007/s40279-014-0152-3.

117. Duncan MJ, Taylor S, Lyons M. The effect of caffeine ingestion on field hockey skill performance following physical fatigue. *Research in Sports Medicine.* 2012;20(1):25–36. http://www.tandfonline.com/doi/abs/10.1080/15438627.2012.634686. doi:10.1080/1543 8627.2012.634686.

118. Duvnjak-Zaknich DM, Dawson BT, Wallman KE, Henry G. Effect of caffeine on reactive agility time when fresh and fatigued. *Medicine and Science in Sports and Exercise.* 2011;43(8):1523–1530. http://www.ncbi.nlm.nih.gov/pubmed/21266929. doi:10.1249/ MSS.0b013e31821048ab.

119. Foskett A, Ali A, Gant N. Caffeine enhances cognitive function and skill performance during simulated soccer activity. *International Journal of Sport Nutrition and Exercise Metabolism.* 2009;19(4):410–423. http://www.ncbi.nlm.nih.gov/pubmed/19827465.

120. Pontifex KJ, Wallman KE, Dawson BT, Goodman C. Effects of caffeine on repeated sprint ability, reactive agility time, sleep and next day performance. *The Journal of Sports Medicine and Physical Fitness.* 2010;50(4):455. http://www.ncbi.nlm.nih.gov/ pubmed/21178933.

121. Ferrauti A, Weber K, Strüder HK. Metabolic and ergogenic effects of carbohydrate and caffeine beverages in tennis. *The Journal of Sports Medicine and Physical Fitness.* 1997;37(4):258. http://www.ncbi.nlm.nih.gov/pubmed/9509824.

122. Lorino AJ, Lloyd LK, Crixell SH, Walker JL. The effects of caffeine on athletic agility. *Journal of Strength and Conditioning Research.* 2006;20(4):851–854. http:// ovidsp.ovid.com/ovidweb.cgi?T=JS&NEWS=n&CSC=Y&PAGE=fulltext&D=ovft &AN=00124278-200611000-00021. doi:10.1519/00124278-200611000-00021.

123. Ishaque S, Shamseer L, Bukutu C, Vohra S. Rhodiola rosea for physical and mental fatigue: A systematic review. *BMC Complementary and Alternative Medicine.* 2012;12(1):70. http://www.ncbi.nlm.nih.gov/pubmed/22643043. doi:10.1186/1472-6882-12-70.

124. Darbinyan V, Kteyan A, Panossian A, Gabrielian E, Wikman G, Wagner H. Rhodiola rosea in stress induced fatigue — A double blind cross-over study of a standardized extract SHR-5 with a repeated low-dose regimen on the mental performance of healthy physicians during night duty. *Phytomedicine: International Journal of Phytotherapy*

and Phytopharmacology. 2000;7(5):365–371. https://www.sciencedirect.com/science/article/pii/S0944711300800550. doi:10.1016/S0944-7113(00)80055-0.

125. Shevtsov VA, Zholus BI, Shervarly VI, et al. A randomized trial of two different doses of a SHR-5 Rhodiola rosea extract versus placebo and control of capacity for mental work. *Phytomedicine.* 2003;10(2):95–105. https://www.sciencedirect.com/science/article/pii/S0944711304702007. doi:10.1078/094471103321659780.

126. Jówko E, Sadowski J, Długołęcka B, Gierczuk D, Opaszowski B, Cieśliński I. Effects of Rhodiola rosea supplementation on mental performance, physical capacity, and oxidative stress biomarkers in healthy men. *Journal of Sport and Health Science.* 2016; 7(4):473–480. https://www.sciencedirect.com/science/article/pii/S2095254616300345. doi:10.1016/j.jshs.2016.05.005.

127. De Bock K, Eijnde BO, Ramaekers M, Hespel P. Acute Rhodiola rosea intake can improve endurance exercise performance. *International Journal of Sport Nutrition and Exercise Metabolism.* 2004;14(3):298–307. http://www.ncbi.nlm.nih.gov/pubmed/15256690.

128. Noreen E, Buckley J, Lewis S, Brandauer J, Stuempfle K. The effects of an acute dose of Rhodiola rosea on endurance exercise performance. *Journal of Strength and Conditioning Research.* 2013;27(3):839–847. http://ovidsp.ovid.com/ovidweb.cgi?T=J S&NEWS=n&CSC=Y&PAGE=fulltext&D=ovft&AN=00124278-201303000-00037. doi:10.1519/JSC.0b013e31825d9799.

129. Hung SK, Perry R, Ernst E. The effectiveness and efficacy of Rhodiola rosea L.: A systematic review of randomized clinical trials. *Phytomedicine.* 2011;18(4):235–244. https://www.sciencedirect.com/science/article/pii/S0944711310002680. doi:10.1016/j.phymed.2010.08.014.

130. Smith I, Williamson EM, Putnam S, Farrimond J, Whalley BJ. Effects and mechanisms of ginseng and ginsenosides on cognition. *Nutrition Reviews.* 2014;72(5):319–333. http://onlinelibrary.wiley.com/doi/10.1111/nure.12099/abstract. doi:10.1111/nure.12099.

131. Dalinger O. Effect of eleutherococcus extract on functional state of cardiovascular system and working capacity of skiers. In: Saratikov AS, ed. *Stimulants of the Central Nervous System.* Tomsk: Tomsk University Publishing Press; 1966:106–111.

132. Kelly SP, Gomez-Ramirez M, Montesi JL, Foxe JJ. L-theanine and caffeine in combination affect human cognition as evidenced by oscillatory alpha-band activity and attention task performance. *The Journal of Nutrition.* 2008;138(8):1572S–1577S. http://www.ncbi.nlm.nih.gov/pubmed/18641209.

133. Foxe JJ, Morie KP, Laud PJ, Rowson MJ, de Bruin EA, Kelly SP. Assessing the effects of caffeine and theanine on the maintenance of vigilance during a sustained attention task. *Neuropharmacology.* 2012;62(7):2320–2327.

134. Twycross-Lewis R, Kilduff LP, Wang G, Pitsiladis Y. The effects of creatine supplementation on thermoregulation and physical (cognitive) performance: A review and future prospects. *Amino Acids.* 2016. http://eprints.brighton.ac.uk/15305/.

135. McMorris T, Mielcarz G, Harris RC, Swain JP, Howard A. Creatine supplementation and cognitive performance in elderly individuals. *Aging, Neuropsychology, and Cognition.* 2007;14(5):517–528. http://www.tandfonline.com/doi/abs/10.1080/13825580600788100. doi:10.1080/13825580600788100.

136. Turner CE, Byblow WD, Gant N. Creatine supplementation enhances corticomotor excitability and cognitive performance during oxygen deprivation. *The Journal of Neuroscience: the Official Journal of the Society for Neuroscience.* 2015;35(4):1773–1780. http://www.ncbi.nlm.nih.gov/pubmed/25632150. doi:10.1523/JNEUROSCI.3113-14.2015.

137. McMorris T, Harris R, Swain J, Corbett J, Collard K, Dyson RJ, Dye L, Hodgson C, Draper N. Effect of creatine supplementation and sleep deprivation, with mild exercise, on cognitive and psychomotor performance, mood state, and plasma concentrations of catecholamines and cortisol. *Psychopharmacology.* 2006;185(1):93–103. http://www.ncbi.nlm.nih.gov/pubmed/16416332. doi:10.1007/s00213-005-0269-z.

138. Ziegenfuss TN, Habowski SM, Sandrock JE, Kedia AW, Kerksick CM, Lopez HL. A two-part approach to examine the effects of theacrine (TeaCrine®) supplementation on oxygen consumption, hemodynamic responses, and subjective measures of cognitive and psychometric parameters. *Journal of Dietary Supplements.* 2017;14(1):9–24. http://dx.doi.org/10.1080/19390211.2016.1178678. Accessed Jul 14, 2017. doi:10.1080/193902 11.2016.1178678.

139. Hoffman JR, Ratamess NA, Tranchina CP, Rashti SL, Kang J, Faigenbaum AD. Effect of protein-supplement timing on strength, power, and body-composition changes in resistance-trained men. *International Journal of Sport Nutrition and Exercise Metabolism.* 2009;19(2):172–185. http://www.ncbi.nlm.nih.gov/pubmed/19478342.

140. Hoffman JR, Ratamess NA, Kang J, Falvo MJ, Faigenbaum AD. Effects of protein supplementation on muscular performance and resting hormonal changes in college football players. *Journal of Sports Science and Medicine.* 2007;6(1):85–92. http://www.ncbi.nlm.nih.gov/pubmed/24149229.

141. Cribb PJ, Hayes A. Effects of supplement timing and resistance exercise on skeletal muscle hypertrophy. *Medicine and Science in Sports and Exercise.* 2006;38(11):1918–1925. http://www.ncbi.nlm.nih.gov/pubmed/17095924. doi:10.1249/01.mss.0000233790.08788.3e.

142. Cribb PJ, Williams AD, Hayes A. A creatine-protein-carbohydrate supplement enhances responses to resistance training. *Medicine and Science in Sports and Exercise.* 2007;39(11):1960–1968. http://www.ncbi.nlm.nih.gov/pubmed/17986903. doi:10.1249/mss.0b013e31814fb52a.

143. Hulmi JJ, Lockwood CM, Stout JR. Effect of protein/essential amino acids and resistance training on skeletal muscle hypertrophy: A case for whey protein. *Nutrition and Metabolism.* 2010;7(1):51. http://www.ncbi.nlm.nih.gov/pubmed/20565767. doi:10.1186/1743-7075-7-51.

144. Cermak NM, Res PT, de Groot LC, Saris WH, van Loon LJC. Protein supplementation augments the adaptive response of skeletal muscle to resistance-type exercise training: A meta-analysis. *The American Journal of Clinical Nutrition.* 2012;96(6):1454–1464. http://www.narcis.nl/publication/RecordID/oai:cris.maastrichtuniversity.nl:publications%2F3abe65a8-00ea-4db4-9c27-2d98e3eada92. doi:10.3945/ajcn.112.037556.

145. Naclerio F, Larumbe-Zabala E. Effects of whey protein alone or as part of a multi-ingredient formulation on strength, fat-free mass, or lean body mass in resistance-trained individuals: A meta-analysis. *Sports Medicine.* 2016;46(1):125–137. http://www.ncbi.nlm.nih.gov/pubmed/26403469. doi:10.1007/s40279-015-0403-y.

146. Morton RW, Murphy KT, McKellar SR, et al. A systematic review, meta-analysis and meta-regression of the effect of protein supplementation on resistance training-induced gains in muscle mass and strength in healthy adults. *British Journal of Sports Medicine.* 2017;52(6):376–384. doi:10.1136/bjsports-2017-097608.

147. Schoenfeld BJ, Aragon AA, Krieger JW. The effect of protein timing on muscle strength and hypertrophy: A meta-analysis. *Journal of the International Society of Sports Nutrition.* 2013;10(1):53. http://www.ncbi.nlm.nih.gov/pubmed/24299050. doi:10.1186/1550-2783-10-53.

148. Pasiakos S, Lieberman H, McLellan T. Effects of protein supplements on muscle damage, soreness and recovery of muscle function and physical performance: A systematic review. *Sports Medicine.* 2014;44(5):655–670. http://www.ncbi.nlm.nih.gov/pubmed/24435468. doi:10.1007/s40279-013-0137-7.

149. Farshidfar F, Pinder MA, Myrie SB. Creatine supplementation and skeletal muscle metabolism for building muscle mass- review of the potential mechanisms of action. *Current Protein and Peptide Science.* 2017;18(12):1273–1287. http://www.eurekaselect.com/openurl/content.php?genre=article&issn=1389-2037&volume=18&issue=12&spage=1273.

150. Rosene J, Matthews T, Ryan C, et al. Short and longer-term effects of creatine supplementation on exercise induced muscle damage. *Journal of Sports Science and Medicine.* 2009;8(1):89–96. http://www.ncbi.nlm.nih.gov/pubmed/24150561.
151. Veggi K FT, Machado M, Koch AJ, Santana SC, Oliveira SS, Stec MJ. Oral creatine supplementation augments the repeated bout effect. *International Journal of Sport Nutrition and Exercise Metabolism.* 2013;23(4):378–387. http://www.ncbi.nlm.nih.gov/pubmed/23349298.
152. Cooke MB, Rybalka E, Williams AD, Cribb PJ, Hayes A. Creatine supplementation enhances muscle force recovery after eccentrically-induced muscle damage in healthy individuals. *Journal of the International Society of Sports Nutrition.* 2009;6(13):1–11. http://www.ncbi.nlm.nih.gov/pubmed/19490606. doi:10.1186/1550-2783-6-13.
153. Kim J, Lee J, Kim S, Yoon D, Kim J, Sung DJ. Role of creatine supplementation in exercise-induced muscle damage: A mini review. *Journal of Exercise Rehabilitation.* 2015;11(5):244–250. http://www.earticle.net/Article.aspx?sn=257772.
154. Wilson JM, Fitschen PJ, Campbell B, et al. International society of sports nutrition position stand: Beta-hydroxy-beta-methylbutyrate (HMB). *Journal of the International Society of Sports Nutrition.* 2013;10(1):6. http://www.ncbi.nlm.nih.gov/pubmed/23374455. doi:10.1186/1550-2783-10-6.
155. Silva VR, Belozo FL, Micheletti TO, Conrado M, Stout JR, Pimentel GD, Gonzalez AM. B-hydroxy-β-methylbutyrate free acid supplementation may improve recovery and muscle adaptations after resistance training: A systematic review. *Nutrition Research.* 2017;45:1–9. https://www.sciencedirect.com/science/article/pii/S0271531717302543. doi:10.1016/j.nutres.2017.07.008.
156. Albert FJ, Morente-Sánchez J, Ortega FB, Castillo MJ, Gutiérrez Á. Usefulness of β-hydroxy-β-methylbutyrate (HMB) supplementation in different sports: An update and practical implications. *Nutrición hospitalaria.* 2015;32(1):20. http://www.ncbi.nlm.nih.gov/pubmed/26262692.
157. Panton LB, Rathmacher JA, Baier S, Nissen S. Nutritional supplementation of the leucine metabolite beta-hydroxy-beta-methylbutyrate (hmb) during resistance training. *Nutrition (Burbank, Los Angeles County, California).* 2000;16(9):734–739. http://www.ncbi.nlm.nih.gov/pubmed/10978853. doi:10.1016/S0899-9007(00)00376-2.
158. Knitter AE, Panton L, Rathmacher JA, Petersen A, Sharp R. Effects of β-hydroxy-β-methylbutyrate on muscle damage after a prolonged run. *Journal of Applied Physiology.* 2000;89(4):1340–1344. http://jap.physiology.org/content/89/4/1340.
159. Beck K, Thomson JS, Swift RJ, von Hurst PR. Role of nutrition in performance enhancement and postexercise recovery. *Open Access Journal of Sports Medicine.* 2015;11(6):259–267. https://doaj.org/article/2d9d5465ce9f4b5fbb51689bf14bb997. doi:10.2147/OAJSM.S33605.
160. Howatson G, Van Someren KA. The prevention and treatment of exercise-induced muscle damage. *Sports Medicine.* 2008;38(6):483–503. http://research.stmarys.ac.uk/43/.
161. Braun WA, von Duvillard SP. Influence of carbohydrate delivery on the immune response during exercise and recovery from exercise. *Nutrition.* 2004;20(7):645–650.
162. Peake JM, Neubauer O, Walsh NP, Simpson RJ. Recovery of the immune system after exercise. *Journal of Applied Physiology.* 2016;122(5):1077–1087. https://search.proquest.com/docview/1898952175. doi:10.1152/japplphysiol.00622.2016.
163. Rahimi MH, Shab-Bidar S, Mollahosseini M, Djafarian K. Branched chain amino acid supplementation and exercise induced muscle damage in exercise recovery: A meta-analysis of randomized clinical trials. *Nutrition.* 2017;42:30–36. https://www.clinicalkey.es/playcontent/1-s2.0-S0899900717300953. doi:10.1016/j.nut.2017.05.005.

164. Burt D, Waldron M, Jeffries O, Howe L, Patterson SD, Whelan K. The effects of acute branched-chain amino acid supplementation on recovery from a single bout of hypertrophy exercise in resistance-trained athletes. *Applied Physiology, Nutrition, and Metabolism*. 2017;42(6):630–636. http://www.nrcresearchpress.com/doi/abs/10.1139/apnm-2016-0569. doi:10.1139/apnm-2016-0569.

165. Børsheim E, Tipton KD, Wolf SE, Wolfe RR. Essential amino acids and muscle protein recovery from resistance exercise. *American Journal of Physiology - Endocrinology and Metabolism*. 2002;283(4):648–657. http://ajpendo.physiology.org/content/283/4/E648. doi:10.1152/ajpendo.00466.2001.

166. Fujita S, Dreyer HC, Drummond MJ, Glynn EL, Volpi E, Rasmussen BB. Essential amino acid and carbohydrate ingestion before resistance exercise does not enhance postexercise muscle protein synthesis. *Journal of Applied Physiology*. 2009;106(5):1730–1739. http://jap.physiology.org/content/106/5/1730. doi:10.1152/japplphysiol.90395.2008.

167. Bird SP, Tarpenning KM, Marino FE. Liquid carbohydrate/essential amino acid ingestion during a short-term bout of resistance exercise suppresses myofibrillar protein degradation. *Metabolism*. 2006;55(5):570–577. https://www.sciencedirect.com/science/article/pii/S0026049505004440. doi:10.1016/j.metabol.2005.11.011.

168. Mitchell CJ, Churchward-Venne TA, Parise G, et al. Acute post-exercise myofibrillar protein synthesis is not correlated with resistance training-induced muscle hypertrophy in young men. *PLOS ONE*. 2014;9(2):e89431. http://www.ncbi.nlm.nih.gov/pubmed/24586775. doi:10.1371/journal.pone.0089431.

9 Intake of Selected Nutrients and Some Morphological and Biochemical Blood Parameters of Professional Athletes

Estera Nowacka-Polaczyk, Teresa Leszczyńska, Aneta Kopeć, and Jerzy Zawistowski

CONTENTS

9.1 Introduction 178
9.2 Material and Methods... 178
    9.2.1 Characteristics of the Studied Population... 178
    9.2.2 Dietary Assessment 178
    9.2.3 Statistical Analysis of Results 179
9.3 Results.. 180
    9.3.1 Dietary Assessment 180
        9.3.1.1 Carbohydrate Intake 180
        9.3.1.2 Mineral Intake 180
    9.3.2 Assessment of Selected Morphological and Biochemical
        Blood Parameters.. 180
    9.3.3 Intake of Selected Nutrients with the Diet versus Some
        Morphological and Biochemical Blood Parameters.......................... 180
9.4 Discussion... 184
    9.4.1 Dietary Pattern.. 184
    9.4.2 Mineral Compounds 186
    9.4.3 Selected Morphological and Biochemical Blood Parameters 187
    9.4.4 Intake of Selected Nutrients within the Diet versus
        Morphological and Biochemical Blood Parameters.......................... 188
9.5 Conclusions... 189
References.. 190

9.1 INTRODUCTION

The diet of athletes should be not only diversified but also properly balanced in terms of quantity and quality. A proper dietary pattern may contribute to the sportsperson's optimal psychophysical performance and may help them to maintain good health status, including appropriate morphological and biochemical blood parameters. This, in turn, may improve their physical performance and ability to maintain the optimal concentration of nutrients under stress and fatigue (Czaja et al., 2008; Durkalec-Michalski et al., 2011; Gacek, 2009; Kasprzak, 2009; Lebiedzińska et al., 2008).

Abnormalities in their nutritional status, including morphological and biochemical blood indices, result from insufficient intake of energy and nutrients. In professional sports disciplines, a proper diet eliminating nutritional mistakes may be a decisive factor in winning a sports competition (Durkalec-Michalski et al., 2011; Jarosz and Bułhak-Jachymczyk, 2008).

The objective of this study was to find the correlation between intakes of some nutrients and selected morphological and biochemical blood parameters in professional athletes.

9.2 MATERIAL AND METHODS

9.2.1 CHARACTERISTICS OF THE STUDIED POPULATION

Female (n = 4) and male (n = 15) athletes practising canoe slalom who had the master international class, master class and first class, along with hockey players (n = 12) from the Champions League and the First League were enrolled in this study. The age of the sportspersons (in the first year of this research) was between 18 and 26 for female canoeists, 16 and 27 for male canoeists and 22 and 23 for hockey players.

In order to be included in this research, athletes also had to complete at least a four-year training period and have a very high level of physical activity (PAL), in the range of 2.0 to 2.4.

9.2.2 DIETARY ASSESSMENT

Dietary intake was evaluated using a 24-h dietary recall which was carried out in 2009 and 2010 for three selected days of the week in spring–summer seasons (canoeists) and in autumn–winter seasons (hockey players), as was previously described (Nowacka et al., 2013, 2016).

The nutritive value of the athletes' diets was estimated using the computer software Diet 4.0, developed by the Polish Food and Nutrition Institute (Warszawa, Poland).

The diets of all athletes were examined for the carbohydrate content. In addition, the diets of female and male canoeists were tested for sodium, potassium, magnesium and iron intake, while hockey players' diets were examined for potassium and iron intakes.

An assessment of the nutrients requirements was conducted by Jarosz and Bułhak-Jachymczyk (2008). Individual dietary requirements for every athlete were set in accordance with the standards/recommendations as outlined below:

- dietary digestible carbohydrates at the level recommended in the prevention of non-communicable diseases, that is, 137–187 g/1000 kcal of recommended energy intake.
- minerals Mg and Fe at the estimated average requirement (EAR) level; Na and K at the adequate intake (AI) level. In addition, the tolerable upper intake level (UL) for Na and Mg was taken into account as determined by the European Union Scientific Committee on Food.

The results of these biochemical analyses, which are presented in this paper, were obtained from athletes in the first and second year of the study. For canoeists, data was collected in the spring–summer season, while for hockey players in the autumn–winter season. For these periods, the convergent validity of the biochemical data and the dietary assessment was determined.

For female and male canoeists, glucose concentration was determined in plasma, while the content of sodium, potassium, magnesium and iron was assessed in serum. For hockey players, potassium content was determined in serum, while haemoglobin concentration and the haematocrit level were measured in whole blood.

The adopted ranges of reference values for particular morphological and biochemical parameters are included in the results printouts.

9.2.3 STATISTICAL ANALYSIS OF RESULTS

Statistical analysis was performed using the Statistica software, version 9.0.

For variables with normal distribution, Pearson's linear correlation coefficient was used, while for variables with non-normal distribution, Spearman's rank correlation coefficient was employed. The lack of correlation between the pairs of appropriate values of recommendations for selected nutrients and the values of selected morphological and biochemical blood parameters was hypostatised, and was verified by Pearson's coefficient.

The correlation between the recommended intake of selected nutrients and the values of selected morphological and biochemical blood parameters was deemed to be statistically significant at $p \leq 0.05$.

The correlation between the lower limit of the recommended carbohydrate intake and glucose concentration in the plasma as well as the recommended intake of dietary sodium, potassium, magnesium, and iron and their concentrations in the serum was investigated in female and male canoeists who underwent biochemical analyses.

The correlation between the recommended intake of dietary potassium and iron and potassium concentration in serum as well as the haemoglobin and haematocrit levels in whole blood was examined in hockey players who underwent morphological and biochemical analyses.

9.3 RESULTS

9.3.1 Dietary Assessment

9.3.1.1 Carbohydrate Intake

Our studies show that in two consecutive years, athletes failed to achieve the daily carbohydrate intake recommended by sports nutritionists (Table 9.1). In both years of study, 100% of both female and male canoeists, as well as hockey players, didn't reach the lowest recommended level of carbohydrate intake, with the exception of 20% of male canoeists in the second year who reached the recommended minimum (Table 9.1).

9.3.1.2 Mineral Intake

The results demonstrated that the upper tolerable level of sodium intake was exceeded by 50% of female and 100% of male canoeists in the first year, and 75% of female and 100% of male canoeists in the second year (Table 9.2).

In the first year, at least 42% of hockey players had adequate potassium intake, while in the second year, only 7% of male canoeists and 50% of hockey players met the AI level for this mineral (Table 9.2).

Our results demonstrated that inadequate magnesium intake was observed in 50% of female and 33% of male canoeists in the first year, as well as in 27% of male canoeists in the following year. However, the average intake of this mineral fully covered the EAR (Table 9.2).

In the first year of the study, deficient iron intake was reported only in 25% of female canoeists (Table 9.2).

9.3.2 Assessment of Selected Morphological and Biochemical Blood Parameters

The levels of glucose and selected minerals as determined in athlete blood were generally in the range of reference values. This was also true for red cell indices consisting of haemoglobin and haematocrit concentration (Tables 9.3 through Table 9.5). The exception was the iron concentration in the serum, which in the second year was too low for 25% of female canoeists. However, the level of iron in the blood serum was higher in both years of study for 13% and 33% of male canoeists, respectively (Tables 9.3 and 9.4). An elevated potassium concentration in serum was observed for 17% of hockey players in the first and second year. Furthermore, 8% of hockey players, regardless of the year of the study, had a below normal haemoglobin concentration, as well as a below normal haematocrit level, the latter only in the first year of study (Table 9.5).

9.3.3 Intake of Selected Nutrients with the Diet versus Some Morphological and Biochemical Blood Parameters

This study showed that meeting the lower recommended carbohydrate intake is positively correlated with glucose concentration in blood plasma of canoeists in both

TABLE 9.1

Intake of Dietary Carbohydrates and Meeting the Recommendations by Slalom Canoeists Both Genders and Hockey Players

Year of study	Season	Intake [g/person/24h] x̄ ± SD	Recommended Daily Intake [g/person/24h] On the Level		Percentage of Persons Which Met the Recommendations ±SD On the Level		Percentage of Persons Which Met the Recommendations ±SD [%] On the Level	
			137 [g/1000 kcal]	187	137 [g/1000 kcal]	187	<137 [g/1000 kcal]	>187
			Female slalom canoeists (FSC)					
2009	SS	231.6 ± 70.1	397.3–452.1	542.3–617.1	54.5 ± 17.0	48.5 ± 13.8	100	0
2010	SS	309.3 ± 34.3	385.0–508.8	525.0–693.8	69.4 ± 10.1	50.9 ± 7.36	100	0
			Male slalom canoeist (MSC)					
2009	SS	354.4 ± 74.9	534.3–678.2	729.3–925.7	61.1 ± 14.	44.8 ± 10.3	100	0
2010	SS	472.5 ± 106.2	536.3–632.5	731.3–862.5	79.3 ± 20.6	58.2 ± 15.1	80	0
			Hockey players (H)					
2009	AW	384.2 ± 69.2	575.4–678.2	785.4–925.7	59.0 ± 10.4	43.2 ± 7.67	100	0
2010	AW	429.6 ± 63.4	618.8–680.2	843.8–928.1	65.5 ± 10.8	48.0 ± 7.86	100	0

SS – summer spring season, AW – autumn-winter season, SD – standard deviation.

TABLE 9.2

Intake of Selected Dietary Minerals by Slalom Canoeists and Hockey Players

Year of study	Season	Intake [mg/person/24h] x̄ ± SD	Recommended Daily Intake [mg/person/24h]	Percentage of Persons Which Met the Recommendations ±SD	Percentage of Persons Which Met the Recommendations ±SD [%]	
Female slalom canoeists (FSC)						
Na					≥AI	>UL
2009	SS	2377 ± 331.1	1500	158.4 ± 22.1	100	50
2010	SS	2938 ± 524.4	1500	195.9 ± 35.0	100	75
K					≥AI	
2009	SS	2523 ± 763.6	4700	53.7 ± 16.2	0	
2010	SS	2764 ± 498.7	4700	58.8 ± 10.6	0	
Mg					<EAR	>UL
2009	SS	399.5 ± 143.7	255.0–300.0	144.9 ± 53.8	50	0
2010	SS	395.5 ± 45.5	255.0–300.0	155.1 ± 17.8	0	0
Fe					<EAR	
2009	SS	11.1 ± 2.38	8.00	138.3 ± 29.8	25	
2010	SS	13.3 ± 0.81	8.00	166.4 ± 10.1	0	
Male slalom canoeist (MSC)						
Na					≥AI	>UL
2009	SS	4845 ± 808.0	1500	323.0 ± 53.9	100	100
2010	SS	5570 ± 1444	1500	371.3 ± 96.3	100	100
K					≥AI	
2009	SS	3091 ± 344.8	4700	65.8 ± 7.34	0	
2010	SS	3504 ± 754.6	4700	74.6 ± 16.1	7	
Mg					<EAR	>UL
2009	SS	357.6 ± 56.3	330.0–340.0	107.3 ± 17.0	33	0
2010	SS	388.1 ± 90.2	330.0–340.0	117.1 ± 27.2	27	0
Fe					<EAR	
2009	SS	16.5 ± 4.94	6.00–8.00	247.7 ± 63.2	0	
2010	SS	27.8 ± 10.2	6.00–8.00	452.8 ± 180.8	0	
Hockey players (H)						
K					≥AI	
2009	AW	4356 ± 730.9	4700	92.7 ± 15.6	42	
2010	AW	4720 ± 1252	4700	100.4 ± 26.6	50	
Fe					<EAR	
2009	AW	19.2 ± 7.04	6.00–8.00	319.1 ± 116.9	0	
2010	AW	30.1 ± 15.6	6.00–8.00	501.2 ± 260.5	0	

SS – spring–summer season, AW – autumn–winter season, SD – standard deviation, AI – adequate intake, UL – tolerable upper intake level, EAR – estimated average requirement.

TABLE 9.3

Results of Biochemical Analyses of Glucose and Selected Minerals in Blood of Female Canoeists

Year	Parameter	Unit of Measure	$\bar{x} \pm SD$	Norm Min.	Norm Max.	< Norm	> Norm
2009	Glucose	mg/dl	82.0 ± 4.24	60.0	105.0	0	0
	Iron	µg/dl	80.8 ± 6.70	60.0	150.0	0	0
	Magnesium	mg/dl	1.90 ± 0.08	1.60	2.50	0	0
	Sodium	mmol/l	141.3 ± 0.50	135.0	148.0	0	0
	Potassium	mmol/l	4.30 ± 0.29	3.70	5.30	0	0
2010	Glucose	mg/dl	80.0 ± 7.26	60.0	105.0	0	0
	Iron	µg/dl	97.8 ± 31.1	60.0	150.0	25	0
	Magnesium	mg/dl	2.00 ± 0.16	1.60	2.50	0	0
	Sodium	mmol/l	138.8 ± 0.96	135.0	148.0	0	0
	Potassium	mmol/l	4.25 ± 0.13	3.70	5.30	0	0

TABLE 9.4

Results of Biochemical Analyses of Glucose and Selected Minerals in Blood of Male Canoeists

Year	Parameter	Unit of Measure	$\bar{x} \pm SD$	Norm Min.	Norm Max.	< Norm	> Norm
2009	Glucose	mg/dl	84.6 ± 5.42	60.0	105.0	0	0
	Iron	µg/dl	113.6 ± 32.3	60.0	150.0	0	13
	Magnesium	mg/dl	1.93 ± 0.14	1.60	2.50	0	0
	Sodium	mmol/l	141.2 ± 1.61	135.0	148.0	0	0
	Potassium	mmol/l	4.57 ± 0.30	3.70	5.30	0	0
2010	Glucose	mg/dl	87.9 ± 6.98	60.0	105.0	0	0
	Iron	µg/dl	123.7 ± 33.6	60.0	150.0	0	33
	Magnesium	mg/dl	2.00 ± 0.08	1.60	2.50	0	0
	Sodium	mmol/l	140.1 ± 1.33	135.0	148.0	0	0
	Potassium	mmol/l	4.41 ± 0.28	3.70	5.30	0	0

TABLE 9.5

Results of Morphological and Biochemical Analyses of Hemoglobin, Hematocrit, and Potassium in Blood of Hockey Players

Year	Parameter	Unit of Measure	$\bar{x} \pm SD$	Norm Min.	Norm Max.	Percentage of Results < Norm	Percentage of Results > Norm
2009	Hemoglobin	g/dl	14.8 ± 0.91	14.0	18.0	8	0
	Hematocrit	%	43.0 ± 2.26	40	54	8	0
	Potassium	mmol/l	4.70 ± 0.29	3.50	5.00	0	17
2010	Hemoglobin	g/dl	15.0 ± 0.71	14.0	18.0	8	0
	Hematocrit	%	43.9 ± 1.78	40	54	0	0
	Potassium	mmol/l	4.81 ± 0.30	3.50	5.00	0	17

years of study ($r = 0.6755$; $p = 0.006$ and $r = 0.7655$; $p = 0.001$, respectively). The recommended dietary iron intake for canoeists was correlated with iron concentration in serum ($r = 0.6879$, $p = 0.005$ and $r = 0.5419$, $p = 0.037$, respectively). In addition, the recommended dietary sodium intake for canoeists was well correlated with sodium concentration in serum ($r = 0.6827$, $p = 0.005$ and $r = 0.7166$, $p = 0.003$, respectively) (Table 9.6).

There was also a high positive correlation between the recommended dietary iron intake and the level of haemoglobin in blood for hockey players in the second year ($r = 0.5902$, $p = 0.043$) in 2010 (Table 9.6).

9.4   DISCUSSION

9.4.1   DIETARY PATTERN

This study revealed that, in most cases, the required intake of carbohydrates was too low for all examined athletes. An increased proportion of meat products in a diet may account for limited intake of carbohydrate-rich food. This is in agreement with literature data which showed that carbohydrate intake was also inadequate in other surveyed groups. Ziegler et al. (2001), who assessed the diets of female and male figure skaters of the American national team, found that their carbohydrate intake was insufficient, being 3.4 and 4.3 g/kg body weight (b.w.)/day, respectively. A similarly low value of carbohydrate dietary intake (4.3 g/kg b.w./day) was also recorded by Durkalec-Michalski et al. (2016) for Polish volleyball players from the Second League.

On the contrary, Szczepanska and co-workers (2009) reported that carbohydrate dietary intake by athletes from the Polish national weightlifting team was 5.4 g/kg b.w./day. Adequate carbohydrate intake (about 6.9 g/kg b.w./day) was also reported in a group of the Brazilian female adventure racers as well as in Japanese and Spanish footballers (Iglesias-Gutiérrez et al., 2008; Noda et al., 2009; Zalcman et al., 2007).

TABLE 9.6

Correlation Coefficients between the Recommendations of Selected Dietary Nutrients and Values of Some Morphological and Biochemical Parameters in Blood of Canoeists and Hockey Players

Paired Dietary Nutrients with Biochemical and Morphological Parameters in Blood	Sport Group							
	Slalom Canoeist (n = 15)				Hockey Players (n = 12)			
	Year of Study							
	2009		2010		2009		2010	
	r	p	r	p	r	p	r	p
C&G	0.6755	0.006	0.7655	0.001	–	–	–	–
Fe&Fe$_b$	0.6879	0.005	0.5419	0.037	–	–	–	–
Mg&Mgb	0.4222	0.177	0.2626	0.344	–	–	–	–
Na&Nab	0.6827	0.005	0.7166	0.003	–	–	–	–
KcRP&Kb	0.0655	0.817	0.6979	0.004	0.2406	0.451	0.3419	0.277
Fe&HGB	–	–	–	–	0.4386	0.154	0.5902	0.043
Fe&HCT	–	–	–	–	0.4523	0.140	0.4008	0.197

C – meeting of requirements for carbohydrates on the level 137 g/100 kcal diet [%]; G – the level of glucose in in blood [mg/dl]; Fe – meeting of requirements for the iron [%]; Feb – the level of iron in the blood [p.g/dl]; Mg – meeting of requirements for the magnesium [%]; Mgb – the level of magnesium in the blood [mg/dl]; Na – meeting of requirements for the for the sodium [%]; Na – the level of sodium in the blood [mmol/l]; K – meeting of requirements for potassium [%]; Kb – the level of potassium in the blood [mmol/l]; HGB – the level of hemoglobin in the blood [g/dl]; HCT – hematocrit; r – correlation coefficient; p – significance level.

9.4.2 MINERAL COMPOUNDS

According to the recommendations of the Polish Food and Nutrition Institute, the value of the upper tolerable level of sodium intake is 2300 mg/ day (Jarosz and Bułhak-Jachymczyk, 2008). The results obtained in this study proved that almost all surveyed athletes exceeded this value. This is congruent with the literature data, which generally report excessive sodium consumption by sportsmen.

Zalcman et al. (2007), who analysed the diets of Brazilian female and male adventure racers, found that consumption of sodium was 236.2% and 295.1% by these athletes, respectively, in excess of the recommended level for sodium. It was observed that sodium intake had a low probability of being inadequate in all examined athletes. Czapska and Ostrowska (2005), who examined Polish female and male students practicing sport, have determined that their diet contains 459.0% for women and 654.0% for men of sodium, well above the minimum recommendation for sodium intake. It is worthwhile to note that sodium intake is around 110.0% for non-athletic women and men, respectively.

Sodium intakes above the recommendation were also found among Polish mountain cyclists (673.1%) (Chalcarz et al., 2008b), Polish judo champions (214.4%) (Wyrostek et al., 2016) and long-distance runners (147.9%) (Durkalec-Michalski et al., 2015), as well as female and male athletes from the Polish national teams in various sports (Lebiedzińska et al., 2008) and Polish football players (Chalcarz et al., 2008a; Kasprzak, 2009).

Inadequate potassium intake was found in the diet of 42% of hockey players in the first year of research and of 7% of canoeists and 50% of hockey players in the second year of research. Our results are in line with data reported by other Polish and foreign researchers. Senior members of the Polish national weightlifting team consumed 86% of the recommended potassium level in a conventional diet, while 31% of other sportspersons showed a low probability of inadequate potassium intake (Szczepańska et al., 2009). Also, Zalcman et al. (2007) noted that Brazilian women and men training for adventure racing consumed 71% and 69% of recommended potassium intake in their diet, respectively. The above authors stated that 17% and 6%, respectively, had a low probability of inadequate intake of this mineral. Insufficient intake of potassium was found in Polish mountain cyclists (60.4%) (Chalcarz et al., 2008b), Polish judo champions (87.7%) (Wyrostek et al., 2016), Polish long-distance runners (74.7%) (Durkalec-Michalski et al., 2015) and French long-distance runners, sprinters and handball players (Garcin et al., 2009).

Findings by Kozłowska and Jurkiewicz (2009) showed that the conventional diets of female and male ice speed skaters from the Polish national team, on the days of group training sessions, met recommendations for potassium intake of 80% and 101%, respectively.

According to our results, 50% of female and 33% of male canoeists in the first year and 27% of male canoeists in the second year had insufficient magnesium intake. This is in agreement with the data of other researchers. Inadequate levels of the recommended magnesium intake were found in the diets of Polish hockey players (97.9%) (Gacek, 2010), Japanese football players (91.8%) (Noda et al., 2009), Polish mountain cyclists (73.7%) (Chalcarz et al., 2008b), athletes from the Polish national team (Czaja et al., 2008), Polish football players (Chalcarz et al., 2008a; Kasprzak, 2009) as well as French sprinters, long distance runners and handball players (Garcin et al., 2009). On the contrary, Zalcman and co-workers (2007) have reported that the intake for magnesium in diets of Brazilian female and male adventure racers was 106.1 and 77.4% of the recommended, respectively. However, intake of this mineral was insufficient for 33% of women and 61% of men. Intake of magnesium by female and male athletes from the Polish national team (Czaja et al., 2008; Lebiedzińska et al., 2008), long-distance runners (Durkalec-Michalski et al., 2015) and judo champions (Wyrostek et al., 2016) fully met the recommendation.

Insufficient iron intake was found for 25% of female canoeists but only in the first year of testing. A deficiency of iron in the athletes' diets was also reported by other authors. Inadequate intake of the recommendation for iron has been determined in diets of Polish mountain cyclists (81.8%) (Chalcarz et al., 2008b)) and Polish football players (Chalcarz et al., 2008a; Kasprzak, 2009). Inadequate intake of iron was reported for 28% of Brazilian women and 2% of Brazilian men. However, assessment of nutritional patterns of Brazilian women and men practising adventure racing showed that the percentage of recommended iron amount was 89.4 and 391.3%, respectively (Zalcman et al., 2007). The full recommended iron amount was reported in the diets of Polish hockey players (138.9%) (Gacek, 2010), Japanese football players (107.1%) (Noda et al., 2009), Polish long-distance runners (Durkalec-Michalski et al., 2015), French long-distance runners, French sprinters and handball players (Garcin et al., 2009), athletes (both genders) from the Polish national team (Lebiedzińska et al., 2008), and judo champions (Wyrostek et al., 2016).

9.4.3 Selected Morphological and Biochemical Blood Parameters

Our data indicates that morphological and biochemical parameters of almost all tested athletes were within the range of reference values, which was comparable with the results of other researchers. For example, the average glucose concentration in blood plasma of Polish girls and boys practicing fencing was 84.1 ± 5.9 and 91.4 ± 9.1 mg/dL, respectively, while the normal blood glucose level was 96% for all girls and boys (Chalcarz and Radzimirska-Graczyk (2009). Furthermore, the mean blood glucose concentrations of Brazilian female and male adventure racers were 86.9 ± 5.6, and 87.3 ± 8.7 mg/dL respectively (Zalcman et al., 2007), and were similar to our results.

Studies by Kalinowska and Przybyłowicz (2010) conducted on female and male members of the Polish national taekwondo team revealed that the average serum iron concentrations in this group were 110.5 ± 76.6, and 107.2 ± 37.7 µg/dL, respectively. The values of iron concentration in serum of Polish junior fencers were 98.6 ± 29.8 (girls) and 101.7 ± 48.6 µg/dL (boys), as was reported by Chalcarz and Radzimirska-Graczyk (2009). The authors also noted the normal iron level in serum of all girls and 89% of boys. The average iron concentration in serum of Brazilian adventure racers was 67.7 ± 19.2 (women) and 101.9 ± 30.5 µg/dL (men) (Zalcman et al., 2007), and was lower compared with our results. The average iron concentration in serum was also investigated by Noda et al. (2009) in Japanese football players (104.0 ± 39.0 µg/dL and by Podgórski et al. (2008) in members of the Polish field hockey team (97.0 µg/dL); the latter value was normal.

As was reported by Chalcarz and Radzimirska-Graczyk (2009), Polish girls and boys training in fencing had magnesium levels of 0.8 ± 0.1, and 0.9 ± 0.2 mmol/dL, respectively. In addition, the adequate level of serum magnesium was reported in 58% of female and 70% male juniors.

Sodium concentration in serum as determined by Chalcarz and Radzimirska-Graczyk (2009) in Polish young female and male fencers, was 141.8 ± 1.2 and 141.7 ± 1.0 mmol/dL, respectively. Furthermore, all examined athletes had a proper level of sodium in the serum, as was also stated in this work.

The level of potassium in serum noted by Chalcarz and Radzimirska-Graczyk (2009) in the aforementioned group of young athletes was 4.2 ± 0.4 mmol/dL (girls) and 4.4 ± 0.3 mmol/dL (boys). It was also reported that all girls and 89% of boys had the proper content of potassium.

The haemoglobin level in blood of girls and boys junior fencers was 14.0 ± 0.8, and 15.2 ± 0.9 g/dL, respectively, as measured by Chalcarz and Radzimirska-Graczyk (2009). In addition, all girls and 93% of boys had an adequate haemoglobin level. The study by Zalcman et al. (2007) showed the concentration of haemoglobin in the blood of Brazilian adventure racers at the level of 15.2 ± 0.9 g/dL (women) and 13.9 ± 1.1 g/dL (men). The haemoglobin level in the blood of Japanese football players was 15.3 ± 0.9 g/dL (Noda et al., 2009), which was very close to our findings.

Assessment of nutritional status of Polish young fencers, which was performed by Chalcarz and Radzimirska-Graczyk (2009), showed that juniors had the haematocrit value in blood at the level of 39.7 ± 2.9% (girls) and 42.0 ± 2.9% (boys); the adequate haematocrit values were found in 92% of female and 96% of male fencers. In addition, Zalcman and co-workers (2007) found that Brazilian adventure racers had the average haematocrit level in blood at the level of 45.6 ± 2.8% for women, and 40.7 ± 3.1% for men, while Noda et al. (2009) demonstrated that the mean haematocrit value for Japanese football players was 49.9 ± 3.0%.

9.4.4 Intake of Selected Nutrients within the Diet versus Morphological and Biochemical Blood Parameters

Assessment of the recommendation for carbohydrates, carried out in this study, showed low dietary intake of these nutrients by a significant percentage of canoeists. However, a good correlation was found between dietary carbohydrate intake and plasma glucose concentration. With increase in the lower recommended value of carbohydrate intake, glucose concentration in blood plasma also increased. At the same time, glucose concentration in blood of athletes was within the range of reference values.

The results our study indicated that all surveyed canoeists consumed enough iron with their diet, regardless of the year of research. A highly positive correlation was found between the values of the recommended dietary iron and concentration of the iron in serum. In addition, 13% and 33% of canoeists in the first year, and the second year, respectively, had serum iron concentration above the upper reference value. The diets of all hockey players were also sufficient in iron, regardless of the year of research. The level of the recommended intake for dietary iron was positively correlated with haemoglobin concentration in blood. However, the level of blood haemoglobin was too low for 8% of hockey players in both years of study. Iron concentration in blood has an effect on the maintenance of the desired psychophysical efficiency of athletes. The content of this element determines the level of haemoglobin (a component of red blood cells), myoglobin, as well as many enzymes, which allow for the optimal oxygen transport in the body (Caquet, 2009).

The assessment of the nutritional behaviour showed that diets of the majority of canoeists were insufficient in dietary magnesium; although, the concentration of magnesium in the athletes' serum was within normal reference values. Magnesium deficiency markedly reduces the athlete's physical performance, leading to general weakness, states of apathy, tremor and painful muscle spasms. The deficiency of this mineral is quite common in the diet of athletes, especially in endurance sports. Magnesium deficiency is not always manifested by its low concentration in serum. In sports practice, the so-called "hidden" shortages of this element frequently occur, characterized by its low level inside cells (Caquet, 2009).

Data from our study has shown all canoeists exceeded the tolerable sodium upper intake level. However, the concentration of sodium in the athlete serum was within the reference values and showed a high positive correlation with the percentage of the recommended dietary sodium. Sodium plays an important role in regulation of the acid/base balance as well as the functioning of the nervous and muscular systems. In the human body, the excessive amounts of sodium are excreted through the urine, and to a lesser extent through faeces and sweat. Moreover, high physical performance promotes the removal of sodium through sweat. Too high sodium dietary intake may increase blood pressure and in turn elevates the risk of developing cardiovascular diseases and diabetes, kidney damage, liver problems, elevated cholesterol content and fatigue (Caquet, 2009).

The results of this work show that potassium intake had a low probability of being insufficient in only a small percentage of the surveyed canoeists. Despite this, potassium content in the serum of athletes was within reference values. Potassium, like sodium, is involved in the regulation of the water and electrolyte balance in the body. It is necessary for the proper functioning of the muscular (including myocardium) and the nervous systems. Potassium also regulates the transport of glucose through the cell membrane, takes part in the process of glycogen storage in the muscles and influences its re-synthesis. It also plays a key role in the mechanism of muscle contraction and in the transmission of nerve impulses. The reduction of potassium ion concentration in muscle cells leads to a disturbance of their motoric functions and an increase in the rate of metabolism (Caquet, 2009).

9.5   CONCLUSIONS

Despite the inadequate dietary intake of digestible carbohydrates, potassium and magnesium, and the excessive sodium intake, concentration of blood glucose, as well as the content of these aforementioned minerals, were generally within the reference values. This suggests that the recommendations for these components may be overestimated in athletes' diets, whereas the recommendation for sodium was too low. The athletes whose diets contained the recommended iron/sodium intake also had higher reference values of these elements in blood.

REFERENCES

Caquet R. 2009. *250 badań laboratoryjnych. Kiedy zalecać. Jak interpretować.* Wydawnictwo Lekarskie PZWL, Warszawa.

Chalcarz W., Markiel S., Mikołajczak A., Nowak E. 2008a. Vitamin and mineral intake in football players on the day before match, the match day and the following day. *Bromatologia i Chemia Toksykologiczna*, 41.3, 681–685 (in Polish).

Chalcarz W., Merkiel S., Tyma M. 2008b. Vitamin and mineral intake in mountain cyclists. *Bromatologia i Chemia Toksykologiczna*, 41.3, 686–689 (in Polish).

Chalcarz W., Radzimirska-Graczyk M. 2009. Nutritional status of students practicing fencing attending sports schools. *Science and Sports*, 24.2, 84–90.

Czaja J., Lebiedzińska A., Szefer P. 2008. Nutritional habits and diet supplementation of Polish middle and long distance representative runners (years 2004–2005). *Roczniki PZH*, 59.1, 67–74 (in Polish).

Czapska D., Ostrowska D. 2005. Evaluation content of chosen minerals in a daily ration food of sport - Practicing students. *Żywienie Człowieka i Metabolizm*, 32.1, 668–671 (in Polish).

Durkalec-Michalski K., Baraniak A., Jeszka J. 2015. Effect of diet balancing on body composition and physical performance in recreational long-distance runners. *Problemy Higieny i Epidemiologii*, 96.3, 662–667 (in Polish).

Durkalec-Michalski K., Suliburska J., Jeszka J. 2011. The assessment of nutritional status and eating habits in a selected group of rowers. *Bromatologia i Chemia Toksykologiczna*, 44.3, 262–270 (in Polish).

Durkalec-Michalski K., Zawieja B., Zawieja E., Podgórski T., Jeszka J. 2016. Assessment of dietary intake, nutritional status and physical capacity in a selected group of male volleyball players. *Problemy Higieny i Epidemiologii*, 97.1, 56–61 (in Polish).

Gacek M. 2009. Evaluation of the level of nourishing ingredients intake in a group of young women doing fitness as recreation. *Roczniki PZH*, 60.4, 375–379 (in Polish).

Gacek M. 2010. Evaluation of consumption of selected nutrients in a group of hockey players during the preparation period. *Roczniki PZH*, 61.3, 259–263 (in Polish).

Garcin M., Doussot L., Mille-Hamard L., Billat V. 2009. Athletes' dietary intake was closer to French RDA's than those of young sedentary counterparts. *Nutritional Research*, 29.10, 736–742.

Iglesias-Gutiérreaz E., Garcia-Rovés P.M., Garcia A., Patterson A.M. 2008. Food preferences do not influence adolescent high-level athletes' dietary intake. *Appetite*, 50.2–3, 536–543.

Jarosz M., Bułhak-Jachymczyk B. (ed.). 2008. Recommendations for human nutrition. Fundamentals of prevention of obesity and non-communicable diseases. Ed. PZWL, Warszawa (in Polish).

Kalinowska K., Przybyłowicz K. 2010. Iron metabolism assessment with reference to selected anthropometric parameters and food-stuffs consumption National Taekwondo Team competitors. *Journal of Combat Sports and Martial Arts*, 2.2, 85–90.

Kasprzak Z. 2009. The evaluation of energy and nutritional values in diet: Energy expenditure of group young football players. *Żywienie Człowieka i Metabolizm*, 36.2, 272–277 (in Polish).

Kozłowska L., Jurkitewicz M. 2009. Assessment of dietary habits of national team in speed skating with regard supplements and special foods. *Żywienie Człowieka i Metabolizm*, 36.1, 95–99 (in Polish).

Lebiedzińska A., Czaja J., Żbikowski R., Szefer P. 2008. Assessment of nutrition of Polish national team of athletes. A comparison of theoretical evaluation and analytical results. Part II. Selected macro- and microelements. *Bromatologia i Chemia Toksykologiczna*, 41.3, 428–432 (in Polish).

Nowacka E., Kopec A., Leszczynska T., Polaszczyk S.Z., Pysz K. 2013. Total fats and fatty acids consumption by canoeists and sports shooters. *Science and Sport*, 28, 41–50.

Nowacka E., Leszczyńska T., Kopeć A., Hojka D. 2016. Nutritional behavior of Polish canoeist's athletes: The interest of nutritional education. *Science and Sports*, 31.4, e79–e91, doi:10.1016/j.scipo.2016.04.002.

Noda Y., Iide K., Reika M., Kishida R., Nagata A., Hirakawa F., Yoshimura Y., Imamura H. 2009. Nutrient intake and blood iron status of male collegiate soccer players. *Asia Pacific Journal of Clinical Nutrition*, 18.3, 344–350.

Podgórski T., Konarski J., Kryściak J., Domaszewska K., Pawlak M. 2008. Influence of exercise on selected parameters of iron metabolism on field hockey player organisms. *Medycyna Sportowa*, 24.3, 159–170 (in Polish).

Szczepańska B., Malczewska-Lenczowska J., Gajewski J. 2009. Is it sensible to administer food supplements to polish elite weightlifters on a training camp? *Żywność. Nauka. Technologia. Jakość*, 4.65, 327–336 (in Polish).

Todhunter E.N. 1970. *A Guide to Nutrition Terminology for Indexing and Retrieval.* National Institutes of Health, Public Health Service, U.S. Department of Health, Education, and Welfare, Bethesda, MD.

Wyrostek J., Wyrostek S., Michalczyk M., Pilch W. 2016. Assessment of dietary intake, nutritional status and physical capacity in a selected group of male volleyball players. *Medical & Health Sciences Review*, 2.3, 113–118.

Zalcman I., Vidigal Guarita H., Ridel Juzwiak C., Aparecida Crispim C., Moreira Antunes H.K., Edwards B., Tufik S., de Mello M.T. 2007. Nutritional status of adventure racers. *Nutrition*, 23.5, 404–411.

Ziegler P.J., Jonnalagadda S.S., Lawrence C. 2001. Dietary intake of elite figure skating dancers. *Nutrition Research*, 21.7, 983–992.

10 Testosterone in Sport
The Androgen Response to Extreme Endurance Exercise

Jake Shelley, Christopher Howe, Hannah Jayne Moir, and Andrea Petróczi

CONTENTS

10.1 Introduction 193
10.2 Androgen Response to Acute Extreme Endurance Exercise........................ 194
10.3 Androgen Response to Ultra-Endurance Exercise in Extreme Conditions........ 196
10.4 Androgen Response to Prolonged Extreme Endurance Training................. 197
10.5 Testosterone as a PED in Extreme Endurance Sport.................................. 199
10.6 Nutritional Strategies, Functional Foods and Dietary Supplements
      for Androgen Augmentation 200
10.7 Conclusions... 201
Bibliography 201

10.1 INTRODUCTION

Testosterone is one of a number of naturally occurring androgens. It is a steroid hormone released primarily by the Leydig cells in the testes, and to a lesser extent by the adrenal cortex (Kadi 2008, 522–528). It serves as the primary male sex hormone and plays a key role in the development of male reproductive tissues and the promotion of secondary sexual characteristics, such as the growth of body hair. The normal range for total testosterone in healthy adult males is approximately 10.4 nmol/L to 34.7 nmol/L (Carnegie 2004, S3–8; Boyce et al. 2004, 881–885).

Endurance exercise is now an extremely popular activity in Western society. A growing subsection wish to go beyond conventional endurance exercise and are seeking extreme endurance challenges, such as ultramarathon running, which is typically defined as a running event longer in distance than a marathon (26.2 miles/42.195 km), or ultra-distance cycling, which is more loosely defined but can cover anything longer than a 100-mile ride.

Testosterone, in the context of sport, is most commonly associated with strength and power-based sports and activities, such as weightlifting and sprinting, given its well-characterised anabolic and muscle-building effects (Griggs et al. 1989, 498–503; Kanayama and Pope 2017, 4–13). There have been many cases of athletes competing in these types of sports using synthetic testosterone to artificially enhance their performance, such as Marion Jones and Ben Johnson. However, there have been an equally high number of cases of endurance athletes using synthetic androgens to enhance performance in endurance sports, such as Lance Armstrong and Tyler Hamilton (Gibson 2012).

The response of testosterone to prolonged endurance exercise appears quite variable, as both increases and decreases have been reported (McMurray and Hackney 2000, 135–161; Viru 1992, 201–209). However, it has been consistently reported that endurance-trained athletes may experience subclinical decreases in basal testosterone levels, together with an increase in basal cortisol levels (Barron et al. 1985, 803–806; Seidman et al. 1990, 421–424). Whether or not these hormonal modulations affect performance remains in question (Hackney and Lane 2015, 293–311; Hloogeveen and Zonderland 1996, 423–428; Tenforde et al. 2016, 171–182).

The aim of this review is to explore the androgen response to one-off extreme endurance events and to prolonged endurance training. The potential physiological basis behind the use of testosterone as a performance enhancing drug (PED) for endurance sports will also be discussed, along with dietary components and functional foodstuffs with putative effects on testosterone levels.

10.2 ANDROGEN RESPONSE TO ACUTE EXTREME ENDURANCE EXERCISE

The hormonal response to endurance exercise has been studied for many years, predominantly using either running or cycling as the mode of exercise. Unsurprisingly, moderate- to high-intensity endurance exercise leads to increases in hormones that typically respond to stressful situations, such as cortisol, growth hormone and the catecholamines (Cadegiani and Kater 2017, 14; Kindermann et al. 1982, 389–399). However, the response of testosterone to an acute bout of endurance exercise is less well characterised. Findings vary in the research, with studies showing increases, decreases or no significant change.

One study examined the levels of testosterone in the blood before, during and after a 110 km ultramarathon (Fournier et al. 1997, 252–256). Testosterone was measured by radioimmunoassay at the start, at 33 km, at 75 km and at the finish, and the authors noted a moderate decrease in testosterone during the course of the race. The observation of ultramarathons triggering a decrease in testosterone has been replicated by several other groups, with the length and the severity of the endurance exercise seemingly influencing the magnitude of the reduction. For instance, another study examined the effects of a 400 km road race around Hawaii, completed over 15 days in a series of stages ranging from 15 km to 34 km in length, on plasma testosterone levels (Dressendorfer and Wade 1991, 954–958). Data were collected from 19 male runners before and after the race and the results demonstrated a 31% decrease in testosterone, from an average of 23.5 ± 1.7 nmol/L to 16.2 nmol/L, as well as an 83% increase in the ratio of cortisol to testosterone. Another group compared and contrasted the effects of an ultramarathon race (104 km) with those of an ultra-endurance swimming race (25 km) (Tauler et al. 2013, 560–565) and found that testosterone decreased significantly following both events. At the lower end of the ultra-running distance spectrum, the effects of a competitive marathon (42.2 km) on serum testosterone have also been extensively investigated (Guglielmini, Paolini, and Conconi 1984, 246–249). In contrast to the studies on longer ultra-endurance events, this study showed an average increase in serum testosterone levels of 44.8% ($p < 0.01$) in participating marathon runners. Furthermore, a small study conducted by a Dutch group (Ponjee, De Rooy, and Vader 1994, 1274–1277) showed an increase in serum testosterone levels in 13 of the 18 participating athletes. However, it must be noted that no consistent conclusions can be drawn about the testosterone changes before and after a marathon from these two studies alone, as there are an equal number of studies indicating that a marathon run causes a fall in testosterone levels. For instance, one Finnish group reported a 20% drop in serum testosterone during a marathon in a study with 20 participants (Kuusi et al. 1984, 527–531), and a second Finnish group also reported a highly significant decrease in average plasma testosterone levels from 23.4 nmol/L to 14.1 nmol/L ($p < 0.001$) following completion of a marathon by 14 amateur runners (Dessypris, Kuoppasalmi, and Adlercreutz 1976, 33–37).

Another classic extreme endurance event that many athletes look to in order to challenge themselves beyond the marathon distance is the Ironman triathlon, which consists of a 3.86 km swim, followed by a 180.25 km bicycle ride and finished off with a marathon (42.2 km run). The response of testosterone following an Ironman triathlon was investigated by taking blood samples from 42 male participants two days before, and immediately after, an Ironman event (Neubauer, König, and Wagner 2008, 417–426). This study showed that testosterone fell from an average of 11.4 nmol/L pre-race to 5.3 nmol/L post-race.

These hormonal responses are also detectable in an elite population. For example, one study examined nine professional cyclists who participated in the 1999 Vuelta a Espana (a 22-day elite cycling stage-race during which participants must cover ~3500 km in daily stages of 150–200 km) by measuring testosterone, luteinizing hormone (LH), cortisol and other hormones before the competition, at the end of the first week, at the end of the second week, and at the end of the race. Testosterone was shown to decrease significantly and consistently throughout the three weeks, whilst remaining within a normal physiological range (Lucia et al. 2001, 424–430).

Reviewing the literature in this field, a general trend is apparent – endurance exercise of ~3 hours duration or less appears to have variable effects on serum testosterone levels, whilst endurance exercise beyond ~3 hours duration tends to decrease circulating testosterone, with the magnitude of the decrease roughly proportional to the distance run. Testosterone levels tend to return to roughly baseline levels following 24–48 hours of recovery after extreme endurance exercise.

Ultra-endurance exercise is clearly an activity that stresses the body to a great degree, as demonstrated by the consistently reported large increases in cortisol levels. These events also create conditions of extreme energetic imbalance and this necessitates trade-offs between competing physiological functions for limited resources. Longman et al. (2018, e23052) sought to investigate the trade-off between reproductive effort and somatic maintenance, using an ultramarathon to create the conditions of energetic stress where such trade-offs are expected to occur (Knechtle, Enggist, and Jehle 2005, 499–503). The 66 participants completed a 165 km run and testosterone was measured from saliva pre- and post-race. As expected, there was a significant decrease in testosterone levels. However, in this study two other variables were also measured: libido and innate immune function. Libido decreased after the run, correlating with the change in testosterone levels, whilst markers of innate immune function increased (Longman et al. 2018, e23052). These results suggest that participating in an ultramarathon causes a reordering of energetic priorities, moving away from reproduction and towards somatic maintenance/defence, which could explain the characteristic drop in testosterone levels observed following the majority of ultra-endurance events.

10.3 ANDROGEN RESPONSE TO ULTRA-ENDURANCE EXERCISE IN EXTREME CONDITIONS

With regards to extreme endurance exercise, it is also important to consider the role the environment plays, as thermal conditions can increase the physical exertion. Athletes, particularly ultra-endurance athletes, often find themselves competing in extreme environmental conditions such as hot and humid or cold and dry climates.

These environments place an enhanced physiological strain on the body and present a profound metabolic challenge to maintain the homoeothermic status of the body at a core temperature of 37°C by tightly regulating heat exchange. Heat exposure can increase total metabolic rate and these demands on metabolic and thermoregulatory control make blood flow difficult to maintain cardiac output. The body is limited by cardiovascular overload and critical temperature.

The Western States Endurance Run (WSER), one the oldest and most prestigious 161-km ultramarathons, is not only reputable for the prolonged duration and mountainous terrain but also for the numerous environmental stresses, such as the heat and altitude of the Sierra Nevada mountain range. A 2014 study (Kupchak et al. 2014, 278–288) examined the disrupted hormonal responses of the hypothalamic-pituitary-gonadal (HPG) axis in males competing in the WSER. The study found significant decreases in testosterone and LH with increased levels of cortisol resulting in a catabolic state, as indicated by the decreased testosterone to cortisol (T:C) ratio for up to 2 days post-race.

While exercising in the cold, the low temperatures cause constriction and dilation of blood vessels to preserve heat, but also stimulate the production of heat through shivering and increased sweating to maintain internal temperatures. Typically, cold environments are not shown to alter testosterone but can increase cortisol secretion.

The impact of a 160-km ultramarathon at over 2000 metres altitude in Alaska (now called the Susitna 100) was investigated (Kraemer et al. 2008, 116–120; discussion 120), with the participants comprising of both cyclists and runners and conditions consisting of a frozen environment with temperatures ranging from −8°C to 4°C. Pre-race testosterone levels were low compared with normal reference values, and the race caused a further reduction. It is suggested that the environmentally stressful conditions contributed to this decrease in testosterone and suppression of the HPG axis, but it is not possible to tease out whether the reduction was primarily caused by the race itself, or the variables such as temperature and altitude. However, given that plasma testosterone levels fell to a markedly low average of 6.96 nmol/L by the end of the race in the running group, it can be concluded that the conditions contributed to the overall stress of the race.

Altitude has also been identified as an area of concern as the low-oxygen environment may cause alterations in the HPG axis when combined with the physiological stress of extreme endurance exercise. Changes in testosterone levels were monitored in one study in which six male athletes completed a marathon in Nepal, starting at an altitude of 3860 m and finishing at 3400 m, after reaching a high point of 5100 m (Marinelli et al. 1994, 225–229). Data were collected pre-travel at sea level, pre-race after a week of acclimatisation at altitude, immediately post-race and 24 hours post-race. There was also a control group, consisting of five healthy males who also participated in the expedition (but not the race) and who were sampled at the same times and under the same conditions. The results showed a drastic decrease in testosterone, much larger than previously described after a marathon run. Total testosterone in the athletes fell from an average of 25.13 ± 6.37 nmol/L at first sampling to 15.10 ± 1.50 nmol/L after acclimatisation, and again fell to 11.57 ± 2.44 nmol/L immediately post-race. Control levels remained steady after acclimatisation, showing the marked effect of the marathon run itself, above and beyond the effects of the altitude alone. The athlete's levels did recover to an average 18.09 ± 2.70 24 hours post-race.

Performing exercise that is less intense than a marathon run at altitude appears to significantly diminish the reduction in testosterone levels. In a study examining hormonal responses to altitude exposure, testosterone levels were measured in seven male mountaineers engaged in a 22-day hiking expedition at altitudes in the range of 5900 m, pre-, during and post-expedition. There was no significant change in testosterone levels measured at the three sampling points (Pelliccione et al. 2011, 28–33).

Combining extreme endurance exercise with challenging environmental conditions can amplify the physiological responses, including the androgen response. All care must be taken by extreme endurance athletes to prepare appropriately when racing in challenging conditions, and adjust the target paces accordingly. Extra recovery post-event may also be required to allow androgen levels to return to baseline levels.

10.4   ANDROGEN RESPONSE TO PROLONGED EXTREME ENDURANCE TRAINING

Having discussed whether a one-off extreme endurance event causes a decrease in testosterone levels, it is also important to consider whether regular high-volume endurance exercise training causes changes in basal testosterone levels.

Significant evidence points to the conclusion that men who run high mileage (defined for this purpose as running a minimum of 100 km/week) have lower basal levels of testosterone when compared to matched sedentary individuals. For instance, this finding is supported by a study that took 10 runners who ran an average of 109.2 km per week and compared them with 10 controls who did less than 1 hour of aerobic activity per week (Arce et al. 1993, 398–404). The runners had an average total testosterone concentration of 14.9 ± 1.3 nmol/L compared to the controls 19.5 ± 0.9 nmol/L ($p = 0.046$). Further to this, a separate research group took 11 runners averaging 108.3 km per week and found that they had resting levels of total testosterone averaging 15.3 ± 1.3 nmol/L. This was in comparison to a group of 10 matched, sedentary controls who had resting levels of 19.5 ± 0.9 nmol/L ($p = 0.008$)

(De Souza et al. 1994, 383–391). A difference in total testosterone was again reported in a study that compared five runners averaging 123.9 k per week with sedentary controls. The runners had testosterone levels of 16.6 ± 2.4 nmol/L whilst the controls had levels of 24.6 ± 4.2 nmol/L ($p = 0.05$) (Hackney, Sinning, and Bruot 1990, 298–303). That is not to say that every study investigating testosterone levels in high-mileage runners shows a reduction in basal levels. MacConnie et al. recruited a group of six highly trained male marathon runners who had consistently run between 125 and 200 km per week for at least five years and found no difference in their baseline testosterone levels when compared with 13 healthy age-matched controls who did not run more than 5 km per week (MacConnie et al. 1986, 411–417).

Whilst the MacConnie study did not show any significant differences between the basal testosterone levels of high-mileage runners and sedentary controls, it did reveal that runners displayed a significantly ($p < 0.05$) reduced frequency of LH pulses (2.2 ± 0.48 vs. 3.6 ± 0.24) as well as a significantly ($p < 0.02$) reduced amplitude of the LH pulse (0.9 ± 0.24 mIU/ml vs. 1.6 ± 0.15 mIU/ml). A pulse of LH results as a direct consequence from a pulse of gonadotropin releasing hormone, and downstream, LH acts on the Leydig cells of the testes, stimulating them to produce testosterone (Rowe et al. 1975, 17–26). Although the basal levels of testosterone levels measured were not reduced compared to controls, the changes in LH pulse frequency and amplitude do indicate that the runners may less strongly stimulate the release of testosterone.

These findings prompted comparisons between highly trained male runners and highly trained female runners, who commonly experience deficiencies in gonadotropin-releasing hormone, which are associated with amenorrhea (i.e. the absence of menstruation in females) (De Souza et al. 2014, 289–298). The authors contested that, though the male runners do not have such an obvious clinical sign (e.g. amenorrhea), they may also have a deficiency of gonadotropin-releasing hormone. This deficiency is postulated to be caused by the regular and repetitive fluctuation of testosterone and other hormones known to suppress gonadotropin-releasing hormone, following daily bouts of long and somewhat intense endurance exercise.

The theory that alterations in LH pulsatile release may be responsible for the decreased basal testosterone levels observed in some extreme endurance trained athletes has been tested and challenged. One study took a group of six endurance runners, with a training volume of at least 80 km per week, and measured LH pulse frequency and amplitude via an intravenous cannula at 15 minute intervals for 6 hours following 24 hours without significant physical activity, as well as measuring resting testosterone levels (Wheeler et al. 1991, 422–425). The basal testosterone levels were again found to be lower than the values from sedentary controls, and LH pulse amplitude was also significantly reduced. However, the frequency of LH pulses was the same in the runners as in the controls.

To better understand whether a reduction in LH pulse frequency and/or amplitude are responsible for the lower basal testosterone levels observed in some high-mileage runners, it would be highly beneficial to study LH pulsatility over a 24 hour period in highly trained extreme endurance athletes.

When considering these changes in basal testosterone levels, it is important to note that in all reported cases of a reduction, the reduction is subclinical, as the values do not fall below the lower limit of the normal range (10–35 nmol/L). However, when dealing with elite athletes, even a subclinical decrease could influence performance, and perhaps that gives a clue as to why testosterone is sometimes used as a PED by elite endurance athletes. The reduced levels of testosterone resulting from participation in endurance exercise training have been termed the "exercise-hypogonadal male condition" (Hackney 2008, 932–938).

10.5   TESTOSTERONE AS A PED IN EXTREME ENDURANCE SPORT

In the late 1990s and early 2000s, there was a well-documented and widespread use of PEDs in the professional cycling peloton (Vest Christiansen 2005, 497–514). The most common methods of doping were the use of autologous blood transfusions, erythropoietin (EPO), testosterone and growth hormone. The use of blood transfusions and EPO is designed to increase the oxygen carrying capacity of the blood by increasing the number of red blood cells, and thereby increase the capacity for aerobic respiration and hence improve endurance performance. Testosterone, on the other hand, is thought to have been used by cyclists to recover more quickly, which is obviously important in the prestigious three-week-long grand tours. Growth hormone is thought to have been used for a similar purpose. Testosterone stimulates protein synthesis and may therefore facilitate more rapid repair of damaged muscle fibres. The choice between using testosterone or growth hormone may have come down to personal preference – Floyd Landis, who was stripped of the Tour de France title for doping, reported that growth hormone didn't make him feel as stiff and bloated as testosterone did (Shen 2011).

The possibility also exists that testosterone was used by cyclists as another method to stimulate erythropoietin release, as the association between androgens and erythropoiesis has long been established (Shahani et al. 2009, 704–716). Androgens act on the hematopoietic system by inducing the release of EPO, increasing bone marrow activity and iron incorporation into red blood cells. When this is combined with the anabolic effect of testosterone to counter the catabolic state induced by extreme endurance cycling (Lucia et al. 2001, 424–430), it becomes clear why testosterone was used by a number of cyclists as a PED.

Although the reduced levels of testosterone observed in chronically extreme endurance-trained athletes are generally still within the normal range, there is some evidence to suggest that the lower resting levels may have some detrimental effects on testosterone-dependent physiological processes. For example, a comprehensive study examining the effects of high-intensity and high-volume treadmill running in 286 male participants demonstrated that such a training regimen can significantly decrease semen concentration, motility and morphology (Safarinejad, Azma, and Kolahi 2009, 259–271), and this finding has been reproduced elsewhere (Brant et al. 2010, 114–120). In contradiction to this, it has also been postulated that the lowering of testosterone in chronically trained endurance athletes may be a functional adaptation rather than a maladaptation, since a decrease in testosterone could lead to a lower overall muscle mass, which in turn could decrease the oxygen requirement and the energy expenditure – an important physiological factor for extreme endurance performance (Bribiescas 1996, 163–188; Lane and Hackney 2014).

10.6 NUTRITIONAL STRATEGIES, FUNCTIONAL FOODS AND DIETARY SUPPLEMENTS FOR ANDROGEN AUGMENTATION

The use of synthetic testosterone or other anabolic-androgenic steroids (AAS), which are prohibited for use in competitive sport by the World Anti-Doping Agency (WADA), is not necessarily the only way of boosting androgen levels that may have been suppressed by chronic endurance training. There is evidence to indicate that a number of herbs, supplements and foodstuffs might increase testosterone levels. For instance, vitamin D supplementation (83 µg per day for one year) led to an increase in testosterone levels from 10.7 ± 3.9 nmol/L to 13.4 ± 4.7 nmol/L; $p < 0.001$ ($n = 31$), compared to no significant change in the placebo group ($n = 23$), in a group of overweight, vitamin D deficient, but otherwise healthy, men (Pilz et al. 2011, 223).

Testosterone is excreted mainly as a glucuroconjugate after glucurondination by uridine diphospho-glucuronosyl transferases (UGT), with UGT2B17 and UGT2B7 being particularly active isoenzymes in the glucurondination of testosterone and epitestosterone, a key step in facilitating their excretion in urine. Green and white tea extracts have an inhibitory effect on UGT2B17 and may therefore increase testosterone levels by decreasing the rate of testosterone excretion (Jenkinson et al. 2012, 691–695). Red wine is another flavonoid-containing foodstuff that has been shown to inhibit UGT2B17 and thereby potentially elevate circulating testosterone levels again by decreasing excretion rate (Jenkinson, Petroczi, and Naughton 2012, 691–695).

In another study, the effects of treatment with Ashwagandha root extract supplementation (675 mg per day for 90 days) on semen parameters and plasma hormone levels were investigated (Ambiye et al. 2013). Ashwagandha is a plant of the nightshade family that has been used as an aphrodisiac to treat male infertility in Ayurvedic medicine. The results of this investigation showed that in the treatment group ($n = 21$), testosterone levels increased significantly ($p < 0.01$) by 17%, whilst the control group who were treated with placebo showed no significant increase. In a similar vein, Peruvian Maca (*Lepidium meyenii*) has been shown to help sexual dysfunction in both males and females (Shin et al. 2010, 44) but studies failed to show a direct link to increased testosterone levels (Bogani et al. 2006, 415–417; Gonzalez et al. 2002, 367–372). Rather, Maca appears to help endurance sport performance by improving oxygen transportation in the body (Stone et al. 2009, 574–576).

Tribulus terrestris (*TT*) is perhaps the most commonly used herbal extract aimed at boosting testosterone levels, and many "performance-enhancing" food supplements contain *TT* extract. To assess the effectiveness of *TT* for this purpose, a systematic review was carried out, which evaluated the findings of 11 studies, and the results suggest that despite the common marketing claims, *TT* is ineffective at increasing testosterone levels in humans (Qureshi, Naughton, and Petroczi 2014, 64–79).

Whilst there is some evidence that certain nutritional supplements and foodstuffs may boost testosterone, further research is required to determine the long-term efficacy, mechanism of action and optimal dose before any firm position can be taken on the potential benefits of these approaches for extreme endurance athletes.

10.7 CONCLUSIONS

Extreme endurance exercise can cause a transient dip in testosterone levels, and over time, this may lead to a subtle lowering in basal testosterone levels in individuals who regularly participate in extreme volumes of endurance exercise. Those individuals must be aware that suppressed levels of testosterone may become counterproductive, although research into the exact performance effect of a subclinical decrease in testosterone levels is sorely lacking. Events such as the Tour de France create enormous physiological demands and inevitably cause perturbations of the endocrine system. The use of testosterone as a doping agent in these events may enhance performance by mitigating any presumed decreases in testosterone levels during the course of the race. The evidence gathered so far indicates that the moderate reductions in resting testosterone levels caused by extreme endurance exercise do not pose any significant risk to health and can be managed by including appropriate amounts of recovery between each bout of exercise. Certain dietary strategies may also help to mitigate testosterone suppression.

BIBLIOGRAPHY

Ambiye, V. R., D. Langade, S. Dongre, P. Aptikar, M. Kulkarni, and A. Dongre. 2013. "Clinical Evaluation of the Spermatogenic Activity of the Root Extract of Ashwagandha (Withania Somnifera) in Oligospermic Males: A Pilot Study". *Evidence-Based Complementary and Alternative Medicine: eCAM* 2013: 571420.

Arce, J. C., M. J. De Souza, L. S. Pescatello, and A. A. Luciano. 1993. "Subclinical Alterations in Hormone and Semen Profile in Athletes". *Fertility and Sterility* 59 (2): 398–404.

Barron, J., T. Noakes, W. Levy, C. Smith, and R. Millar. 1985. "Hypothalamic Dysfunction in Overtrained Athletes". *The Journal of Clinical Endocrinology and Metabolism* 60 (4): 803–806.

Bogani, P., F. Simonini, M. Iriti, M. Rossoni, F. Faoro, A. Poletti, and F. Visioli. 2006. "Lepidium Meyenii (Maca) Does Not Exert Direct Androgenic Activities". *Journal of Ethnopharmacology* 104 (3): 415–417.

Boyce, M. J., K. J. Baisley, E. V. Clark, and S. J. Warrington. 2004. "Are Published Normal Ranges of Serum Testosterone Too High? Results of a Cross-sectional Survey of Serum Testosterone and Luteinizing Hormone in Healthy Men". *BJU International* 94 (6): 881–885.

Brant, W. O., J. B. Myers, D. T. Carrell, and J. F. Smith. 2010. "Male Athletic Activities and Their Effects on Semen and Hormonal Parameters". *The Physician and Sportsmedicine* 38 (3): 114–120.

Bribiescas, R. G. 1996. "Testosterone Levels among Aché Hunter-Gatherer Men". *Human and Nature* 7 (2): 163–188.

Cadegiani, F. A., and C. E. Kater. 2017. "Hormonal Aspects of Overtraining Syndrome: A Systematic Review". *BMC Sports Science, Medicine and Rehabilitation* 9 (1): 14.

Carnegie, C. 2004. "Diagnosis of Hypogonadism: Clinical Assessments and Laboratory Tests". *Reviews in Urology* 6 (6 Suppl): S3–8.

De Souza, M. J., J. C. Arce, L. S. Pescatello, H. S. Scherzer, and A. A. Luciano. 1994. "Gonadal Hormones and Semen Quality in Male Runners". *International Journal of Sports Medicine* 15 (7): 383–391.

De Souza, M. J., A. Nattiv, E. Joy, M. Misra, N. I. Williams, R. J. Mallinson, J. C. Gibbs, M. Olmsted, M. Goolsby, and G. Matheson. 2014. "2014 Female Athlete Triad Coalition Consensus Statement on Treatment and Return to Play of the Female Athlete Triad:

1st International Conference Held in San Francisco, California, May 2012 and 2nd International Conference Held in Indianapolis, Indiana, May 2013". *British Journal of Sports Medicine* 48 (4): 289.

Dessypris, A., K. Kuoppasalmi, and H. Adlercreutz. 1976. "Plasma Cortisol, Testosterone, Androstenedione and Luteinizing Hormone (LH) in a Non-Competitive Marathon Run". *Journal of Steroid Biochemistry* 7 (1): 33–37.

Dressendorfer, R. H., and C. E. Wade. 1991. "Effects of a 15-D Race on Plasma Steroid Levels and Leg Muscle Fitness in Runners". *Medicine and Science in Sports and Exercise* 23 (8): 954–958.

Fournier, P. E., J. Stalder, B. Mermillod, and A. Chantraine. 1997. "Effects of a 110 Kilometers Ultra-Marathon Race on Plasma Hormone Levels". *International Journal of Sports Medicine* 18 (4): 252–256.

Gibson, O. 2012. "Lance Armstrong Case: The Different Drugs Taken and How They Were Used". *The Guardian*. 11th October, 2012.

Griggs, R. C., W. Kingston, R. F. Jozefowicz, B. E. Herr, G. Forbes, and D. Halliday. 1989. "Effect of Testosterone on Muscle Mass and Muscle Protein Synthesis". *Journal of Applied Physiology* 66 (1): 498–503.

Gonzales, G. F., A. Cordova, K. Vega, A. Chung, A. Villena, C. Góñez, and S. Castillo. 2002. "Effect of Lepidium Meyenii (MACA) on Sexual Desire and Its Absent Relationship with Serum Testosterone Levels in Adult Healthy Men." *Andrologia* 34 (6): 367–372.

Guglielmini, C., A. R. Paolini, and F. Conconi. 1984. "Variations of Serum Testosterone Concentrations after Physical Exercises of Different Duration". *International Journal of Sports Medicine* 5 (5): 246–249.

Hackney, A. C. 2008. "Effects of Endurance Exercise on the Reproductive System of Men: The "Exercise-Hypogonadal Male Condition". *Journal of Endocrinological Investigation* 31 (10): 932–938.

Hackney, A. C., and A. R. Lane. 2015. "Exercise and the Regulation of Endocrine Hormones". *Progress in Molecular Biology and Translational Science* 135: 293–311.

Hackney, A. C., W. E. Sinning, and B. C. Bruot. 1990. "Hypothalamic-Pituitary-Testicular Axis Function in Endurance-Trained Males". *International Journal of Sports Medicine* 11 (4): 298–303.

Hloogeveen, A. R., and M. L. Zonderland. 1996. "Relationships between Testosterone, Cortisol and Performance in Professional Cyclists". *International Journal of Sports Medicine* 17 (6): 423–428.

Jenkinson, C., A. Petroczi, and D. P. Naughton. 2012. "Red Wine and Component Flavonoids Inhibit UGT2B17 in vitro". *Nutrition Journal* 11 (1): 67.

Jenkinson, C., A. Petroczi, J. Barker, and D. P. Naughton. 2012. "Dietary Green and White Teas Suppress UDP-Glucuronosyltransferase UGT2B17 Mediated Testosterone Glucuronidation". *Steroids* 77 (6): 691–695.

Kadi, F. 2008. "Cellular and Molecular Mechanisms Responsible for the Action of Testosterone on Human Skeletal Muscle. A Basis for Illegal Performance Enhancement". *British Journal of Pharmacology* 154 (3): 522–528.

Kanayama, G., and H. G. Pope Jr. 2017. "History and Epidemiology of Anabolic Androgens in Athletes and Non-Athletes". *Molecular and Cellular Endocrinology* 464: 4–13.

Kindermann, W., A. Schnabel, W. M. Schmitt, G. Biro, J. Cassens, and F. Weber. 1982. "Catecholamines, Growth Hormone, Cortisol, Insulin, and Sex Hormones in Anaerobic and Aerobic Exercise". *European Journal of Applied Physiology and Occupational Physiology* 49 (3): 389–399.

Knechtle, B., A. Enggist, and T. Jehle. 2005. "Energy Turnover at the Race Across America (RAAM)-A Case Report". *International Journal of Sports Medicine* 26 (6): 499–503.

Kraemer, W. J., M. S. Fragala, G. Watson, J. S. Volek, M. R. Rubin, D. N. French, C. M. Maresh, et al. 2008. "Hormonal Responses to a 160-km Race Across Frozen Alaska". *British Journal of Sports Medicine* 42 (2): 116–120; discussion 120.

Kupchak, B. R., W. J. Kraemer, M. D. Hoffman, S. D. Phinney, and J. S. Volek. 2014. "The Impact of an Ultramarathon on Hormonal and Biochemical Parameters in Men". *Wilderness and Environmental Medicine* 25 (3): 278–288.

Kuusi, T., E. Kostiainen, E. Vartiainen, L. Pitkanen, C. Ehnholm, H. J. Korhonen, A. Nissinen, and P. Puska. 1984. "Acute Effects of Marathon Running on Levels of Serum Lipoproteins and Androgenic Hormones in Healthy Males". *Metabolism: Clinical and Experimental* 33 (6): 527–531.

Lane, A. R., and A. C. Hackney. 2014. "Reproductive Dysfunction from the Stress of Exercise Training Is Not Gender Specific: The "Exercise-Hypogonadal Male Condition". *Journal of Endocrinology and Diabetes* 1 (2): 4.

Longman, D. P., S. P. Prall, E. C. Shattuck, I. D. Stephen, J. T. Stock, J. C. K. Wells, and M. P. Muehlenbein. 2018. "Short-Term Resource Allocation during Extensive Athletic Competition". *American Journal of Human Biology* 30 (1): e23052.

Lucia, A., B. Diaz, J. Hoyos, C. Fernandez, G. Villa, F. Bandres, and J. L. Chicharro. 2001. "Hormone Levels of World Class Cyclists during the Tour of Spain Stage Race". *British Journal of Sports Medicine* 35 (6): 424–430.

MacConnie, S. E., A. Barkan, R. M. Lampman, M. A. Schork, and I. Z. Beitins. 1986. "Decreased Hypothalamic Gonadotropin-Releasing Hormone Secretion in Male Marathon Runners". *New England Journal of Medicine* 315 (7): 411–417.

Marinelli, M., G. S. Roi, M. Giacometti, P. Bonini, and G. Banfi. 1994. "Cortisol, Testosterone, and Free Testosterone in Athletes Performing a Marathon at 4,000 M Altitude". *Hormones* 41 (5–6): 225–229.

McMurray, R. G., and A. C. Hackney. 2000. "Endocrine Responses to Exercise and Training". In Garrett, Jr., W. E., and Kirkendall, D. T., (Eds.), *Exercise and Sport Science*, Philadelphia: Lippincott Williams & Wilkins, pp. 135–161.

Neubauer, O., D. König, and K. H. Wagner. 2008. "Recovery After an Ironman Triathlon: Sustained Inflammatory Responses and Muscular Stress". *European Journal of Applied Physiology* 104 (3): 417–426.

Pelliccione, F., V. Verratti, A. D'Angeli, A. Micillo, C. Doria, A. Pezzella, G. Iacutone, F. Francavilla, C. Di Giulio, and S. Francavilla. 2011. "Physical Exercise at High Altitude Is Associated with a Testicular Dysfunction Leading to Reduced Sperm Concentration but Healthy Sperm Quality". *Fertility and Sterility* 96 (1): 28–33.

Pilz, S., S. Frisch, H. Koertke, J. Kuhn, J. Dreier, B. Obermayer-Pietsch, E. Wehr, and A. Zittermann. 2011. "Effect of Vitamin D Supplementation on Testosterone Levels in Men". *Hormone and Metabolic Research* 43 (3): 223–225.

Ponjee, G. A., H. A. De Rooy, and H. L. Vader. 1994. "Androgen Turnover during Marathon Running". *Medicine and Science in Sports and Exercise* 26 (10): 1274–1277.

Qureshi, A., D. P. Naughton, and A. Petroczi. 2014. "A Systematic Review on the Herbal Extract Tribulus terrestris and the Roots of Its Putative Aphrodisiac and Performance Enhancing Effect". *Journal of Dietary Supplements* 11 (1): 64–79.

Rowe, P. H., P. A. Racey, G. A. Lincoln, M. Ellwood, J. Lehane, and J. C. Shenton. 1975. "The Temporal Relationship between the Secretion of Luteinizing Hormone and Testosterone in Man". *The Journal of Endocrinology* 64 (1): 17–26.

Safarinejad, M. R., K. Azma, and A. A. Kolahi. 2009. "The Effects of Intensive, Long-Term Treadmill Running on Reproductive Hormones, Hypothalamus-Pituitary-Testis Axis, and Semen Quality: A Randomized Controlled Study". *The Journal of Endocrinology* 200 (3): 259–271.

Seidman, D. S., E. Dolev, P. A. Deuster, R. Burstein, R. Arnon, and Y. Epstein. 1990. "Androgenic Response to Long-Term Physical Training in Male Subjects". *International Journal of Sports Medicine* 11 (6): 421–424.

Shahani, S., M. Braga-Basaria, M. Maggio, and S. Basaria. 2009. "Androgens and Erythropoiesis: Past and Present". *Journal of Endocrinological Investigation* 32 (8): 704–716.

Shen, A. 2011. "Landis/Kimmage". *NYvelocity*, January 31st, 2011.

Shin, B. C., M. S. Lee, E. J. Yang, H. S. Lim, and E. Ernst. 2010. "Maca (L. Meyenii) for Improving Sexual Function: A Systematic Review". *BMC Complementary and Alternative Medicine* 10 (1): 44.

Stone, M., A. Ibarra, M. Roller, A. Zangara, and E. Stevenson. 2009. "A Pilot Investigation into the Effect of Maca Supplementation on Physical Activity and Sexual Desire in Sportsmen". *Journal of Ethnopharmacology* 126 (3): 574–576.

Tauler, P., S. Martinez, C.Moreno, P. Martínez, and A. Aguilo. 2013. "Changes in Salivary Hormones, Immunoglobulin A, and C-Reactive Protein in Response to Ultra-Endurance Exercises". *Applied Physiology, Nutrition, and Metabolism* 39 (5): 560–565.

Tenforde, A. S., M. T. Barrack, A. Nattiv, and M. Fredericson. 2016. "Parallels with the Female Athlete Triad in Male Athletes". *Sports Medicine* 46 (2): 171–182.

Vest Christiansen, A. 2005. "The Legacy of Festina: Patterns of Drug Use in European Cycling Since 1998". *Sport in History* 25 (3): 497–514.

Viru, A. 1992. "Plasma Hormones and Physical Exercise". *International Journal of Sports Medicine* 13 (3): 201–209.

Wheeler, G. D., M. Singh, W. D. Pierce, W. F. Epling, and D. C. Cumming. 1991. "Endurance Training Decreases Serum Testosterone Levels in Men without Change in Luteinizing Hormone Pulsatile Release". *The Journal of Clinical Endocrinology and Metabolism* 72 (2): 422–425.

11 Physical Performance and Antioxidants

Wataru Aoi and Yuji Naito

CONTENTS

11.1 Introduction 205
11.2 Behavior of Exercise-Induced Oxidative Stress 206
11.3 Antioxidants and Exercise-Induced Muscle Damage...................................207
11.4 Antioxidants and Energy Metabolism..208
11.5 Antioxidants and Muscle Mass/Strength.. 211
11.6 Antioxidants and Excitation–Contraction Coupling Fatigue 211
11.7 Perspective.. 212
References.. 213

11.1 INTRODUCTION

Reactive oxygen species (ROS) are generated under various conditions in the living body. A small percentage of the oxygen utilized in the mitochondria is converted to superoxides during the electron transport chain reaction. The skeletal muscle, being a large metabolic organ, is a major source of ROS production. It is known that oxygen consumption during aerobic exercise is elevated 10- to 20-fold in the body, and over 100-fold more in the skeletal muscle alone. Furthermore, the endothelium and invaded phagocytes also produce ROS in muscle tissues catalyzed by enzymes including xanthine oxidase, NADPH oxidase, and myeroperoxidase. Over the past two decades, the impact of ROS on physiological functions and physical performance has been recognized (Figure 11.1).

Various anti-oxidizing factors such as vitamins, carotenoids, and polyphenols are present in natural foods. Previously, the effects of these antioxidants were examined in athletic sports. Intake of certain antioxidants suppresses the exercise-generated oxidative stress, which could potentially attenuate fatigue and improve muscle strength. In contrast, recent studies have shown that a high dose of antioxidants can suppress exercise-induced metabolic benefits. As the generated ROS can act as an activating signal for energy metabolism and protein anabolism, scavenging these ROS may not necessarily benefit athletic performance. Moreover, the effect of antioxidants can vary between the kind and amount of exercise. Thus, it is important to understand how ROS generated during/after exercise act in organs and how individual antioxidant supplements consumed orally can influence the living body.

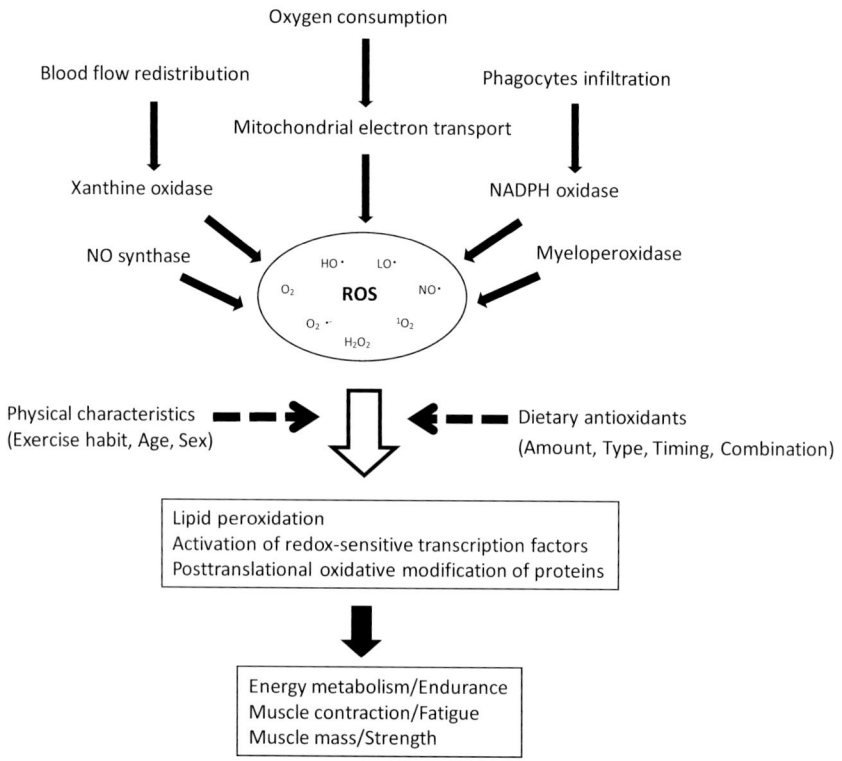

FIGURE 11.1 Exercise-induced oxidative stress and physical modification. Exercise changes several physiological events that produce reactive oxygen species (ROS) in skeletal muscle tissues. According to the amount of ROS, antioxidant capacity, and physical characteristics, muscles are exposed to oxidative stress and cellular components such as DNA, lipids, and proteins are oxidized. Such oxidative stress can also cause transcriptional and post-translational regulation of key proteins and affect their functionality. Consequently, oxidative stress modifies nutrient metabolism and contractile capacity, which can regulate endurance, fatigue, and strength.

11.2 BEHAVIOR OF EXERCISE-INDUCED OXIDATIVE STRESS

During physical exercise, when ROS are generated in quantities beyond the protective capacity of antioxidants, they induce oxidative stress in muscle tissues. Cellular components such as lipids, proteins, and DNA are easy targets for ROS; an accumulation of oxidative products of these components is observed under oxidative stress conditions.

Numerous post-translational modifications can result from direct modifications of the amino acid residues or from the formation of reactive intermediates via the oxidation of other cellular components (Naito and Yoshikawa 2009). Various modifications of the 20 different amino acids play a key role in the function of many proteins. The modifications can be subdivided into two general forms: reversible and irreversible. Some of the lipid peroxidation products exhibit a facile reactivity with proteins, generating a variety of intra- and inter- molecular covalent adducts such as 4-hydroxy-2-nonenal (4-HNE), N^ε-(hexanoyl) lysine (HEL), and carbonylation. It has been shown that cysteine can frequently be oxidized to sulfenic, sulfinic, and sulfonic acids, which in turn, can often be enzymatically reduced. Other frequently detected modifications include nitration, chlorination, and bromination of the target proteins by reactive nitrogen species, hypochlorous acid, and hypobromous acid, respectively.

In contrast to reversible modifications, an irreversible modification is a difficult-to-control chemical reaction that leads to the production of abnormal proteins. Therefore, in many cases, as the abnormal proteins cannot be repaired, the oxidized protein must be catabolized in the proteasome. The modification may occur on constitutive proteins and enzymatic proteins, which regulate various cellular signal transductions. Therefore, the inactivation of upstream proteins in a signal transduction cascade, via oxidative modification, can induce an abnormal cellular response. Much evidence has demonstrated the irreversible post-translational modification of membrane transporters, enzymes, and chaperone proteins in several types of cells. These modifications can be associated with tissue dysfunction and the onset of various common diseases (Bidasee et al. 2004; Hill and Bhatnagar 2012; Oya-Ito et al. 2011).

Oxidative stress also affects gene expression via the regulation of transcription factors. It has been suggested that exercise-induced ROS can activate a series of upstream kinases, such as mitogen-activated protein kinase (MAPK), I-kappa B kinase, protein kinase C, and phosphatidylinositol 3-kinase (PI3K). These kinases can then activate NF-κB by phosphorylation-mediated degradation of I-kappa Bα (Ji et al. 2007; Pianetti et al. 2001). Activated upstream kinases may also phosphorylate p65, the active subunit of NF-κB. Activated NF-κB, in the form of the p65-p50 heterodimer, is translocated to the nucleus, where it binds to the κB sequences located in the promoter of the target gene. Alternatively, MAPKs can activate AP-1 components c-Jun and c-Fos, leading to AP-1 binding to the cyclic AMP response element (CRE) sequences of the target promoter gene (Meyer et al. 1993). Such signaling cascades could mechanistically explain the delayed-onset muscle damage and fatigue.

11.3 ANTIOXIDANTS AND EXERCISE-INDUCED MUSCLE DAMAGE

Unaccustomed and strenuous exercise causes muscle damage—clinically manifested as muscular pain—and involves protein degradation and ultrastructural changes in the muscle. The release of soluble muscle enzymes, most notably creatine kinase (CK), leads to the disruption of the sarcomere architecture (Fridén et al. 1983) and damages the surface membrane (Schwane et al. 1983). Muscle damage usually occurs sometime after exercise (rather than during or immediately after exercise), peaks at about 24–48 h, and is called delayed-onset muscle damage (Maughan et al. 1989). Muscle-damaging exercise leads to phagocytic infiltration into the muscle tissue and this inflammatory response induces the delayed-onset muscle damage (Tidball 1995). Previous studies have shown that delayed-onset muscle damage is induced primarily by not only mechanical stress (Newham et al. 1983; Proske and Morgan 2001), but also oxidative stress (Aoi et al. 2004). Prolonged acute exercise causes neutrophil invasion-mediated muscle damage on the following day. Therefore, delayed-onset muscle damage after exercise is a secondary inflammatory response to ROS. NF-κB and AP-1 activation mediate phagocyte infiltration, transiently activated by a single bout of exercise (Aoi et al. 2004; Hollander et al. 2001).

Previous studies have demonstrated that consuming a diet containing antioxidant vitamins and carotenoids can decrease muscle damage and the accompanying circulating oxidative damage induced by intense exercise (Aoi et al. 2004; Kanter et al. 1993). In contrast, the markers of delayed-onset muscle damage are not always attenuated by these supplements. Overall, in contrast to eccentric exercise and resistance exercise, antioxidants can more easily influence the muscle damage associated with prolonged endurance exercise, as oxidative stress mediates initiation of the muscle damage cascade via activating redox-sensitive transcription. Eccentric and resistance exercises rather cause elevated levels of mechanical stress (likely the major inducer of inflammatory response), rendering it difficult for antioxidants to prevent the initial onset of the inflammatory cascade leading to delayed-onset muscle damage.

Under the conditions of exercise-induced muscle damage, oxidative stress can transiently decrease insulin-stimulated glucose uptake in skeletal muscle. A euglycemic-hyperinsulinemic clamp study (Kirwan et al. 1992) reported that reduced insulin sensitivity and elevated circulating CK levels persist up to 48 h after eccentric exercise in human subjects. It has been shown that the impairment of insulin sensitivity is caused by reduced insulin-dependent glucose uptake signal in the damaged muscle in both mice and humans (Aoi et al. 2012; Del Aguila et al. 2000). In addition to proinflammatory cytokines (such as TNF-α, interleukin-1β, and interleukin-6), the accumulation of 4-HNE—a lipid peroxidation product that covalently modifies proteins on cysteine, histidine, and lysine residues—was observed in the damaged muscle and blood after acute running (Aoi et al. 2012; Liu et al. 2005). Particularly, 4-HNE modification of insulin receptor substrate-1 might mediate the impairment of insulin signal transduction in the damaged muscle (Aoi et al. 2012).

Lactobacillus-fermented milk has various benefits including the promotion of health and prevention of diseases. We have shown that milk fermented with a starter culture containing *Lactobacillus helveticus* and *Saccharomyces cerevisiae* prevents exercise-induced muscle damage in skeletal muscles by inducing the expression of antioxidative enzymes (Aoi et al. 2007). We also found that supplementing *Lactobacillus helveticus*-fermented milk improved glucose metabolism and alleviated muscle soreness after high-intensity exercise in young healthy men (Iwasa et al. 2013). Peptides from fermented milk may act as a signaling factor associated with specific physiological functions. In addition, milk casein hydrolysate (MCH), developed using an *Aspergillus oryzae* protease and including common fermented milk peptides, alleviated muscle soreness and improved glucose metabolism following downhill walking in middle-aged to elderly men (Iwasa et al. 2015). This may increase the level and activity of antioxidant enzymes.

11.4 ANTIOXIDANTS AND ENERGY METABOLISM

Most of the ATP production in muscular mitochondria relies on the consumption of oxygen and, simultaneously, this metabolic process generates ROS. Thus, mitochondrial components can be a major target of oxidative stress. Because mitochondria are the aerobic metabolism centers for glucose/glycogen and fatty acid, their oxidative damage can directly disturb energy metabolism. These disturbances may include reduced energy expenditure, reduced fatty acid oxidation, and accelerated glycogen depletion. Previously, we reported post-translational oxidative modification of a mitochondrial membrane protein in exercised muscles (Aoi et al. 2008). The HEL moiety, a novel adduct formed from the reaction of linoleic acid hydroperoxide and lysine, is a marker of lipid peroxidation-derived protein modification in the initial stages after oxidative stress (Kato et al. 1999; Osawa and Kato 2005). Immediately after exercise, HEL-mediated modification of carnitine palmitoyltransferase I (CPT I), a rate-limiting protein in fatty acyl-CoA entry into the mitochondria (McGarry and Brown 1997), by HEL was increased (Aoi et al. 2008). In contrast, astaxanthin, an antioxidant that accumulates in the mitochondrial membrane, prevented the modification of CPT I by HEL in the exercised muscle, leading to its increased interaction with fatty acid translocase. Several studies have shown that dietary astaxanthin increased fat utilization during exercise, improved endurance, and reduced fat mass (Aoi et al. 2008; Ikeuchi et al. 2006). This may result from the interaction between CPT I and FAT.

Another key modulator of aerobic metabolism in the skeletal muscle is peroxisome proliferator-activated receptor gamma coactivator-1 alpha (PGC-1α), a family of transcriptional co-activators. The activation of PGC-1α alters the metabolic phenotype through its interaction with the nuclear respiratory factor and peroxisome proliferator-activated receptor α (PPARα) (Baar 2004; Patti et al. 2003). This, in turn, improves lipid metabolism, elevates mitochondrial biogenesis, and facilitates a fast-to-slow fiber type switch. Therefore, the activation or expression of PGC-1α is associated with athletic endurance performance (Calvo et al. 2008) and prevention and treatment of obesity and related metabolic diseases such as diabetes (Besseiche et al. 2015). We showed that astaxanthin supplementation increases PGC-1α and mitochondrial contents in mouse skeletal muscle, which may be another mechanism underlying the accelerated lipid metabolism (Liu et al. 2014). The flavonoids catechin and quercetin exist abundantly in fruits and vegetables including onions, apples, and various kinds of teas, and can activate aerobic metabolism and accelerate increased PGC-1α-associated mitochondrial biogenesis (Gahreman et al. 2015; Henagan et al. 2014; Murase et al. 2006). In addition, it has recently been shown that glutathione, a natural food component (including fruit and vegetables), accelerates the aerobic metabolism via mitochondrial biogenesis in skeletal muscle (Aoi et al. 2015). This factor is abundantly synthesized in the human body, although dietary intake can lead to effects different from that produced by the endogenous factor. Other antioxidants, α-lipoic acid and anthocyanins, have beneficial effects on insulin-dependent and -independent glucose metabolism in the muscle (Henriksen 2006).

In some human clinical studies, several antioxidants have been reported to exert positive effects for physical performance (Table 11.1). As found in animal studies, daily supplementation of astaxanthin, quercetin, catechin, and anthocyanins-enriched Black currant improved endurance and VO$_{2max}$ (Cook et al. 2015; Davis et al. 2010; Daneshvar et al. 2013; Earnest et al. 2011; Richards et al. 2010). Intake of glutathione suppressed fatigue-related parameters in cycling exercise (Aoi et al. 2015).

TABLE 11.1

Benefit Findings of Dietary Antioxidants for Physical Performance in Clinical Studies

Compound	Subject	Intake	Efficacy	References
Anthocyanin	Trained	105 mg/day, 7 days	Cycling endurance ↑	Cook et al. (2015)
	Trained	820 mg/day, 6 days	Swimming endurance →	McCormick et al. (2016)
Astaxanthin	Trained	4 mg/day, 4 weeks	Cycling endurance ↑	Earnest et al. (2011)
	Trained	20 mg/day, 4 weeks	Cycling endurance →	Res et al. (2013)
Epigallocatechin-3-gallate	Untrained	405 mg/day, 3 days	VO_{2max} ↑	Richards et al. (2010)
	Trained	270 mg/day, 6 days	Cycling endurance →	Dean et al. (2009)
Glutathione	Untrained	1000 mg/day, 14 days	Fatigue parameters ↓	Aoi et al. (2015)
Quercetin	Untrained	1000 mg/day, 7 days	VO_{2max} ↑	Davis et al. (2010)
	Trained	1000 mg/day, 8 weeks	Cycling endurance ↑	Daneshvar et al. (2013)
	Untrained	1000 mg/day, 6 weeks	VO_{2peak} →	Scholten and Sergeev (2013)

In contrast, other studies have shown that those antioxidants did not have any positive effects (Dean et al. 2009; McCormick et al. 2016; Res et al. 2013; Scholten and Sergeev 2013). Although the exact reason for the discrepancy between studies is unclear, the effectiveness of the compounds may differ according to gender, individual characteristics, and mode of ingestion. Recently, we showed that daily intake of antioxidant-rich foods containing catechin, astaxanthin, quercetin, and anthocyanin could benefit training-induced aerobic metabolism of carbohydrates and fats during rest and exercise in healthy young subjects (Takami et al. 2018). This suggests that those antioxidants may exert the benefit by combined additive effect, even a small amount of individual compound.

Several studies demonstrate that ROS impair insulin-mediated glucose uptake and storage by disrupting signaling control points, such as glycogen synthase kinase-3, Akt phosphorylation, and actin remodeling (Irrcher et al. 2009; Petersen et al. 2003). As mentioned above, muscle damage-induced oxidants suppress insulin-induced glucose uptake and glucose transporter 4 (GLUT4) translocation by impairing insulin receptor activation and PI3-K/Akt signaling (Aoi et al. 2012; Del Aguila et al. 2000). Dietary antioxidants can potentially improve the suppressed glucose metabolism resulting from muscle damage after exercise.

11.5 ANTIOXIDANTS AND MUSCLE MASS/STRENGTH

ROS accelerate muscle atrophy via several pathways. It is well known that ROS stimulate protein degradation via activation of the ubiquitin-proteasome pathway. Polyubiquitinated proteins accumulate in muscle tissues during muscle atrophy (Ikemoto et al. 2001; Tawa et al. 1997). *In vitro* studies also reported that addition of oxidants to muscle cells increased protein degradation via an increased ubiquitination of proteins and expression of major ubiquitin-proteasome pathway proteins (Gomes-Marcondes and Tisdale 2002; Onishi et al. 2005). NF-κB can regulate the ubiquitin-proteasome proteolytic pathway through induction of a ubiquitin ligase, muscle ring finger 1, and proteasome expression (Wyke and Tisdale 2005). Furthermore, it has been shown that the 20S proteasome can selectively degrade oxidatively modified proteins, even without ubiquitination (Grune et al. 2003). These observations suggest that protein degradation could be the link between oxidative stress and muscle atrophy. Alternatively, the intracellular production of ROS could play a key role in the disturbance of calcium homeostasis (Gutierrez-Martin et al. 2004), which could activate the calpain proteolytic system. Intake of several dietary antioxidants may be effective for an improvement in age-related muscle dysfunction. In animal models, vitamin E has been shown to contribute to the maintenance of muscle mass, prior to and during the early phase of immobilization (Appell et al. 1997; Servais et al. 2007). Moreover, other carotenoids and flavonoids could also prevent muscle atrophy (Mukai et al. 2016; Ogawa et al. 2013; Shibaguchi et al. 2016).

In contrast, the effect of oxidative stress on protein synthesis is unclear. Nevertheless, some factors have been shown to stimulate muscular protein synthesis. Protein synthesis is triggered by the insulin-like growth factor-1 (IGF-1) signaling pathway, which in turn activates the mTOR/p70S6K pathway, a protein anabolic signal. Oral administration of β-carotene, a carotenoid, for 14 days increased muscle mass by activating the IGF-1-mediated protein anabolic signaling in mouse skeletal muscle (Kitakaze et al. 2015). Resveratrol, a polyphenol, has also been shown to stimulate the IGF-1-mediated signaling and promote hypertrophy in cultured muscle cells (Montesano et al. 2013).

11.6 ANTIOXIDANTS AND EXCITATION–CONTRACTION COUPLING FATIGUE

It is well established that excess ROS have a negative influence on force generation in the skeletal muscle. The effect of oxidative stress on the sarcoplasmic reticulum (SR)—a subcellular organelle that controls the contractile state of the muscle by regulating the calcium concentration in the cytosol—is associated with force reduction (Andersson et al. 2011; Anzueto et al. 1992). Muscle contraction is performed by increasing intracellular calcium concentrations. Calcium ions are released from the SR via the ryanodine receptor (RyR) calcium-release channel following action potentials during the excitation-contraction coupling process. Afterward, calcium is immediately taken into the SR via the SR calcium-dependent ATPase (SERCA), which relaxes the muscle. It has been known that RyR and SERCA are sensitive to oxidative stress (Daiho et al. 1994; Sun et al. 2001). Consequently, oxidation of RyR and SR proteins tends to increase cytosolic calcium levels, which prevents muscle relaxation.

A study using spin traps and vitamin E in animals demonstrated that scavenging ROS in muscles during exercise delays the onset of muscular fatigue (Novelli et al. 1990). Moreover, several reports have shown that the administration of the antioxidant N-acetylcysteine (NAC), a reduced thiol donor supporting glutathione re-synthesis, delays muscular fatigue during a variety of submaximal exercise including cycling and repetitive handgrip exercise in humans (Cobley et al. 2011; Matuszczak et al. 2005; McKenna et al. 2006; Reid et al. 1994).

11.7   PERSPECTIVE

Exercise-induced oxidative stress plays an important role in improving metabolism adaptation through exercise. This exercise-induced effect does not occur in the absence of oxidative stress, as recognized in the theory of hormesis (Ji et al. 2006). Therefore, there is much debate concerning the intake of dietary antioxidants during exercise. Previously, it has been suggested that a moderate level of oxidative stress caused by low-to-moderate intensity exercise (which does not cause muscle damage) is important for cellular signal transduction.

ROS-induced defense systems include antioxidant enzymes and thiol reductants. These are predominantly regulated by a transcription factor Nrf2 (nuclear erythroid 2-related factor 2), which translocates to the nucleus and binds to the antioxidant-responsive element (ARE)-containing gene (Ding et al. 2008). Exercise induces expression of various antioxidant enzymes via the activation of Nrf2 in human muscles, presumably resulting from moderate oxidative stress in response to exercise (Safdar et al. 2010). NF-κB and MAPK pathways in the skeletal muscle have also been shown to enhance the gene expression of several antioxidant enzymes, such as manganese superoxide dismutase (MnSOD) (Gomez-Cabrera et al. 2008b). Despite ambiguities, moderate exercise can lead to the mild activation of NF-κB and MAPK (without inflammation and with phagocyte infiltration) via moderate oxidative stress, which contributes to the up-regulation of antioxidant capacity.

In contrast, a high-dose of dietary antioxidants, combined with a dietary-exercise regimen, can counteract the oxidative stress that induces beneficial effects of moderate exercise. Therefore, there is some debate about the intake of dietary antioxidants during exercise. Gomez-Cabrera et al. (2008a) demonstrated, in a human double-blind study, that oral administration of vitamin C (1 g/d) suppresses the adaptation of endurance capacity with exercise training for 8 weeks. In this case, the expression of a key modulator of mitochondria biogenesis, PGC-1α, was found to be suppressed. Ristow et al. (2009) also reported that administration of vitamin C (1000 mg/d) and vitamin E (400 IU/d) with a 4-week training intervention significantly ameliorated improvements in glucose infusion rates during a hyper-insulinemic, euglycemic clamp, along with the down-regulation of PGC-1α and Mn-SOD. Therefore, the negative effects of antioxidant vitamins would result from their capacity to reduce the exercise-induced expression of key transcription factors involved in nutrient metabolism and oxidation. Therefore, the effectiveness of the compounds may differ according to gender, individual characteristics, and mode of ingestion. The optimum method of intake, the quantity and quality of the foods to be ingested, and the timing of their intake need to be established in accordance with the purpose of using each food product or component and the physiological changes caused by exercise.

REFERENCES

Andersson, D.C., Betzenhauser, M.J., Reiken, S., et al. 2011. Ryanodine receptor oxidation causes intracellular calcium leak and muscle weakness in aging. *Cell Metab*, 14: 196–207.

Anzueto, A., Andrade, F.H., Maxwell, L.C., et al. 1992. Resistive breathing activates the glutathione redox cycle and impairs performance of rat diaphragm. *J Appl Physiol*, 72: 529–34.

Appell, H.J., Duarte, J.A., Soares, J.M. 1997. Supplementation of vitamin E may attenuate skeletal muscle immobilization atrophy. *Int J Sports Med*, 18: 157–60.

Aoi, W., Naito, Y., Nakamura, T., et al. 2007. Inhibitory effect of fermented milk on delayed-onset muscle damage after exercise. *J Nutr Biochem*, 18: 140–5.

Aoi, W., Naito, Y., Takanami, Y., et al. 2004. Oxidative stress and delayed-onset muscle damage after exercise. *Free Radic Biol Med*, 37: 480–7.

Aoi, W., Naito, Y., Takanami, Y., et al. 2008. Astaxanthin improves muscle lipid metabolism in exercise via inhibitory effect of oxidative CPT I modification. *Biochem Biophys Res Commun*, 366: 892–97.

Aoi, W., Naito, Y., Tokuda, H., et al. 2012. Exercise-induced muscle damage impairs insulin signaling pathway associated with IRS-1 oxidative modification. *Physiol Res*, 61: 81–8.

Aoi, W., Ogaya, Y., Takami, M., et al. 2015. Glutathione supplementation suppresses muscle fatigue induced by prolonged exercise via improved aerobic metabolism. *J Int Soc Sports Nutr*, 12: 7.

Baar, K. 2004. Involvement of PPAR gamma co-activator-1, nuclear respiratory factors 1 and 2, and PPAR alpha in the adaptive response to endurance exercise. *Proc Nutr Soc*, 63: 269–73.

Besseiche, A., Riveline, J.P., Gautier, J.F., et al. 2015. Metabolic roles of PGC-1α and its implications for type 2 diabetes. *Diabetes Metab*, 41: 347–57.

Bidasee, K.R., Zhang, Y., Shao, C.H., et al. 2004. Diabetes increases formation of advanced glycation end products on Sarco(endo)plasmic reticulum Ca2+-ATPase. *Diabetes*, 53: 463–73.

Calvo, J.A., Daniels, T.G., Wang, X., et al. 2008. Muscle-specific expression of PPARgamma coactivator-1alpha improves exercise performance and increases peak oxygen uptake. *J Appl Physiol*, 104: 1304–12.

Cobley, J.N., McGlory, C., Morton, J.P., Close, G.L. 2011. N-acetylcysteine's attenuation of fatigue after repeated bouts of intermittent exercise: Practical implications for tournament situations. *Int J Sport Nutr Exerc Metab*, 21: 451–61.

Cook, M.D., Myers, S.D., Blacker, S.D., Willems, M.E.T. 2015. New Zealand blackcurrant extract improves cycling performance and fat oxidation in cyclists. *Eur J Appl Physiol*, 115: 2357–65.

Daiho, T., Kanazawa, T. 1994. Reduction of disulfide bonds in sarcoplasmic reticulum Ca^{2+}-ATPase by dithiothreitol causes inhibition of phosphoenzyme isomerization in catalytic cycle: This reduction requires binding of both purine nucleotide and Ca^{2+} to enzyme. *J Biol Chem*, 269: 11060–4.

Daneshvar, P., Hariri, M., Ghiasvand, R., et al. 2013. Effect of eight weeks of quercetin supplementation on exercise performance, muscle damage and body muscle in male badminton players. *Int J Prev Med*, 4(Suppl 1): S53–7.

Davis, J.M., Carlstedt, C.J., Chen, S., et al. 2010. The dietary flavonoid quercetin increases VO(2max) and endurance capacity. *Int J Sport Nutr Exerc Metab*, 20: 56–62.

Dean, S., Braakhuis, A., Paton, C. 2009. The effects of EGCG on fat oxidation and endurance performance in male cyclists. *Int J Sport Nutr Exerc Metab*, 19: 624–44.

Del Aguila, L.F., Krishnan, R.K., Ulbrecht, J.S., et al. 2000. Muscle damage impairs insulin stimulation of IRS-1, PI 3-kinase, and Akt-kinase in human skeletal muscle. *Am J Physiol Endocrinol Metab*, 279: E206–12.

Ding, Y., Choi, K.J., Kim, J.H., et al. 2008. Endogenous hydrogen peroxide regulates glutathione redox via nuclear factor erythroid 2-related factor 2 downstream of phosphatidylinositol 3-kinase during muscle differentiation. *Am J Pathol*, 172: 1529–41.

Earnest, C.P., Lupo, M., White, K.M., Church, T.S. 2011. Effect of astaxanthin on cycling time trial performance. *Int J Sports Med*, 32: 882–8.

Fridén, J., Sjöström, M., Ekblom, B. 1983. Myofibrillar damage following intense eccentric exercise in man. *Int J Sports Med*, 4: 170–6.

Gahreman, D., Wang, R., Boutcher, Y., Boutcher, S. 2015. Green tea, intermittent sprinting exercise, and fat oxidation. *Nutrients*, 7: 5646–63.

Gomes-Marcondes, M.C., Tisdale, M.J. 2002. Induction of protein catabolism and the ubiquitin-proteasome pathway by mild oxidative stress. *Cancer Lett*, 180: 69–74.

Gomez-Cabrera, M.C., Domenech, E., Romagnoli, M. et al. 2008a. Oral administration of vitamin C decreases muscle mitochondrial biogenesis and hampers training-induced adaptations in endurance performance. *Am J Clin Nutr*, 87: 142–9.

Gomez-Cabrera, M.C., Domenech, E., Viña, J. 2008b. Moderate exercise is an antioxidant: Upregulation of antioxidant genes by training. *Free Radic Biol Med*, 44: 126–31.

Grune, T., Merker, K., Sandig, G., Davies, K.J.A. 2003. Selective degradation of oxidatively modified protein substrates by the proteasome. *Biochem Biophys Res Commun*, 305: 709–18.

Gutiérrez-Martín, Y., Martín-Romero, F.J., Iñesta-Vaquera F.A., et al. 2004. Modulation of sarcoplasmic reticulum Ca^{2+}-ATPase by chronic and acute exposure to peroxynitrite. *Eur J Biochem*, 271: 2647–57.

Henagan, T.M., Lenard, N.R., Gettys, T.W., Stewart, L.K. 2014. Dietary quercetin supplementation in mice increases skeletal muscle PGC1α expression, improves mitochondrial function and attenuates insulin resistance in a time-specific manner. *PLOS ONE*, 9: e89365.

Henriksen, E.J. 2006. Exercise training and the antioxidant alpha-lipoic acid in the treatment of insulin resistance and type 2 diabetes. *Free Radic Biol Med*, 40: 3–12.

Hill, B.G., Bhatnagar, A. 2012. Protein S-glutathiolation: Redox-sensitive regulation of protein function. *J Mol Cell Cardiol*, 52: 559–67.

Hollander, J., Fiebig, R., Gore, M., et al. 2001. Superoxide dismutase gene expression is activated by a single bout of exercise in rat skeletal muscle. *Pflug Arch*, 442: 426–34.

Ikemoto, M., Nikawa, T., Takeda, S., et al. 2001. Space shuttle flight (STS-90) enhances degradation of rat myosin heavy chain in association with activation of ubiquitin-proteasome pathway. *FASEB J*, 15: 1279–81.

Ikeuchi, M., Koyama, T., Takahashi, J., Yazawa, K. 2006. Effects of astaxanthin supplementation on exercise-induced fatigue in mice. *Biol Pharm Bull*, 29: 2106–10.

Irrcher, I., Ljubicic, V., Hood, D.A. 2009. Interactions between ROS and AMP kinase activity in the regulation of PGC-1α transcription in skeletal muscle cells. *Am J Physiol Cell Physiol*, 296: C116–23.

Iwasa, M., Aoi, W., Mune, K., et al. 2013. Fermented milk improves glucose metabolism in exercise-induced muscle damage in young healthy men. *Nutr J*, 12: 83.

Iwasa, M., Aoi, W., Nakayama, A., et al. 2015. Milk casein hydrolysate alleviates muscle soreness and fatigue after downhill walking exercise in middle-aged to elderly men. *Ann Sports Med Res*, 2: 1045.

Ji, L.L., Gomez-Cabrera, M.C., Vina, J. 2006. Exercise and hormesis: Activation of cellular antioxidant signaling pathway. *Ann N Y Acad Sci*, 1067: 425–35.

Ji, L.L., Gomez-Cabrera, M.C., Vina, J. 2007. Role of nuclear factor kappaB and mitogen-activated protein kinase signaling in exercise-induced antioxidant enzyme adaptation. *Appl Physiol Nutr Metab*, 32: 930–5.

Kato, Y., Mori, Y., Makino, Y., et al. 1999. Formation of Nepsilon-(hexanonyl)lysine in protein exposed to lipid hydroperoxide. A plausible marker for lipid hydroperoxide-derived protein modification. *J Biol Chem*, 274: 20406–14.

Kanter, M.M., Nolte, L.A., Holloszy, J.O. 1993. Effects of an antioxidant vitamin mixture on lipid peroxidation at rest and postexercise. *J Appl Physiol 1985*, 74: 965–9.

Kirwan, J.P., Hickner, R.C., Yarasheski, K.E., et al. 1992. Eccentric exercise induces transient insulin resistance in healthy individuals. *J Appl Physiol*, 72: 2197–202.

Kitakaze, T., Harada, N., Imagita, H., et al. 2015. β-carotene increases muscle mass and hypertrophy in the soleus muscle in mice. *J Nutr Sci Vitaminol (Tokyo)*, 61: 481–7.

Liu, P.H., Aoi, W., Takami, M., et al. 2014. The astaxanthin-induced improvement in lipid metabolism during exercise is mediated by a PGC-1α increase in skeletal muscle. *J Clin Biochem Nutr*, 54: 86–9.

Liu, J.F., Chang, W.Y., Chan, K.H., et al. 2005. Blood lipid peroxides and muscle damage increased following intensive resistance training of female weightlifters. *Ann N Y Acad Sci*, 1042: 255–61.

Matuszczak, Y., Farid, M., Jones, J., et al. 2005. Effects of N-acetylcysteine on glutathione oxidation and fatigue during handgrip exercise. *Muscle Nerve*, 32: 633–8.

Maughan, R.J., Donnelly, A.E., Gleeson, M., et al. 1989. Delayed-onset muscle damage and lipid peroxidation in man after a downhill run. *Muscle Nerve*, 12: 332–6.

McCormick, R., Peeling, P., Binnie, M., et al. 2016. Effect of tart cherry juice on recovery and next day performance in well-trained water polo players. *J Int Soc Sports Nutr*, 13: 41.

McGarry, J.D., Brown, N.F. 1997. The mitochondrial carnitine palmitoyltransferase system. From concept to molecular analysis. *Eur J Biochem*, 244: 1–14.

McKenna, M.J., Medved, I., Goodman, C.A., et al. 2006. N-acetylcysteine attenuates the decline in muscle Na+,K+-pump activity and delays fatigue during prolonged exercise in humans. *J Physiol*, 576: 279–88.

Meyer, M., Schreck, R., Baeuerle, P.A. 1993. H2O2 and antioxidants have opposite effects on activation of NF-kappa B and AP-1 in intact cells: AP-1 as secondary antioxidant-responsive factor. *EMBO J*, 12: 2005–15.

Montesano, A., Luzi, L., Senesi, P., et al. 2013. Resveratrol promotes myogenesis and hypertrophy in murine myoblasts. *J Transl Med*, 11: 310.

Mukai, R., Matsui, N., Fujikura, Y., et al. 2016. Preventive effect of dietary quercetin on disuse muscle atrophy by targeting mitochondria in denervated mice. *J Nutr Biochem*, 31: 67–76.

Murase, T., Haramizu, S., Hase, T., et al. 2006. Green tea extract improves running endurance in mice by stimulating lipid utilization during exercise. *Am J Physiol Regul Integr Comp Physiol*, 290: R1550–6.

Naito, Y., Yoshikawa, T. 2009. Oxidative stress-induced posttranslational modification of proteins as a target of functional food. *Forum Nutr*, 61: 39–54.

Newham, D.J., McPhail, G., Mills, K.R., Edwards, R.H.T. 1983. Ultrastructural changes after concentric and eccentric contractions of human muscle. *J Neurol Sci*, 61: 109–22.

Novelli, G.P., Bracciotti, G., Falsini, S. 1990. Spin-trappers and vitamin E prolong endurance to muscle fatigue in mice. *Free Radic Biol Med*, 8: 9–13.

Ogawa, M., Kariya, Y., Kitakaze, T., et al. 2013. The preventive effect of β-carotene on denervation-induced soleus muscle atrophy in mice. *Br J Nutr*, 109: 1349–58.

Onishi, Y., Hirasaka, K., Ishihara, I., et al. 2005. Identification of mono-ubiquitinated LDH-A in skeletal muscle cells exposed to oxidative stress. *Biochem Biophys Res Commun*, 336: 799–806.

Osawa, T., Kato, Y. 2005. Protective role of antioxidative food factors in oxidative stress caused by hyperglycemia. *Ann N Y Acad Sci*, 1043: 440–51.

Oya-Ito, T., Naito, Y., Takagi, T., et al. 2011. Heat-shock protein 27 (Hsp27) as a target of methylglyoxal in gastrointestinal cancer. *Biochim Biophys Acta*, 1812: 769–81.

Patti, M.E., Butte, A.J., Crunkhorn, S., et al. 2003. Coordinated reduction of genes of oxidative metabolism in humans with insulin resistance and diabetes: Potential role of PGC1 and NRF1. *Proc Natl Acad Sci USA*, 100: 8466–71.

Petersen, K.F., Befroy, D., Dufour, S. 2003. Mitochondrial dysfunction in the elderly: Possible role in insulin resistance. *Science*, 300: 1140–2.

Pianetti, S., Arsura, M., Romieu-Mourez, R., et al. 2001. Her-2/neu overexpression induces NF-kappaB via a PI3-kinase/Akt pathway involving calpain-mediated degradation of IkappaB-alpha that can be inhibited by the tumor suppressor PTEN. *Oncogene*, 20: 1287–99.

Proske, U., Morgan, D.L. 2001. Muscle damage from eccentric exercise: Mechanism, mechanical signs, adaptation and clinical applications. *J Physiol*, 537: 333–45.

Reid, M.B., Stokic, D.S., Koch, S.M., et al. 1994. N-acetylcysteine inhibits muscle fatigue in humans. *J Clin Invest*, 94: 2468–74.

Res, P.T., Cermak, N.M., Stinkens, R., et al. 2013. Astaxanthin supplementation does not augment fat use or improve endurance performance. *Med Sci Sports Exerc*, 45: 1158–65.

Richards, J.C., Lonac, M.C., Johnson, T.K., et al. 2010. Epigallocatechin-3-gallate increases maximal oxygen uptake in adult humans. *Med Sci Sports Exerc*, 42: 739–44.

Ristow, M., Zarse, K., Oberbach, A., et al. 2009. Antioxidants prevent health-promoting effects of physical exercise in humans. *Proc Natl Acad Sci USA*, 106: 8665–70.

Safdar, A., deBeer, J., Tarnopolsky, M.A. 2010. Dysfunctional Nrf2-Keap1 redox signaling in skeletal muscle of the sedentary old. *Free Radic Biol Med*, 49: 1487–93.

Scholten, S.D., Sergeev, I.N. 2013. Long-term quercetin supplementation reduces lipid peroxidation but does not improve performance in endurance runners. *Open Access J Sports Med*, 4: 53–61.

Schwane, J.A., Johnson, S.R., Vandenakker, C.B., Armstrong, R.B. 1983. Delayed-onset muscular soreness and plasma CPK and LDH activities after downhill running. *Med Sci Sports Exerc*, 15: 51–6.

Servais, S., Letexier, D., Favier, R., et al. 2007. Prevention of unloading-induced atrophy by vitamin E supplementation: Links between oxidative stress and soleus muscle proteolysis? *Free Radic Biol Med*, 42: 627–35.

Shibaguchi, T., Yamaguchi, Y., Miyaji, N., et al. 2016. Astaxanthin intake attenuates muscle atrophy caused by immobilization in rats. *Physiol Rep*, 4: e12885.

Sun, J., Xu, L., Eu, J.P., et al. 2001. Classes of thiols that influence the activity of the skeletal muscle calcium release channel. *J Biol Chem*, 276: 15625–30.

Takami, M., Aoi, W., Terajima, H., et al. 2018. Effect of dietary antioxidant-rich foods combined with aerobic training on energy metabolism in healthy young men. *J Clin Biochem Nutr* 64: 79–85.

Tawa, N.E. Jr., Odessey, R., Goldberg, A.L. 1997. Inhibitors of the proteasome reduce the accelerated proteolysis in atrophying rat skeletal muscles. *J Clin Invest*, 100: 197–203.

Tidball, J.G. 1995. Inflammatory cell response to acute muscle injury. *Med Sci Sports Exerc*, 27: 1022–32.

Wyke, S.M., Tisdale, M.J. 2005. NF-kappaB mediates proteolysis-inducing factor induced protein degradation and expression of the ubiquitin-proteasome system in skeletal muscle. *Br J Cancer*, 92: 711–21.

Section IV

Olympic Sports and Evolution
of Current Extreme Sports

12 Greek Olympic Sports
The Beginning of Modern Extreme Sports

Sourya Datta and Debasis Bagchi

CONTENTS

12.1 History of Greek Olympic Sports 220
12.2 Description of Categories of Greek sports 221
12.3 Types of Greek Olympic Sports 221
    12.3.1 Boxing 221
    12.3.2 Wrestling 221
        12.3.2.1 Current Wrestling Rules 221
        12.3.2.2 Greek Wrestling Rules 221
    12.3.3 Equestrian 222
    12.3.4 Running/Foot Race 222
    12.3.5 Long Jump 222
    12.3.6 Pentathlon 222
    12.3.7 Discus Throw, Javelin Throw and Pankration 223
12.4 Other Events in Ancient Greece 223
    12.4.1 Ball Games 223
    12.4.2 Team Sports 223
12.5 Other Extensions 224
    12.5.1 Gladiator Games 224
    12.5.2 Wild Animal Hunting 224
    12.5.3 Chariot Games 225
12.6 Criteria for Being an Olympic Sportsperson 225
12.7 Who Took Part in These Diverse Sports/Games and Why 225
12.8 Training of Athletes 225
12.9 Athletes in Ancient Greece 226
    12.9.1 Nutrition 226
    12.9.2 Doping 226
    12.9.3 Sports and Medicine 226
    12.9.4 Sports and Education 226
    12.9.5 Wounds 226
    12.9.6 Skin Care 227
    12.9.7 Self-Control and Discipline 227
    12.9.8 Gymnasiums and Training 227
    12.9.9 Event Location/Map 227
12.10 Food, Nutrition Requirements and Training of Ancient Greek Athletes 227

12.10.1   Diet 227
12.10.2   Grain 228
12.10.3   Meat 228
12.10.4   Drink/Water 228
12.10.5   Dessert 228
12.10.6   Doping 228
12.11   Differences between Current Athletes from Ancient Olympics in
        Terms of Food Habits 228
12.12   Details on Food and Nutrition in Ancient Greek Society and
        How It Differed for Athletes 229
12.13   Which Modern Foods Would Ancient Greek Athletes Use for Their
        Nutritional Requirements? 230
        12.13.1   Category: Racing 230
        12.13.2   Category: Combat Sports 231
        12.13.3   Category: Pentathlon 232
12.14   Comparison of Ancient Greek Athletes with Modern Athletes ... 233
        12.14.1   Diet Comparisons for Normal People 233
        12.14.2   Athlete Training Comparison 233
12.15   Modern Athletes' Food Requirements 234
12.16   End of the Olympic Games 234
12.17   Transition from the Greek Olympic Games to the Modern Olympic
        Games 234
12.18   Conclusion 235
References 235

Famous Quotes from Olympic and world sports athletes: [1]

"He who is not courageous enough to take risks will accomplish nothing in life"

Muhammad Ali

"I've missed more than 9,000 shots in my career ... I've failed over and over and over again in my life. And that is why I succeed."

Michael Jordan

"We all have dreams. But in order to make dreams come into reality, it takes an awful lot of determination, dedication, self-discipline, and effort."

Jesse Owens

12.1   HISTORY OF GREEK OLYMPIC SPORTS

The ancient Olympic games started in Olympia, which is located in the southwest of Greece. [2] Greek and ancient sports started as only one-day games, and later extended to three-day events from around 776 BC. The ancient games gave rise to the modern Olympic games, which started in 1896. The ancient games were held in honor of Zeus who was king of the gods. The oath ceremony of the athletes was one of a kind where oaths were sworn on slices of boar's flesh. [3]

The ancient Greek Olympics actually continued for a long time (started from 776 BC and continuing until the late fourth century AD). It was so enormous and vital that a sacred truce was created every four years during the games for safe passage for all travelers including athletes, coaches and spectators through all different states. Only free men were allowed to participate. The price for winning might not seem very grand in modern times, but at that time it had a lot of value, not just money and food but also the recognition and honour of being an Olympic champion, which came with top-tier recognition and immense pride. The athletes were crowned with a crown made of olive leaves, which were specially cut from the Zeus grove.

12.2   DESCRIPTION OF CATEGORIES OF GREEK SPORTS [3]

The Greek event would start in summer and initially there were no winter events. There were no tracks for running and water sports were non-existent. Women older than 18 were barred from entering and there were no women involved in these sport events. However, for equestrian events, the winner was not just the jockey but also the owner, who could often be a woman. Team sports were also missing, and there was no concept of second or third place.

12.3   TYPES OF GREEK OLYMPIC SPORTS

In the early stages, there were seven specific types of games.

12.3.1   BOXING

Boxers had to wear straps for strengthening the fingers and hands. Instead of soft wraps, boxers started using hard wraps which would disfigure the opponent's face. This was legal in the early Greek Olympics.

12.3.2   WRESTLING

Wrestling is very similar to the current format in the Olympic games. Wrestling, just like today's games, did not include weapons.

12.3.2.1   Current Wrestling Rules

Wrestling matches consist of three periods and the length of the periods vary as per different age group. A winner is declared if any one of the wrestlers is able to pin the other wrestler or if there is a difference of 14 points between the two wrestlers. If either of the options mentioned above don't happen, the wrestler who has accumulated more points than the other by the end of third period is declared the winner. If there is a tie by the end of three rounds, it goes to overtime where one wrestler emerges victorious.

12.3.2.2   Greek Wrestling Rules

Greek wrestling rules were slightly different, and the modern wrestling has evolved from Greek wrestling. It was a point system. A total of three points was required to win the match, however the wrestler could also win outright. The three different ways of winning are:

    a. Creating a pin down or submissive hold over the opponent
    b. Forcing opponent out of wrestling area
    c. Winning by points

Points were collected when the other player would touch the ground – in this case the touch was considered as a point loss only when the upper body (back, hip, shoulder) touched the ground.

The competitions were all elimination style and only one wrestler will emerge victorious.

12.3.3   Equestrian

Equestrian games were of mainly two types:

    i. Horse race
   ii. Chariot race

12.3.4   Running/Foot Race

Three different types of races were contested in early Greek sports:

    i. Short distance (stade race)
   ii. Middle distance (diaulos)
  iii. Long distance (dolichos)

Short distance, middle distance and long distance were based on the distance covered.

Short distance: 200 m-foot race. This covered one stade, which is one Olympic track end to end.

Middle distance: 400 m-foot race. This covered two stades, which is one Olympic track end to end twice

Long Distance: Varied, this could range between 7 to 24 stades.

The Greek Marathon actually led to the modern Olympics.

12.3.5   Long Jump

Long jumps were of two different types:

    i. Use of a stone weight
   ii. Use of a lead weight

The concept of the long jump was the same as the present version. Athletes could use either stone or lead for propelling themselves for the jump.

12.3.6   Pentathlon

The pentathlon contained five contests (long jump, discus throwing, javelin throwing, running and wrestling).

The long jump, wrestling and running are described above. Discus throw and javelin throw are very similar to their versions in the current Olympic games.

12.3.7 Discus Throw, Javelin Throw and Pankration

i. Discus Throw

In terms of technique, the discus throw event of the ancient Greek Olympicsis very similar to the version in today's Olympic games. The discus was made of iron initially, then lead was used and finally bronze.

ii. Javelin Throw

Not much is different for the javelin throw; it too is similar to today's version.

iii. Pankration

Pankration was a combination of wrestling and boxing. Everything was allowed apart from biting and eye gouging. Athletes wore light boxing gloves to protect their hands and not necessarily the face of their opponents. A decision on the winner was made when an athlete gave up or could not continue any further and was recognized as unable to do so by the judges.

12.4 OTHER EVENTS IN ANCIENT GREECE: [4]

The games described below were not part of the Greek Olympic games but had a major influence on defining the modern Olympic games.

12.4.1 Ball Games

Ball games or ball sports were not part of any professional event. Ball games, popularly called ball sports, were played by both males and females. Girls played mostly at home, in the courtyard or in their rooms. The 'horse with rider' game was extremely popular and mostly played by two people at a time. Two girls would throw the ball at the target and whoever's ball was closer to the target would win. The losing girl would carry the winner on their back and go to fetch the ball.

Boys played ball games in the gymnasium and such games were apart of their physical education. There were two kinds of games—in one game the ball was soft and small while the other had a harder bouncing ball. For the 'horse with rider' game, the trainer would throw the ball and each of the boys would try to catch. Another popular game was 'ball on the line' where the ball was positioned on a line in the middle of the field. On both sides of the line there was a small field and the goal of the game was to throw the ball from the middle beyond the square of the opponent so that the opponent's team couldn't catch it.

12.4.2 Team Sports

Even though there were no concepts of team sports in ancient Greece, there were a few games that were played not as a part of a competition but more to improve community spirit. One extremely popular game was the torch race, which was nothing but a relay race. Team members carried a torch which was relayed through the team and the goal was to finish before all other relay teams. Boat races were also common, where boats were operated by a team.

Apart from these few team games, almost all games were individual. Greeks were extremely competitive and hence the concept of team games was almost non existent. One person wanted to be the best. However, once the Romans captured Greece, more team games started and Romans brought in their own games.

12.5   OTHER EXTENSIONS

Roman sports also became very popular within a few years of the Roman conquest and a few specific games were extremely popular. A list of Roman games are described below.

12.5.1   GLADIATOR GAMES: [4]

Gladiator combat games used to take place in the afternoon following public executions in the morning and wild animal hunting. The gladiator fights were not organized by state like horse races but by private persons who had a lot of money. There were different types of gladiators:

Based on their knowledge of fighting:

i. Gauls and Thracians: native region fighters. These were considered the top category of fighters.
ii. Slaves: slaves were trained as gladiators due to a limited availability of people.

Based on the types of weapons used:

i. Thracian/Thraex: short shield and a short, curved sword.
ii. Murmillo: longer shield and a long sword. the helmet used was long and wide and had a vertical rim.
iii. Secutor: similar to Murmillo. A special helmet protected the face.
iv. Retiarius: the body wasn't protected and gladiators used a net and trident for fighting.

Gladiator contests were a big occasion and doctors were associated with most of the events, but if the gladiator lost, then his life depended on the mercy of the emperor and the grace of the public.

12.5.2   WILD ANIMAL HUNTING

Wild animal hunt started in the morning within the amphitheater. There were different activities at different times. The following table shows the details of activities that took place at different times.

Activity Sequence	Activities
First Activity	Fights between animals (e.g. lion _versus_ leopard, bull versus elephant)
Second Activity	Intermezzo (tricks performed by tamed animals)
Third Activity	Fight between trained men and wild animal • One man against one animal • Group of men against group of animal
Lunch time Activity	Public Execution • Citizens killed with sword • Slaves were crucified • Defenseless prisoners thrown in front of wild animals

12.5.3 CHARIOT GAMES: [5]

There was a basic difference between the Greek way of visualizing and performing games and the Roman way of seeing and performing in the games. Greeks believed in competition and enjoyment and to them spectator/viewership was secondary. To the Romans, however, the entertainment of spectators was primary. Romans had two horse- and four-horse chariots but there were no races which involved drivers. In almost all cases, participants were slaves and not free men. One of the most important distinguishing features in the Roman chariot games as compared to the Greek version was that there was not a single owner of the horse as well as the horse and jockey not belonging to a single owner and not running to increase the owner's prestige. There were four stables and factions—red, white, blue and greens, all of which participated in chariots. The Roman crowd supported a color but not a particular owner.

12.6 CRITERIA FOR BEING AN OLYMPIC SPORTSPERSON: [5]

There were three main criteria for a person to be able to participate in Olympic sports. The athlete needed to be male, of Greek origin and free. If any of the criteria were not met, then the athlete was not allowed to participate in the games. Foreigners, slaves and women were not allowed to participate, however, women, as said, could own horses.

12.7 WHO TOOK PART IN THESE DIVERSE SPORTS/GAMES AND WHY

i.   The competitors/athletes went on their own to take part and they spent their own money, but there was a screening before they were allowed to participate. [6]

ii. The training required three important factors—time, money and instruction—and there were no concepts of government backing or subsidy at that time.

iii. Even though the wreath crown had no monetary value, it would be unwise to think that athletes were not material thinkers. The athletes were rewarded immensely after their win by the city/state that they represented and in the sixth century Athenian Olympians who came out victorious were given 500 drachmas (close to $300,000). This was not a 'one-off' situation, and more often than not the victorious athlete would be given food and grand rewards.

12.8 TRAINING OF ATHLETES

All the participants had to train for at least 10 months and the training for the final month was carried out at Elis, a city that was very close to Olympia. Training at Elis was an extremely important phase since an athlete could be debarred from entering the main competition if they were not given a 'go-ahead' by the judges, who held enormous power. A number of things changed from the sixth century BC. Athletes started becoming more trained, gave more importance to training, food and diet and even started hiring personal coaches. [7]

Greek athletes were not only trained in gymnasia but also at places called palaestrae, which were distinct from the gymnasia. The head of a gymnasium was called the gymnasiarch and these were the superintendents of the gymnasia.

12.9 ATHLETES IN ANCIENT GREECE

12.9.1 NUTRITION

Initially, athletes were more focused on carbohydrate diets but later realized the importance of protein. Most athletes consumed protein, which was not readily available to other sectors of society in Greece. Details of food and nutrition are covered in this chapter. [8]

12.9.2 DOPING: [9]

Doping in older forms did exist, just as it exists in today's world. In ancient Greece, professional athletes had trainers and attendants. Trainers were extremely powerful and had a lot of say in the life of ancient Greek athletes. Each trainer created a strict schedule for the athletes. They created the diet and set of remedies—not always very scientific, and sometimes based on belief as well. It has been claimed that every trainer considered themselves a great doctor and the trainers would sometimes provide herbal potions and also use potions for wounds. The effect and impact of real doping is not very clear, especially since there were no rules and nothing was specifically forbidden. Most plants that can actually enhance performance are from South America, so there was no access to them for the Greeks. Black magic was prohibited, though sometimes ancient Greek athletes tried to curse their opponents.

12.9.3 SPORTS AND MEDICINE: [10]

Sports were always considered healthy. Exercise was considered extremely beneficial for healthy living. At the same time, extreme conditioning and training were not supported, and were condemned by doctors.

12.9.4 SPORTS AND EDUCATION: [11]

Sports were extremely important in the life of ancient Greeks, and a number of ancient well-to-do Greeks didn't just spend their lives being spectators but actively participated in the games. Education had a huge impact behind the scenes of sports. There were three types of teachers who were each responsible for specific areas:

  i. Intellectual education for reading and writing
  ii. Cultural upbringing for music and dance
  iii. Sports training (athletics)

Training was provided from an early age and made the young boys ready for the Olympics early in their lives. For girls, however, there were not so many options, and only Spartan girls received sports training and education.

12.9.5 WOUNDS: [12]

Athletes would be wounded, and in most cases this would happen in combat sports. The face would be often battered for boxers since this is where most punches would fall. Another area where the boxers would show signs of being battered would be the ears, which would show huge lumps, known as 'cauliflower ears'. Boxers would use leather straps so that punches could become harder. Unlike today's boxing gloves, which have some amount of protection due to the soft padding, ancient Greek boxers only used hard straps and this often resulted in the disfigurement of opponent's faces.

12.9.6 SKIN CARE: [13]

Skin and hygiene care was a big concern for ancient Greek athletes. After training, the athletes would use pure olive oil and apply it on the skin. This had three main purposes: a. to make the skin glossy and supple, b. to protect against too much heat and/or too much cold, and c. for esthetic reasons. After applying oil, dust was sprinkled on top of the skin. After the entire process, athletes used an iron scraper to scrape the dirt off and after a shower of cold and warm water, re-applied oil. This helped in rehydration of the skin.

12.9.7 SELF-CONTROL AND DISCIPLINE: [14]

Self-control and discipline was one of the major requirements for ancient Greek athletes. Abstinence from sex was extremely important since sperm was an indication of strength and masculinity, and both needed to be shown during the Olympic games.

12.9.8 GYMNASIUMS AND TRAINING: [15]

Ancient Greek athletes used to train naked and hence the name gymnasiums, which comes from the Greek term *gymnós*, meaning naked. The gymnasium was moved from outside the city to the city center and developed as a secondary marketplace. The gymnasium had multiple rooms—a wrestling pit, a room with punching bags, a room with sand for wrestling, a dressing room, a running track, a room for baths, a room for body care, a room for messages, a dining room and a library, to name a few.

12.9.9 EVENT LOCATION/MAP: [16]

The event location was spectacular. The main stadium was grand and at that time had all the ingredients (in the concept of an Olympic village) that later developed into the current Olympic village.

12.10 FOOD, NUTRITION REQUIREMENTS AND TRAINING OF ANCIENT GREEK ATHLETES

12.10.1 DIET

The diet of most common people in ancient Greece consisted of bread, vegetables and fruits. Fish was also an integral part of the diet, mainly due to the close proximity of the sea. However, early athlete diets were completely different from the diets of modern athletes. One of the major differences between current and ancient Greek athletes was their social stature. Most Greek Olympians came from upper class of society and hence were able to get more meat instead of vegetables, fruits and breads. The initial diets of athletes were food and vegetable based but slowly changed to meat based. Nuts and dried figs were also very popular with Greek athletes and wine was used both for cooking and drinking.

12.10.2 GRAIN

The most important grain was barley. [2]

Barley was considered to have some important characteristics that were better than wheat. Barley was considered by ancient Greek athletes and coaches to give more energy and make athletes feel stronger and healthier than wheat. Wheat was always considered a secondary food item and was looked down upon, and even held responsible for an athlete's poor performance. Early 600 BC saw strict guidelines for food, and a mostly vegetarian diet was administered consisting of barley and nuts, as well as dried figs, bread and cheese. Cheese was actually extremely famous and was either moist or a newer cheese was available called turoi [17] At a later date, athletes started consuming wheat known as puroi.

12.10.3 MEAT

Meat became quite popular for Greek athletes and in most cases was important for athletes who were involved in the games which required either endurance or strength. The table below shows the type of sport along with the preferred meat corresponding to the type of activity.

Type of Sports	Type of Meat
Boxers	Bull meat
Wrestlers	Pork and pork fat
Jumpers	Goat meat
Runners	Goat meat

12.10.4 DRINK/WATER

In almost all cases, water was regular and cold water wasn't allowed. Wine was allowed only on a number of occasions during the day.

12.10.5 DESSERT

Most or all dessert was forbidden, especially the very popular honey cake or penmata.

12.10.6 DOPING

Doping, just like today, was prevalent in this period, although perhaps not to such a scale as it is now. A very common form of doping was using raw animal testicles. There was not a strict program which would check for an athlete's purity, nor any formal process to evaluate athletes' progress.

12.11 DIFFERENCES BETWEEN CURRENT ATHLETES FROM ANCIENT OLYMPICS IN TERMS OF FOOD HABITS [26,27]

The diets of recent athletes have changed a lot from where they started initially. Let's discuss how food has evolved through different times.

Early Greek/Roman Food: diets were mostly vegetarian and based primarily on fruits, vegetable, cereals, nuts and wine. Dried fig was also very popular. Meat came much later and was made popular in ancient Greece by Milo of Croton (who won wrestling in five Olympics from 532 BC to 516 BC). He was a huge proponent of meat and according to Greek texts he ate 20 lbs of meat every day. It is difficult to get more detailed explanation of earlier Greek food habits.

Past Olympic games: the 1952 Olympic games showed that the diets of most Olympic athletes were a combination of high protein, high fat and high energy. An average daily intake of 19,000kJ (kilojoules)* of daily energy were consumed by Olympians and 40% of this came from fat, 40% from carbohydrate and 20% from protein. The dietary intake varied from country to country and it ranged from as low as 7700 to 25,000 KJ. The percentage of fat varied from 29% to 49%, carbohydrate ranged from 33% to 57% and protein ranged from 12% to 26%.

Current Olympic games: Current Olympic games have seen another change in food habit and restrictions. The options have increased tremendously and food is prepared not only based on exclusively dietary requirements but is based on country, ethnicity and other related factors. Many more choices in types of meat, cheese, and food ranging from South American cuisine to Asian along with unique fruits from all over the world are part of the menu.

12.12 DETAILS ON FOOD AND NUTRITION IN ANCIENT GREEK SOCIETY AND HOW IT DIFFERED FOR ATHLETES

There were differences between ancient Greek athletes and other people in general society. [18] Food habits varied vastly and the table here captures the diet of normal people and Greek athletes.

Normal People	Ancient Greek Athletes
Daily food consisted of corn-porridge or bread and a side dish. The side dish could be one of the following: • Fresh vegetables • Cheese • Dried Figs • Olives	Food consisted of enough proteins for muscle growth. Most of the athletes needed a lot of meat and fish.
Protein came from fish as it was more common than meat, which was eaten rarely, mostly during an occasion.	Protein was obtained through meat and fish.
Normal people were poor so they would go for cheaper food options and meat was a delicacy.	Athletes in ancient Greece were in general rich and so could afford to pay more for food.
Normal people were allowed to eat sweets and there weren't very strict protocols about the quantity and frequency of such consumption.	Generally, athletes were not allowed to eat sweets, or there were strict protocols about the quantity of sweet consumption.

* 1000 KJ = 239 calories, 19,000 KJ = ~4500 Calories

Quantity of food consumed was normal.

Often, athletes have been referred to as 'gluttons'. Since there was no weight limit criteria, and there were no weight categories, the heavier an athlete's weight, the more advantages they had. This was especially true for athletes in combat sports while, on the other hand, runners needed to be more careful since they needed to be more agile and in better shape.

12.13   WHICH MODERN FOODS WOULD ANCIENT GREEK ATHLETES USE FOR THEIR NUTRITIONAL REQUIREMENTS? [19]

12.13.1   CATEGORY: RACING

Racing would include three distance running events (stade, diaulos and dolichos) and two special events (races in armor and the torch-race). For racing, the following types of food would be important—fat, carbohydrates, herbal extracts, electrolytes, liquids and other supplemental food.

Fats: provide energy
Time for consumption: part of regular diet
Types of food providing necessary nutrition: meats, fish, nuts
Extensions: regular food (generally non-specific)
Ingredients: regular food
Carbohydrates: store glycogen in liver and muscles
Time for consumption:
   a.   An hour before exercise
   b.   For longer workouts, small amount of carbs to be taken at mid-point of exercise
Types of food providing necessary nutrition: pasta, potatoes, oatmeal, bananas, fruits
Extensions: energy bars and drinks, gels
Ingredients: glucose, maltodextrin, cyclic dextrin

Herbal Extracts: increase blood flow through the muscle and used to burn fat
Time for consumption: before exercise
Types of food providing necessary nutrition: green tea, black tea, black coffee
Extensions: drink supplements
Ingredients: caffeine, quercetin

Electrolytes: replenish electrolytes in the body
Time for consumption: during strenuous workout
Types of food providing necessary nutrition: sports drinks
Food product extensions: electrolyte tablets
Ingredients: sodium, magnesium, potassium

Liquids: keep body hydrated

Time for consumption: before workout, during workout and after workout (ideally 10–15 minutes during workout)

Types of food providing necessary nutrition: regular water, coconut water and fruit juice

Extensions: sports drinks

Ingredients: regular water, juice

12.13.2 Category: Combat Sports

Combat sports would include wrestling, boxing and pankration

For combat sports, different types of food are extremely important - protein, carbohydrates, minerals, Omega-3 fatty acids and glucosamine

Protein: helps muscle repair

Time for consumption: half an hour before and after exercise

Types of food providing necessary nutrition: egg, chicken, red and black beans

Extensions: protein bars, energy bars, drink, supplements

Ingredients: soy protein, whey protein, L-Glutamine, amino acids

Carbohydrate: replenishes glycogen

Time for consumption: one hour before exercise and one hour after exercise

Types of food providing necessary nutrition: chicken, meat, nuts, seeds

Extensions: protein powder

Ingredients: glucose, maltodextrin, trehalose, cyclic dextrins

Minerals: make muscle health better

Time for consumption: no particular time (part of diet)

Types of food providing necessary nutrition: meat (Red meat), beans, green vegetables

Extensions: supplements

Ingredients: zinc, iron, calcium

Omega-3 fatty acids: reduces muscle soreness

Time for consumption: after workout

Types of food providing necessary nutrition: fish

Extensions: supplements

Ingredients: combination of alpha-linolenic acid (ALA), eicosapentaenoic acid (EPA) and docasahexaenoic acid (DHA), which is basically long-chain polyunsaturated fatty acids (LC-PUFAs) [20]

Glucosamine: relieves joint pain

Time for consumption: after workout

Types of food providing necessary nutrition: shrimp, lobster, crab and crawfish

Extensions: supplements

Ingredients: glycosylated proteins, lipids

12.13.3 Category: Pentathlon

Type of food and nutrition required for the two sports would be discussed: discus throwing and javelin throwing

Mainly six different types of food are extremely important—protein, vitamins, herbal extracts, glutamine, probiotics and fish oil

Protein: used for muscle repair
Time for consumption: both before and after workout
Types of food providing necessary nutrition: meat (red meat), beans, green vegetables
Extensions: protein powder
Ingredients: soy protein, whey protein

Vitamins: used for improving bone health and muscle function
Time for consumption: part of regular diet
Types of food providing necessary nutrition: apart from food, sunlight is a great source
Extensions: supplements
Ingredients: Vitamin C and D

Herbal extracts: reduces inflammation and provides oxidation
Time for consumption: part of regular diet
Types of food providing necessary nutrition: dark color vegetables and fruits
Extensions: supplements
Ingredients: green tea extract, quercetin

Glutamine: improves immunity and gut health
Time for consumption: Part of regular diet and also important after workout
Types of food providing necessary nutrition: spinach, parsley
Extensions: supplements
Ingredients: L-glutamine

Probiotics: Improves immunity and gut health
Time for consumption: part of regular diet and also after workout
Types of food providing necessary nutrition: yogurt and curd
Extensions: supplements
Ingredients: live bacteria

Fish Oil: improves immunity and also reduces inflammation
Time for consumption: part of regular diet
Types of food providing necessary nutrition: fish
Extensions: supplements
Ingredients: Omega-3 [21]

12.14   COMPARISON OF ANCIENT GREEK ATHLETES WITH MODERN ATHLETES: [22]

12.14.1   Diet Comparisons for Normal People

Ancient Greek Diet	Modern Diet
Diet was based on cereals (carbohydrates), olive oil (fat) and wine.	Diet is more wholesome, consisting of protein, carbohydrate and fat.
Protein was obtained from cheese	Protein is obtained from different sources: on one hand, protein is obtained from lean white meats, e.g., fish or chicken. Red meat is also another source of protein, though is less healthy than the lean meats.
Fiber and carbohydrate needs were satisfied but diet was inadequate for protein and vitamins.	A more balanced diet and approach has been set up. Adequate amounts of protein, carbohydrate, fat and vitamins are obtained.

Diet Comparisons for Athletes

Ancient Greek Diet	Modern Diet
High carbohydrate diet.	Combination of high carbohydrate and high protein diet.
Cheese along with wheat formed the basis of diets,with vegetables also forming an important part. A number of vegetables were common, including beans, onions, beets, garlic and peas.	Diet is determined depending on the type of sport. A good mix of vegetables, fish, chicken and meat is provided for optimum health.
The most common fruits included dried figs, dates, apples and pears.	There is more fruit, both in quantity and options.
Meat was introduced much later in the diet. Diets in later times included higher amounts of red meat and involved meat from deer, oxen, bulls and goats.	Meat has long been a part of diet. Lean meat is preferred over red meat.
Trainers took on the responsibility of providing diet and nutritional advice, and the concept of physicians came in much later.	Trainers take care of only the training part. Physicians are responsible for food and diet along with doctors.

12.14.2   Athlete Training Comparison

Greek Athletes	Modern Athletes
Athletes took part in military training. The ancient Olympic games consisted of games that included combat, archery, discus and javelin throwing, wrestling, boxing and running.	Modern athletes are generally categorized in two groups: 1. Endurance athletes 2. High intensity, short duration athletes
More importance was given to strength and most of the games were tests of strength.	Endurance athletes need a lot of energy and often need carbohydrates to allow glycogen absorption. These athletes need 'carbohydrate loading'.

High intensity athletes use glycogen as the primary energy source. High carbohydrate diets for a week prior to actual activity result in better performance.

Two specific types of training were administered: one type of game required frequent use of arm and leg muscles, while the other type of game required the use of different body parts and a lot of strength. These two groups were treated differently. The first group were involved in chariot racing while the second group were involved in wrestling and pankration.

Training has become more versatile and, depending on the type of sport and competition, training methods are changed.

12.15   MODERN ATHLETES' FOOD REQUIREMENTS: [23]

Currently, nutritionists and athletes' trainers/coaches recommend diets which have a combination of appropriate protein, carbohydrates, fat, vitamins, amino acids and minerals—the quantity of each ingredient depends on the nature of the game and the participant.

12.16   END OF THE OLYMPIC GAMES: [24]

Rome conquered Greece in 146 BC, which caused the demise of the Olympic games. 393 AD marked the year in which Emperor Theodosius I abolished most of the Olympic games centers, which resulted in the demise of the Olympic games going forward after their one thousand years of history. All the sites were slowly destroyed and earthquakes and flooding intensified the destruction. Finally, in 1875, Germans with the approval of Greek authorities excavated the location and discovered ancient Olympia.

12.17   TRANSITION FROM THE GREEK OLYMPIC GAMES TO THE MODERN OLYMPIC GAMES: [25]

The ancient Olympic games originally allowed only Greeks to participate, while non-Greeks were termed as barbarians and not even allowed to apply to participate. There was no concept of second or third place and there was only one winner. Women weren't allowed to participate and the only time when a woman could win was when she would be the owner of the chariot which won the race. There was very limited team games and almost no importance given to the viewers of the Olympic games; it was all about the participants and the winner. Things completely changed when the Romans conquered Greece and forced Greece to allow Romans to compete. Romans changed the format of the games and more team games were introduced. Viewer quality was also thought about for the first time.

Every four years, the Romans held the games and this continued until 393 AD when Theodosius I came into power. Nero even pushed the Olympic date forward two years so that he could participate. Even though he fell from his chariot and was a complete failure, he was still awarded the crown. However, after that the games continued and every four years the games were played at different locations, which has continued to date.

12.18   CONCLUSION

Overall, the world has come a long way with the introduction of diverse games, varied and difficult athletic performances, cutting-edge techniques, highly trained athletes, superior training personnel and well-developed nutritional supplements, along with technology which helps in developing the participation of new athletes in diverse sporting activities.

REFERENCES

1. Coles T. Famous Olympic Quotes to Get Inspired About the Games. https://www. huffingtonpost.ca/2014/02/07/famous-olympic-quotes_n_4745472.html(AccessedJune 16, 2018)

2. Medrano K. The Ancient Olympian Diet Was Pretty Tame; 2016. https://www.inverse. com/article/19074-2016-rio-olympics-ancient-olympian-diet-food (Accessed June 18, 2018)

3. Kyle, D.G. Winning at Olympia; 2004. http://archive.archaeology.org/online/features/ olympics/olympia.html (Accessed June 16, 2018)

4. Clarysse W., Remijsen S., Haiying Y., Jing W., Xiang W. Ancient Olympics; 2012. http: //ancientolympics.arts.kuleuven.be/eng/TC000EN.html (Accessed June 20, 2018)

5. International Olympic Committee. Factsheet. The Olympic Games of Antiquity; 2012. https://stillmed.olympic.org/media/Document%20Library/OlympicOrg/Factsheets -Reference-Documents/Games/OG-of-Antiquity/Factsheet-The-Olympic-Games-of-A ntiquity-May-2012.pdf#_ga=1.183844385.629319118.1487433097 (Accessed May 20, 2018)

6. Archaeological Institute of America. Ancient Olympics Guide; 2004. http://archive. archaeology.org/online/features/olympics/olympia.html (Accessed May 30, 2018)

7. Kyle D.G. *Athletics in Ancient Athens*. Leiden: E.J. Brill; rev. ed., 1993 (Accessed May 30, 2018)

8. Faculty of Arts, Department of Ancient History, Belgium. Ancient Olympics, Nutrition; 2012. http://ancientolympics.arts.kuleuven.be/eng/TC023EN.html (Accessed May 30, 2018)

9. Faculty of Arts, Department of Ancient History, Belgium. Ancient Olympics, Doping; 2012. http://ancientolympics.arts.kuleuven.be/eng/TC024EN.html (Accessed May 30, 2018)

10. Faculty of Arts, Department of Ancient History, Belgium. Ancient Olympics, Sport and Medicine; 2012. http://ancientolympics.arts.kuleuven.be/eng/TC027EN.html (Accessed May 30, 2018)

11. Faculty of Arts, Department of Ancient History, Belgium. Ancient Olympics, Sport and Education; 2012. http://ancientolympics.arts.kuleuven.be/eng/TD029EN.html (Accessed May 30, 2018)

12. Faculty of Arts, Department of Ancient History, Belgium. Ancient Olympics, Wounds; 2012. http://ancientolympics.arts.kuleuven.be/eng/TC026EN.html (Accessed May 30, 2018)

13. Faculty of Arts, Department of Ancient History, Belgium. Ancient Olympics, Hygiene and Care of Skin; 2012. http://ancientolympics.arts.kuleuven.be/eng/TC025EN.html (Accessed May 30, 2018)

14. Faculty of Arts, Department of Ancient History, Belgium. Ancient Olympics, the Self-Control of Athletes, an Ascetic Ideal; 2012. http://ancientolympics.arts.kuleuven.be/eng/TC022EN.html (Accessed May 30, 2018)

15. Faculty of Arts, Department of Ancient History, Belgium. Ancient Olympics, the Gymnasion; 2012. http://ancientolympics.arts.kuleuven.be/eng/TC028EN.html (Accessed May 30, 2018)

16. Shepherd, W.R. Map of Olympia, the Historical Atlas; 1923. http://www.hellenicaworld.com/Greece/Geo/en/OlympiaMap.html (Accessed May 30, 2018)

17. Kyle, D.G. *Sport and Spectacle in the Ancient World*, 1st edition, London: Wiley-Blackwell; 2007.

18. Faculty of Arts – Department of Ancient History, Belgium. Ancient Olympics, Hygiene and Care of Skin; 2012. http://ancientolympics.arts.kuleuven.be/eng/TC023EN.html (Accessed June 18, 2018)

19. Faculty of Arts – Department of Ancient History, Belgium. Ancient Olympics, Greek Sport: The Events and the Athletes; 2012. http://ancientolympics.arts.kuleuven.be/eng/TC000EN.html (Accessed June 18, 2018)

20. Toops, D. Understanding Omega-3 Fatty Acids; 2009. https://www.foodprocessing.com/articles/2009/augustwellnessomega/ (Accessed June 18, 2018)

21. Four String Farm. The Ideals of the Ancient Olympians; 2014. https://fourstringfarm.com/tag/food-of-ancient-olympics/(Accessed June 18,2018)

22. Harrison, A. & Bartels E.M. A Comparison of Ancient Greek and Roman Sports Diets with Modern Day Practices; 2016. https://www.researchgate.net/publication/309453257_A_Comparison_of_Ancient_Greek_and_Roman_Sports_Diets_with_Modern_Day_Practices (Accessed June 18, 2018)

23. Harrison, A. & Bartels E.M. Sports Nutrition and Therapy; 2016. https://www.researchgate.net/publication/309453257_A_Comparison_of_Ancient_Greek_and_Roman_Sports_Diets_with_Modern_Day_Practices (Accessed June 18, 2018).

24. International Olympic Committee. The Olympic Games of the Antiquity: the Athlete; 2012. https://stillmed.olympic.org/media/Document%20Library/OlympicOrg/Factsheets-Reference-Documents/Games/OG-of-Antiquity/Factsheet-The-Olympic-Games-of-Antiquity-May-2012.pdf#_ga=1.183844385.629319118.1487433097 (Accessed June 18, 2018)

25. BBC News. How Much Were the Original Olympics Like the Modern Games?; 2012. http://www.bbc.com/news/magazine-18611638 (Accessed June 18, 2018)

26. Walker C. Ancient Olympians Followed "Atkins" Diet; 2004 https://news.nationalgeographic.com/news/2004/08/0810_040810_olympic_food.html (Date accessed: May 23, 2018)

27. Grandjean A.C. Diets of Elite Athletes: Has the Discipline of Sports Nutrition Made an Impact?; 1997. J Nutr. 127: 874S – 877S. https://doi.org/10.1093/jn/127.5.874S (Date accessed: May 23, 2018)

13 An Overview of Extreme Sports

Sourya Datta and Debasis Bagchi

CONTENTS

13.1 What Are Extreme Sports 239
13.2 Evolution and History of Extreme Sports 239
    13.2.1 Skiing 239
    13.2.2 Ice Canoeing 239
    13.2.3 Surfing 239
    13.2.4 Hang Gliding 240
    13.2.5 Kite Surfing 240
    13.2.6 Skateboarding 240
    13.2.7 Windsurfing 240
    13.2.8 Snowboarding/'Snurfing' 240
    13.2.9 Base jumping and Bungee jumping 240
    13.2.10 BMX (bicycle motocross) 240
    13.2.11 Inline Skating 241
13.3 Broad Classification of Extreme Sports 241
    13.3.1 Earth/Land 241
    13.3.2 Water 241
    13.3.3 Snow and Ice 241
    13.3.4 Air 241
13.4 Deep Dive on Extreme Sports 241
    13.4.1 Skateboarding 242
    13.4.2 Longboarding 242
    13.4.3 Sandboarding 242
    13.4.4 Mountainboarding 242
    13.4.5 Drifting 243
    13.4.6 BMX 243
    13.4.7 Motocross 243
    13.4.8 FMX 243
    13.4.9 Inline Skating 244
    13.4.10 Mountain Biking 244
    13.4.11 Caving 244
    13.4.12 Slacklining 244
    13.4.13 Abseiling 244
    13.4.14 Rock Climbing 245
    13.4.15 Free Climbing 245

13.4.16 Bouldering...245
13.4.17 Mountaineering...245
13.4.18 Parkour..245
13.4.19 Landkiting..245
13.4.20 Zorbing...245
13.5 Another Approach of Land Based Extreme Sports...................................246
13.6 Market Size, People's Interest and Future Prospects.............................246
    13.6.1 Market Size for Land Based Extreme Sports..............................246
    13.6.2 Growth of Extreme Sports:...246
    13.6.3 Difference in the Food Habits of Millennials with Other
           Generations...247
           13.6.3.1 Definition of 'Healthy'.....................................247
           13.6.3.2 'Food with Ethics'..247
           13.6.3.3 Avoid the Tag of 'Fast Food Eater'..........................248
           13.6.3.4 Fast Service..248
13.7 Reason for Growth/Evolution of Land Based Extreme Sports........................248
13.8 Difference between Regular and Extreme Sports...................................249
    13.8.1 Difference between Two Types of Sports:................................249
    13.8.2 Difference in Athletes Involved with Extreme Sports versus
           Traditional Sports..249
    13.8.3 Traditional Sports and Amateur Sportsperson Requirements...............250
13.9 Who Does Extreme Sports?...250
13.10 Demographics of Land Based Extreme Sports.....................................250
13.11 Top 10 Land Based Extreme Sports in USA Based on Number of
      Participants..250
13.12 Food Requirements for Athletes to be Successful...............................251
    13.12.1 Protein Need..251
    13.12.2 Carbohydrate Need...251
    13.12.3 Fat Requirements..252
    13.12.4 Energy Requirement..252
    13.12.5 Fluid Requirement...253
13.13 Food and Nutrition Requirements for Different Types of
      Extreme Sports..253
    13.13.1 Category: Racing..253
    13.13.2 Category: Combat Sports..254
    13.13.3 Other Types of Extreme Sports..255
13.14 Popular Markets for Land Based Extreme Sports.................................255
13.15 Risks of Extreme Sports..256
13.16 Future of Extreme Sports...256
13.17 Conclusion...256
References...257

13.1   WHAT ARE EXTREME SPORTS [1]

The definition of *'Extreme'* is execution of activity that needs to be extremely challenging, exciting and thrilling (extremely good), otherwise there is or could be major impact. *'Sports'* is defined as activity where a participant must show both mental and physical skills. 'Extreme Sports' is a type of activity that gives an adrenaline rush to individuals who are part of the 'community of extreme sportsmen'. It could also be defined as a type of sport where the adrenaline rush and excitement are felt by both performers and avid sports enthusiasts.

Extreme sports are a set of two words that involves danger. In most cases, extreme sports include intense speed and high level of risk. Often time, extreme sports provide excitement to other enthusiasts. Extreme sports has two components; one side is physical and the other side is psychological. In some cases, extreme sports could be fatal, but not everything that could be fatal will fall under the category of extreme sports.

13.2   EVOLUTION AND HISTORY OF EXTREME SPORTS

It is difficult to pinpoint the exact time when the concept of extreme sports was initiated. It probably started around late 1960 or early 1970 with short and long distance marathons.

There are a few views as to the start of extreme sports. But early 1970 showed a high interest in marathons on one side and rock climbing on the other side. [2]

Different extreme sports had different phases of starting and it is quite possible that rodeo could have been the oldest form of extreme sports. [3]

Initially, riding on horses and covering distances were much faster and easier than other modes of transportation and horse riding gradually gave rise to rodeo which was completely different from just riding a horse. As time progressed, some sports that had started differently slowly morphed into more traditional sports while other sports transformed into the category of 'Extreme'. [4]

Some games started as early as 600 BC which later evolved into modern games.

13.2.1   SKIING

Skiing initially started with the concept of travelers traveling on sticks as early as 6000 BC in China and 5000 BC in Russia. At that time, this activity was purely for moving from one place to another. Only in the 1800s did skiing become a sport.

13.2.2   ICE CANOEING

Canoeing also started as a mode of transportation between two places. As early as the 1600s people were canoeing across Saint Lawrence River in Canada.

13.2.3   SURFING

Surfing in some form started as early as 1769. Early surf boards were made from wiiwii or koa'ulu. Initially surfboards were used barefoot and 1960s saw manufacturers coming to market with professional surf boards. Surfboards became immensely popular thereafter and the sport continues to be one of the most sought after sports in the world now.

13.2.4 HANG GLIDING

The first basic structure for hang gliding was created as early as 1880s. German aviator Otto Lilienthal created the grip bar and frames, and he went on to undertake more than 2000 flights. The 1970s brought back gliding as sport and it became popular in the years after.

13.2.5 KITE SURFING

Inventor Samuel Cody created a 'man-lifting-kite' for the first time in 1903 and the sport was made popular in late 1970s once the French Legaignoux brothers created more suitable kites.

13.2.6 SKATEBOARDING

Skateboarding is a more recent phenomenon and began around the 1940s by surfers.

13.2.7 WINDSURFING

Windsurfing was made a sport around late 1940s by Newman Darby who came up with a sail and rig. The rider could control the board by shifting the body weight.

13.2.8 SNOWBOARDING/'SNURFING'

Snowboarding was initially called 'snurfing' and around 1977 it became a full-fledged sport when Jake Burton Carpenter added foot bindings to the board.

13.2.9 BASE JUMPING AND BUNGEE JUMPING

Base jumping was made a sport by Carl Boenish who photographed jumpers who were free falling from El Capitan in Yosemite National park.

Bungee jumping was started in 1979 when two members of 'Oxford University Dangerous Sports Club' jumped from Clifton Suspension Bridge in Bristol, England. They also jumped from Golden Gate Bridge and later from Royal Gorge Bridge.

13.2.10 BMX (BICYCLE MOTOCROSS)

BMX was started around the 1970s when kids started using wheelie bikes. Manufacturers later started creating special bikes designed for off road racing. This was followed by the National Bicycle League and the American Bicycle Association in 1980, as well as International BMX Federation in 1981 and the first world championship in 1982.

13.2.11 INLINE SKATING

Inline skateboarding started gaining popularity around early 1990s when Rollerblade, Inc released new skates with wheels. The national inline Skate series was started in 1995 and then Inline skating became extremely popular through the X-Games featured on ESPN.

13.3 BROAD CLASSIFICATION OF EXTREME SPORTS [5]

Extreme Sports could be classified based on a number of factors but one of the popular methods of classification is based on the elements defined below. The following list is not exhaustive but covers most of the popular games.

13.3.1 EARTH/LAND

a. Different types and variations of pedal games: skateboarding, mountain boarding, sandboarding, long boarding
b. Racing: BMX, motocross, FMX
c. Climbing: rock climbing, bouldering, mountaineering, free climbing, abseiling
d. Others such as aggressive inline skating, slacklining caving, drifting, caving, zorbing, parkour, sand kiting

13.3.2 WATER

Based on the second element of water, there are a number of extreme sports. Some popular sports include surfing, kitesurfing, windsurfing, waterskiing, paddle surfing, kayaking (extreme kayaking), cliff jumping, skim boarding, fly boarding, body boarding, wakeboarding, knee boarding, flow boarding, cave diving, coasteering, scuba diving, whitewater fafting and jet skiing,

13.3.3 SNOW AND ICE

Ice games like snowboarding, snowblading, snowmobiling skiing, ice climbing, snow kiting and monoskiing.

13.3.4 AIR

Air based extreme sports include sky diving, base jumping, wing suiting, bungee jumping, high-lining, paragliding and hang gliding.

13.4 DEEP DIVE ON EXTREME SPORTS

The above method is one way of classifying extreme sports and when we take a deeper look at extreme sports, we can provide multiple examples of some very popular sports. The goal is not to cover all extreme sports but to give a flavour of the most popular.

13.4.1 SKATEBOARDING

Skating with the help of a board. Skateboarding has its root in surfing. Surfers would consider using a skateboard as sidewalk surfing. Boarders ride on a wooden board with wheels attached to the bottom and with the help of one's foot, they push the board forward.

Skateboarding by itself is a simple sport but the complexity can be increased by the terrain where skateboarding takes place or when it involves different tricks, such as

   a. Ollie: Skateboarders push at the back of the skateboard and control the upward movement of board with their front foot.
   b. Flip: Different flips are performed – these could be kickflips, backside flips or heel flips.
   c. Grinds: Skateboarders jump onto certain object like handrail and slide along the rail.
   d. Aerials: Boarders perform tricks like twists or flips while airborne.

Skills required: Airborne control, landing control on raw asphalt, balance

13.4.2 LONGBOARDING

Form of skateboarding involving downhill gliding, taking turns based on the curves of a road. Originally developed in the 1960s to replicate surfing or snowboarding without snow (paved surfaces). Boarding Performing various tricks like ollies and flips is more difficult with a longboard and longboard enthusiasts typically use fast turns and cover long distances. This sport has grown in popularity and currently has more than 750,000 active participants in the United States alone.

Unlike skateboarding, the terrain could make longboarding could make it extremely dangerous. Riding downhill at a pace of 10–15 miles/hour or even higher makes this sport very challenging. Added to the speed is the terrain where the terrain often contains cracks, boulders or even obstacles that make longboarding challenging.

Skills required: Ability to manage speed, ability to maneuver around cliffs and various road conditions

13.4.3 SANDBOARDING

An alternative to skating, surfing and snowboarding; or it could be defined as a combination of surfing, skateboarding and snowboarding. This is also a board sport where one stands on the board and travels down a sand dune. Modern sandboarding first started around the 1960s and expanded rapidly in the 1970s. Longer boards were used on big hills and shorter boards were used on small hills.

Skills required: Ability to manage extreme weather conditions, managing steep dunes

13.4.4 MOUNTAINBOARDING

Alternative to skating and snowboarding. The inception of mountainboarding was extremely interesting; a few snowboarders added four tires to a snowboard and started going down the slopes of offseason ski resorts. This initial format has still not changed apart from the modification of the board and the terrain.

Skills required: High jumps in the air, 900-degree spins and landing 50 feet /15.2 meters down the hill, the ability to maneuver between rocks or obstacles, maintaining good balance over center of gravity

13.4.5   DRIFTING

Drifting is a more recent phenomenon compared to other sports. Drifting started around the 1990s in Japan where drivers would drive the car across a track in the midst of heavy smoke and burning tires. The drivers force the cars to drift sideways and drivers are able to control when the tires are above the ground and are not gripping the road. While racing across a track, and when drivers turn at high speed, the tires would lose control and the rear end of the car will swing out and the driver has to bring the car back under control.

Skills required: The ability to bring the car back under control after losing control for at high speed

13.4.6   BMX

The use of bikes to reach high in the air and then land safely on the ground. The premise of BMX is built on the fact it is a sport where the bicycle, smaller than a mountain/road bike is used to ride on dirt. The bike has 20-inch wheels, good tires for traction on dirt and handlebars with crossbars and rear wheel brakes. BMX has evolved as a sport and could be of the following:

    a.   Flatland BMX: performed on flat surfaces with no ramps.
    b.   Street BMX: In urban surroundings, terrain could be creative which could have stairs and handrails.
    c.   Park: Terrain is man-made and could be done in skate parks or other terrains specifically built for the purpose.
    d.   Dirt: Mostly done on dirt race tracks.

Skills required: Ability to jump over high ramps and managing a difficult course on one hand and at the same time doing tricks on dirt and mud

13.4.7   MOTOCROSS

This is a type of off-road motorcycle racing which is held in closed circuits. Driving bikes in muddy roads and in bad terrain is the name of the game.

Skills required: Extremely high speed, high control, ability to speed and slow down effectively within seconds

13.4.8   FMX

Freestyle motocross is the acrobatic version of motocross. Motorists jump on the air and provide multiple stunts. It's often called motocross on drugs.

There are two types:

Freestyle Motocross: The motorist gives two performances and each performance could last as long as 14 minutes. Courses vary in length and participants are scored on a scale of 0 to 100 with higher scores given when there are difficult tricks and different variations of tricks performed.

Big Air: In this format, participants performs two jumps; starting from a ramp covered with dirt. The highest jump of one motorist is compared with the other motorist's jump and the motorist with the highest jump wins.

Skills required:

Risks: Higher airtime, better control, reaching heights and dangerous spins in the air

13.4.9 INLINE SKATING

Inline skating developed from ice skating. Inline skating was modified later to become a set of skates with a single line of wheels and no brakes.

Skills required: Performing spins in the air, control in the air and on land and landing on surfaces

13.4.10 MOUNTAIN BIKING

This is a sport where a bicycle is driven over difficult terrain and off-road conditions. Driving a bike across muddy hills and mountains at extremely high speed gives a special thrill which is absent in normal biking

Skills required: Coordination between speed and turns, high speed and maneuvering around multiple cliffs

13.4.11 CAVING

Caving is exploring caves around the world. It involves climbing through deep abysses, avoiding dangerous falling rocks, and difficult terrain and handling any kind of weather to reach the end.

Skills required: Keeping track of routes; sense of direction and ability to continue for long times without water

13.4.12 SLACKLINING

Slacklining is a phenomenon which involves the art of moving, walking and balancing on a tight flat webbing that is held between two points. Slacklining in the normal form itself is extremely difficult but it becomes extreme when athletes perform a number of tricks including spins while traversing through the path from one end to the other.

Skills required: High degree of balance l

13.4.13 ABSEILING

Also known as rappelling or house running, abseiling involves climbing down a mountain using a rope. The descent down varies in degree of difficulty and the difficulty level depends on how vertical the rock surface is.

Skills required: Speed, managing safety, ability to increase friction of rope, managing weight

13.4.14 ROCK CLIMBING

Climbing rocks to reach to a certain point. Rocks come in different shapes and sizes and rock climbing could mean climbing up or climbing down or climbing across natural rock walls.

Skills required: Balance, control of the body, ability to grab and leave surface

13.4.15 FREE CLIMBING

Skills required: Extremely high drop, laser like focus. High level of patience

13.4.16 BOULDERING

This is another version of rock climbing, but the only difference between bouldering and other forms of rock climbing is that bouldering has a pre-installed course.

Skills required: Balance, control of the body, high concentration and strength

13.4.17 MOUNTAINEERING

Hiking and climbing mountains and glaciers within a set span of time (speed is important and a big factor in this sport). It's a form of sport that involves climbing mountains. It includes a number of activities like climbing, hiking, skiing etc. Mountaineering is the sport that covers anything related to climbing and/or mountains.

Skills required: Ability to face blizzards and storms on one hand and deep abysses on the other, overall ability to survive extreme conditions

13.4.18 PARKOUR

Overcome obstacles within a set span of time. This form of sport had its origins from military training and was developed from obstacle trainings in military. Just like mountaineering, this involves a number of various events. It includes climbing, running, jumping, vaulting and crawling to reach from one point to the other.

Skills required: Maintaining balance and pace between obstacles

13.4.19 LANDKITING

Using a board or on a board while holding a kite handle and doing multiple stunts in the air. This game is also called kitesurfing or flyboarding.

Skills required: Ability to perform tricks at different heights

13.4.20 ZORBING

Zorbing started as more of a fun game and evolved into a race. Overall, it's still considered as a recreational sport and is a type of game where one goes inside a transparent plastic and rolls down the hill.

Zorbing can also be done on water. Even though it's still considered a recreational sport, more recent competitions are coming up with innovative ways of making this sport more complex by changing the route to be more complicated. It's still not in a category of extreme sports but zorbing could be made extreme by tweaking the format and the course.

Skills required: More of a fun game but does need balance and control of the body

13.5 ANOTHER APPROACH OF LAND BASED EXTREME SPORTS

Another way to divide land based extreme sports would be the specific type of activity [6].

a. Racing
   i.   Adventure Race; ii. Endurance Race; iii. Trail Run; iv. Triathlon Race; v. Obstacle Race
b. Climb
   i.   Mountaineering; ii. Rock Climbing; iii. Ice Climbing; iv. Mixed Climbing; v. Abseiling (or Rappelling); vi. Free Climbing; vii. Bouldering; I. Slacklining
c. Wheel
   i.   Mountain Biking; ii. Cycling; iii. Unicycling; iv. Bicycle Polo; v. Motocross; vi. Motorcycle Racing; vii. BMX; viii. Skateboarding; ix. Longboarding; x. Mountainboarding (or All-Terrain Boarding); xi. Rallying; xii. Inline Skating; xiii. Street Luging
d. Other
   i.   Sepak Takraw; ii. Jai Alai; iii. Tricking; iv. Paintball; v. Parkour; vi. Sandboarding; vii. Train Surfing; viii. Bossaball
e. Fun based
   i.   Leisure Diving; ii. Extreme Ironing; iii. Planking

13.6 MARKET SIZE, PEOPLE'S INTEREST AND FUTURE PROSPECTS [7]

13.6.1 MARKET SIZE FOR LAND BASED EXTREME SPORTS:

It is extremely difficult to determine the market size of extreme sports due to the open nature of its definition. People have tried to define and come up with the market size from various aspects but it has never been a full proof verifiable answer. An alternative way of identifying the market size could be to understand the 'adventure travel' market size in the world.

13.6.2 GROWTH OF EXTREME SPORTS:

Approximately twenty percent has been the annual growth rate in extreme sports since 2000. Even though there is a very high growth in extreme sports, the market is very volatile and also evolves very rapidly. One of difficulties in determining the growth of extreme sports is how to define exactly what falls under the category of extreme sports. Two important factors are responsible for the volatility and evolution in extreme sports.

   a. Extreme sports could be influenced by what is 'in fashion'. Few sports lose charm with change in popularity.

   b. Non extreme sports could be made extreme. Running a half marathon or scuba diving in the Arctic are great examples of traditional sporting events moved into the category of extreme. Running a half marathon or even a full marathon might not be part of 'Extreme Sports' but doing the same in the Arctic could push it towards extreme. At the same time an extreme sport could be made simpler with a change of rules. For example, the complexity of the Spartan race could be made simpler by making the terrain and obstacles easier and also allowing the contestants to clear obstacles by giving the option of an easier alternative to do so.

13.6.3   Difference in the Food Habits of Millennials with Other Generations:

One of the most important factors in understanding the future growth of extreme sports will be to see what millennial are thinking and understanding their food habits. The basic difference in food habits between millennial and Gen X and/or Baby Boomers are extremely important to understand so as to consider people's interest in extreme sports in the long run. [8]

If we do a deep-dive, we will understand the difference between various groups and what could be used in understanding the current interest in the sports and how interests could evolve in the future.

13.6.3.1   Definition of 'Healthy' [7]

It's extremely important to understand the definition of 'healthy' for each groups. Both Gen X and Baby Bloomers consider healthy food as food which has less calories. But the millennial definition of 'healthy' food is different. Food is considered healthy if it satisfies three basic criteria:

   a. Least processed
   b. Less artificial/external entities added
   c. Fresh

Restaurants that give fresh vegetables and provide less processed food have a better chance of being liked by millennials due to being seen as in the 'healthy' quotient.

13.6.3.2   'Food with Ethics'

Millennials are commonly seen as looking for companies that have better social ethics than what Gen X or Baby Boomers would look at (although this is still debatable). In general, this criterion still has a lower impact than other criteria but has potential of becoming more important in the future.

13.6.3.3   Avoid the Tag of 'Fast Food Eater'

Millennials don't want to get associated with fast food chains like McDonald's. McDonald's is still one of the most popular fast food outlets but often millennials don't want to associate themselves with a fast food place, mainly for two reasons:

a. Social stature
b. Food taste and quality

13.6.3.4   Fast Service

Millennials look for three important factors when eating outside:

a. Speed of service
b. Quality (good, at least decent, definition is very broad since the terms could be viewed alternatively by different people)
c. Good price

All three factors mentioned above have become extremely important for millennials in choosing the type of food and restaurants.

These differences in food habits are also applicable in sportspersons and extreme sports as well. The presence of functional food and beverages have made a huge difference in the eating habits of millennial versus previous generations. An extremely important example is that of energy drinks. Energy drinks have become extremely popular and along with energy bars have changed the sports industry in general. Availability of functional food and beverages, huge demand, ease of access and functional and nutritional beverages have made huge differences in the sports industry especially in the extreme sports sector.

13.7   REASON FOR GROWTH/EVOLUTION OF LAND BASED EXTREME SPORTS [7]

The reason or answer to the above question could be due to the impact of and interests of millennials in extreme sports. Food is also an important factor and millennials are more willing to try new functional food, beverages and energy drinks as compared to generation X and/or baby boomers. In addition, availability and demand are other factors that have led to the growth of the sports. Below are a few reasons behind the growth of extreme sports.

- Increased safety of modern life: Absence of 'feeling of danger'
- Improved sports medicine and healing
- Improved sports technology
- Movies, televisions, magazines
  a.   Advent of Summer and Winter Olympics
- Combination of two sports
      For example, two normal sports are often combined to make a new sport which is more challenging:

   a. Snowboarding = skateboarding + surfing [9]
   b. sky surfing = snowboarding + skydiving
* Conversion of regular sports into extreme sports
       Another important factor behind the growth of extreme sports has been
   the modifications of regular sports into more difficult sports
   a. Regular bike riding was converted to dirt biking
   b. BMX (bicycle motocross) turned into Extreme BMX (bicycle motocross)
* Obesity and other diseases have had an enormous impact on the minds of
   normal people and more so sports enthusiasts
* The idea and zeal to not only stay alive longer but lead a much more active
   lifestyle

13.8   DIFFERENCE BETWEEN REGULAR AND EXTREME SPORTS [7]:

13.8.1   DIFFERENCE BETWEEN TWO TYPES OF SPORTS:

Traditional/Regular Sports	Extreme Sports
Most traditional sports are played and viewed by young people in their 20s as well as in their 30s, 40s, 50s and those who ar even older. Viewers range from young o older ages	Played by young athletes and mostly viewed by young audiences
Formal coaching/training are provided to improve players' skills and stamina	Less formal training and coaching than traditional sports
Less dynamic and players practice to lower the risk of unseen and uncontrollable factors as much as possible	More dynamic and uncontrollable factors involved
Performance judged on pre-set and specific parameters	More qualitative factors than quantitative for judging performance (completing the sport is the end goal most of the time)
Sportspersons are more careful and often times they determine the time to peak	High adrenaline rush and effect of hormones throughout
In most cases, it is a team sport or people involved in a group	Extreme sports are more individualistic

13.8.2   DIFFERENCE IN ATHLETES INVOLVED WITH EXTREME SPORTS VERSUS TRADITIONAL SPORTS:

   a. It has been determined from some studies that extreme athletes are more
       of the types of *Introversion, Perceiving, and Sensation* than traditional ath-
       letes in general.
   b. Extreme athletes are in general found to be more flexible, spontaneous, and
       adaptive than traditional athletes.
   c. In most cases, people are moving to individual sports and extreme sports
       can now be seen as an individual sport.

13.8.3 TRADITIONAL SPORTS AND AMATEUR SPORTSPERSON REQUIREMENTS:

For people aged below 30, carbohydrates are important and herbal supplements help in high intensity sports, but as people age more muscle degeneration (Sarcopenia) happens and fat storage increases. Studies show that chromium supplements may minimize the impact of muscle degeneration. [10]

For traditional sports, studies have shown the importance of copper, silver and gold which we will cover in detail under 'Food requirements for athletes'.

13.9   WHO DOES EXTREME SPORTS? [11]

There is no specific set of people who like to perform extreme sports. In most cases of extreme sports, it has been determined that completing the mark is the goal or the key for extreme sports enthusiasts and not necessarily the competition itself or winning against others. Achieving the final mark in extreme sports gives a sense of pride and identity along with the high adrenaline factor. Added to this is the fact that extreme sports enthusiasts want to push harder and faster - they are not satisfied with achieving something, they want to achieve more and achieve faster. A record is meant to be broken and there is pride in breaking that record.

13.10   DEMOGRAPHICS OF LAND BASED EXTREME SPORTS

Generally speaking, the age group for extreme sports enthusiasts has been determined to be young. In most cases, people in the age group of 20–35 years take part in extreme sports. However, that trend is slowly changing since people above 40 and 50 years of age are taking keen interest and taking part in extreme sports, a trend which seems to have changed from 2013 onwards.

13.11   TOP 10 LAND BASED EXTREME SPORTS IN USA BASED ON NUMBER OF PARTICIPANTS

Based on data collected in 2004, statistics show the following for extreme sports in USA.

Note*: Number of participants are based on the fact that participants participated at least once in the year 2004

Rank	Sport	Number of participants	Comments
1	Inline Skating	17M	
2	Skateboarding	11.5M	Average number days of participation
3	Paintball	9.6M	Participation has grown by 60% over a period of 6 years
4	Artificial Wall climbing	7.6M	Average age is 21 years
5	Snowboarding	7.1M	Average is 8 days of participation
6	Trail Running	6.4M	25% increase in participation

7	Mountain Biking	5.3M	Average age is 25 years
9	BMX Bicycle	2.6M	Average age is 25 years
10	Mountain/Rock Climbing	2.1M	Average age is 23 years
11	Roller Hockey	1.7M	Mostly male dominated game

13.12 FOOD REQUIREMENTS FOR ATHLETES TO BE SUCCESSFUL

To understand the food requirement of extreme sports athletes, we would need to understand the body type and the type of activity the athlete will perform. General food requirements are detailed below:

13.12.1 PROTEIN NEED:

Type of Training	Daily Needs Per Pound bodyweight (in grams)
Low	0.55
Moderate	0.8
High	1.0

In general, it has been determined that extreme sports athletes need 1.4 gm/Kg body weight/day of protein. On a strenuous weight day, it has been determined that 2 gm/kg of body weight/day is needed. [12]

13.12.2 CARBOHYDRATE NEED:

Type of Training	Daily Needs Per Pound body weight (In grams)
Low	2.3–3.3
Moderate	3–4.5
High	3.5–5.5

It is also important to note that it is extremely important to have not just carbohydrates but good carbohydrates - whole wheat is a great example. Another great example of superfood is quinoa. [13]

The importance of quinoa is listed below:

- Highly protein rich
  - Contains amino acids
- Has iron [14, 15]
  - Iron is important for red blood cells
  - Iron carries oxygen from cell to cell and improves brain function
  - Iron helps in maintaining energy metabolism

- Great source of fiber [16]
  - Fiber helps in reducing constipation
  - Helps in managing or controlling diabetes
  - Lowers cholesterol and helps in reducing weight
  - Has lesser calories for same amount/quantity/volume of food
- Lysine
  - Helps in tissue growth and tissue repair
- Magnesium
  - Reduces migraine
  - Helps in controlling blood sugar
  - Helps in growth and formation of teeth and bone
  - Maintains body temperature
  - Produces energy
- Manganese
  - Protects all cells including red blood cells from injury
  - Prevents mitochondrial damage
- Riboflavin (B2)
  - Used to convert carbohydrate to glucose. In other words, converts food to fuel and thus helps in producing energy. [17]

13.12.3   FAT REQUIREMENTS: [18]

There is no particular level of fat intake that is ideal since the amount of fat intake differs in various sports. However, it's been proven that high fat diets ranging from 42%-55% that maintain adequate carbohydrate levels provide more endurance [19] in both male and female sportspersons than a low fat intake of 10%-15% diet. Researchers and sports medicine nutritionists have determined baseline diets to contain 30% fat, 30% carbohydrate, 20% protein and 20% distributed between carbohydrate and fat based on duration and intensity of the sport in question. It has been determined that diet should have fat content between 20% - 40% of total kilocalories for sportspersons. [20]

One of the most important characteristics during exercise is the way the source of energy in the body shifts from carbohydrate to fat in order to fuel the activities of a sportsperson. If it is a longer duration but low intensity activity, the source of fuel for the activity changes from carbohydrate to fat once the activity time increases by more than thirty minutes. [20]

It has been determined that out of the total calorie requirement, 25%-30% should come from fat. Out of the 30%, 10% should be from monounsaturated sources, another 10% from polyunsaturated sources and no more than 10% from saturated (should be kept the lowest). Research has shown that there is no benefit from a diet that includes meeting more than 70% of energy through fat.

13.12.4   ENERGY REQUIREMENT

Smaller athletes need 2000–2500 calories per day while larger athletes with high levels of training need 5000–5500 calories per day.

For a high intensity run or activity, e.g. Iron Man, Tough Mudder race or Spartan Race, typically athletes would need to eat 65% of their calories from carbohydrates to increase their performance. It also depends on the way 'Carbohydrate-loading' is done. Often times, it is advisable to eat carbohydrates 2–3 days before the actual race/event. This is before the race but athletes need to eat well after the race as well.

13.12.5 FLUID REQUIREMENT

In general, the fluid requirements for athletes is higher than normal adults and for extreme sports athletes it could be even higher. After a race/workout/activity, the fluid lost due to sweat should be replaced by the same amount of fluid; in short, the fluid intake should match the fluid outflow due to sweat during and after exercise.

Another good measure of fluid intake is based on the following formula:

Fluid Intake = Athlete's body weight before activity – Athlete's body weight after activity

Along with water, another important intake is that of electrolytes. It has been determined by the National Research Council that daily water intake for adults should be 1.5 ml water/kcal energy, which means 2500 Kcal energy spent would need 2.5 liters of water on a daily basis. This, however, is not the best measure and depending on the body type and the activity, water intake requirement could be even higher. If weight drops more than 1 lb. from the previous day in an extreme sport athlete then this shows that more fluid intake is necessary.

Dietary guidelines have set up definitions given below:

a. EAR Estimated Average requirement
b. RDA Recommended Dietary Allowances
c. AI: Adequate Intake
d. UL: Tolerable Upper limit

13.13 FOOD AND NUTRITION REQUIREMENTS FOR DIFFERENT TYPES OF EXTREME SPORTS [21]

Extreme sports can be divided into a number of broad categories. Even though most categories of extreme food require almost all types of food some food types might vary. Based on the broad categories, food and nutrient requirements are broadly classified as described below. Each type of category has details of type of food along with benefits of the particular type of food.

13.13.1 CATEGORY: RACING

Racing includes pure running like marathons, half marathons but also includes swimming, Spartan Race, Tough Mudder, Iron Man and other related races. For racing, three different types of food are extremely important: fat, carbohydrates and other supplemental food.

Fats: used for energy
When to take: should be part of regular diet
Which types of food provide necessary nutrition: meats, fish, nuts
Food product extensions: regular food (generally nonspecific)
Ingredients: regular food

Carbohydrates: used for storing glycogen in liver and muscles
When to take:
  a. An hour before exercise
  b. If workout lasts more than an hour, small amount of carbs could be
      taken during the exercise (at mid-point of exercise)
Which types of food provide necessary nutritive value:
  a. Before exercise: pasta, potatoes, oatmeal, bananas
  b. During exercise: bananas, fruits
Food product extensions: energy bars, gels, energy drinks
Ingredients: glucose, maltodextrin, cyclic dextrin

Herbal Extracts: used for fat burning and helps in blood flow through the
    muscle
When to take: before exercise
Which types of food provide necessary nutrition: green tea, black tea, black
    coffee
Food product extensions: drink supplements
Ingredients: caffeine, quercetin

13.13.2 CATEGORY: COMBAT SPORTS

Combat sports would include boxing, mixed martial arts, wrestling and even sword
fighting
   For combat sports, different types of food are extremely important - protein, carbohydrates, minerals Omega-3 fatty acids and glucosamine

Protein: used for repairing muscle
When to take:
  a. Half an hour before exercise
  b. Half an hour after exercise
Which types of food provide necessary nutrition: egg whites, chicken, red
    beans beans and black beans
Even though bananas don't fall under high protein rich food, they ar extremely
    beneficial for any tissue repair
Food product extensions: protein bars, energy bars, drink, supplements
Ingredients: soy protein, whey protein, L-Glutamine, amino acids

Carbohydrate: used for replenishing glycogen
When to take:
  a. One hour before exercise
  b. Half an hour/one hour after exercise
Which types of food provide necessary nutrition: chicken, meat, nuts, seeds
Food product extensions: protein powder
Ingredients: glucose, maltodextrin, trehalose, cyclic dextrins

Minerals: used for supporting muscle and in general increase muscle health
When to take: no particular time (part of diet)

Which types of food provide necessary nutrition: meat (red meat), beans, green vegetables
Food product extensions: supplements
Ingredients: zinc, iron, calcium

Omega-3 fatty acids: used for helping muscle soreness
When to take: after workout
Which types of food provide necessary nutrition: fish
Food product extensions: supplements, nutrition drinks
Ingredients: collection of different nutrients, most notably EPA and DHA, and found in salmon, tuna, trout (lake trout), mackerel, anchovies and fish and algal oils

Glucosamine: relieves pain from joints [5]
When to take: after workout
Which types of food provide necessary nutrition: shellfish (shells and tails of shrimp, crab, lobster contains minute amount, not the flesh itself)
Food product extensions: supplements
Ingredients: shells of shellfish

13.13.3 OTHER TYPES OF EXTREME SPORTS

Apart from the extreme sports mentioned above, there are a number of extreme sports and in general a number of sports that require hydration. For hydration purposes, mainly liquids and electrolytes are used.

Electrolytes: used for replenishing electrolytes in the body
When to take: mainly during workout; when workout is strenuous it is important to have electrolytes in the body
Which types of food provide necessary nutrition: sports drinks
Food product extensions: electrolyte tablets
Ingredients: sodium, magnesium, potassium

Liquids: used for water storage and keeping body hydrated
When to take: before workout, during workout and after workout (ideally 10–15 minutes during workout)
Which types of food provide necessary nutrition: regular water, coconut water and fruit juice
Food product extensions: sports drinks

13.14 POPULAR MARKETS FOR LAND BASED EXTREME SPORTS [7]

In general, the extreme sports market could be divided into two categories based on countries:

a. Main markets include USA, Germany, Italy, United Kingdom, Scandinavia, Australia, New Zealand, Canada
b. Secondary or emerging markets include Czech Republic, Croatia, Hungary, Poland, Brazil

13.15   RISKS OF EXTREME SPORTS [22, 23]

Even though it is a common theory that extreme sports are performed by adventurists who take high degree of risks, this might not always be that case. An in-depth study by a group of scientists on extreme sports enthusiasts has determined there are and could be two separate sets of people who perform extreme sports:

  a. According to the traditional thought: extreme sports enthusiasts are the group of people who enjoy taking risks and enjoy performing acts that could be fatal
  b. According to another set of research, it has been determined that extreme sports enthusiasts take more precautions so that risks for any and all activities are minimized

13.16   FUTURE OF EXTREME SPORTS

There is no stopping extreme sports in the future and their popularity will only increase, with multiple reasons behind this rise. Three different trends/factors will be responsible for the future increase in popularity of extreme sports:

  a. Technology trends
     i.   New technologies that have elevated the entire experience of extreme sports
     ii. Online streaming
     iii. Social media
  b. Economic trends
     i.   Increase in commercialization
     ii. Generation 'Y' is more ready than ever
     iii. Demographics with more disposable income
     iv. Marketing techniques that generate more enthusiasm and interest
  c. Social trends
     i.   Increase in the use of social media
     ii. Industry going mainstream
     iii. Increase in tourism around the world and specially adventure tourism
The impact of climate change, however, may change location and the way water and snow sports are organized around the world.

The only other parallel sports that are related to extreme sports are in the Olympics and Paralympics. Paralympics [24] might not be an extreme sport in a true form but has a number of challenges for the Paralympic athletes that makes it extremely challenging.

The future will be interesting as people will continue to push the horizon and develop new and harder obstacles to cross!

13.17   CONCLUSION

Overall, land-based extreme sports need lots of enthusiasm, focus and attention, as well as a strong desire to achieve the goal. A significant promise has been demonstrated especially in people between the ages of 20–35. There are two sets of extreme sports enthusiasts – one set of people who don't have a background and are inspired due to the thrill of the sports and the other set comprising sportspersons and people who have a sporting background. A more recent phenomenon in the increase in popularity of extreme sports is due to the high involvement of army and navy veterans; an active lifestyle along with food habits that include appropriate nutrition provide them the necessary motivation, strength and desire to participate. We have provided a detailed review of the nutritional requirements for the individuals engaged in land-based extreme sports. Further research studies are in progress to unveil the mechanism of how personalized nutrition can help the athletes engaged in diverse land-based extreme sports.

REFERENCES

1. Reuter A., Holder J. Traditional vs. Extreme Athletes: An Exploration of Personality Indicators (Ursidae: The Undergraduate Research Journal at the University of Northern Colorado), 2013; 2, Article 5; https://digscholarship.unco.edu/urj/vol2/iss3/5/ (Date accessed: May 22, 2018)
2. Grivetti L.E., Applegate E.A. From Olympia to Atlanta: A Cultural-Historical Perspective on Diet and Athletic Training. *The Journal of Nutrition,* 1997. 127: 860S–868S.
3. Williamson M. The History of Extreme Sports, 2007; https://www.catalogs.com/info/sports/history-of-extreme-sports.html (Date accessed: May 22, 2018)
4. EXTREME. Types of Extreme Sports by Brand EXTREME (an Iconic Lifestyle Brand Fueled by the Passion, Creativity and Freedom of Action), 2017; https://www.extremesportscompany.com/extreme-about-us (Date accessed: February 8, 2018)
5. i. List of Extreme Sports. Expression through Action. Extreme: Founders of the Extreme Sports Channel, 1995; https://www.extremesportscompany.com/list-of-extreme-sports (Date accessed: May 20, 2018); ii. Active Sports and Active Cities. Active Cities blog, 2013; http://activecities.com/blog/ (Date accessed: May 20, 2018)
6. Perlman A. Nerve Rush. Extreme Sports Statistics, 2009; http://www.nerverush.com/extreme-sports-list/ (Date accessed: May 20, 2018)
7. Dunbar D. Extreme Dreams, 2002; www.extremedreams.co.uk; Extreme Sports Niche Markets, 2005; http://www.onecaribbean.org/content/files/ExtremeSportCaribbeanNicheMarkets.pdf
8. Lutz A. 5 Ways Millennials' Dining Habits Are Different from Their Parents (Business Insider), 2015; https://www.businessinsider.com/millennials-dining-habits-are-different-2015-3 (Date accessed: May 20, 2018)
9. Rahmat M. Strength and Conditioning Components for Elite Snowboarders, 2016; https://breakingmuscle.com/fitness/strength-and-conditioning-components-for-elite-snowboarders (Date accessed : May 22, 2018)
10. Office of Dietary Supplements. National Institutes of Health (Chromium Fact Sheet), 2013; https://ods.od.nih.gov/factsheets/Chromium-HealthProfessional (Date accessed: May 7, 2018)
11. Hatfield H. Extreme Sports: What's the Appeal? (WebMD) 2006; pp. 4–5; https://www.webmd.com/fitness-exercise/features/extreme-sports-whats-appeal#1 (Date accessed: May 20, 2018)
12. Christianson A. Essential Nutrients for Endurance Athletes (Nutrition Science), 1999; https://chiro.org/nutrition/FULL/Essential_Nutrients_for_Endurance_Athletes.shtml (Date accessed: May 22, 2018)

13. Trulio A. Timeline: The History of Extreme Sports (Therapeutic Characteristics of Sports), 2017; https://blogs.uoregon.edu/atruliof13gateway/timeline/ (Date accessed: October 20, 2017)

14. Grandjean A.C. Diets of Elite Athletes: Has the Discipline of Sports Nutrition Made an Impact. *The Journal of Nutrition*, 1997. 127: 874S–877S.

15. Scripa D. Ancient Olympians Followed "Atkins" Diet, 2004; https://www.boxingscene.com/weight-loss/15387.php (Date accessed: May 22, 2018)

16. Mellentin J. Key Trends in Functional Foods & Beverages for 2016 – Nutraceuticals World (Nutrition), 2016; https://www.nutraceuticalsworld.com/issues/2015-11/view_features/key-trends-in-functional-foods-beverages-for-2016 (Date accessed: May 07, 2018)

17. Ehrlich S. Vitamin B2 (Riboflavin) (University of Maryland: Medical Center), 2015; http://www.umm.edu/health/medical/altmed/supplement/vitamin-b2-riboflavin (Date accessed: May 7, 2018)

18. Pendergast D.R., Leddy J.J., Venkatraman J.T. A Perspective on Fat Intake in Athletes. *Journal of the American College of Nutrition*, 2001. 19: 345–350 (Date accessed: May 7, 2018)

19. Misner W. The Endurance Diet, 2006; https://www.hammernutrition.com/knowledge/endurance-library/the-endurance-diet/ (Date accessed: May 22, 2018)

20. Lowery L. Dietary Fat and Performance (National Strength and Conditioning Association), 2004; https://www.ncbi.nlm.nih.gov/pmc/articles/PMC3905293/ (Date accessed: May 7, 2018)

21. Bomgardner M. Athletes Look To Sports Nutrition Products To Improve Performance, 2016; https://cen.acs.org/articles/94/i6/Athletes-Look-Sports-Nutrition-Products.html (Date accessed: May 7, 2018)

22. Dahl M. What Motivates Extreme Athletes to Take Huge Risks? 2015; http://nymag.com/scienceofus/2015/05/what-motivates-extreme-athletes.html (Date accessed: May 7, 2018)

23. Woodman T., Barlow M., Bandura C., Hill M., Kupciw D., MacGregor A. Not All Risks Are Equal: The Risk Taking Inventory for High-Risk Sports. *Journal of Sport & Exercise Psychology*, 2013. 35: 479–492.

24. Olympic Games (Paralympic Games) Official Page: Paralympic Games https://www.olympic.org/paralympic-games (Date accessed: May 22, 2018)

14 An Overview of Challenging Mountain and High Altitude Sports

Sourya Datta and Debasis Bagchi

CONTENTS

14.1 Extreme Sports and Evolution of High Altitude Extreme Sports 260
14.2 Broad Classification of High Altitude Extreme Sports 261
14.3 Snow and Ice and Air Sports 261
    14.3.1 Deep Dive on Snow and Ice Based Sports 261
        14.3.1.1 Snowboarding 261
        14.3.1.2 Snowblading 261
        14.3.1.3 Snowmobiling 262
        14.3.1.4 Skiing 262
        14.3.1.5 Ice Climbing 262
        14.3.1.6 Snow Kiting 262
        14.3.1.7 Monoskiing 262
    14.3.2 Deep Dive on Air Based Sports 262
        14.3.2.1 Skydiving 263
        14.3.2.2 Base Jumping 263
        14.3.2.3 Wing Suiting 263
        14.3.2.4 Bungee Jumping 263
        14.3.2.5 High-Lining 263
        14.3.2.6 Paragliding 263
        14.3.2.7 Hang Gliding 264
14.4 Day to Day Activities for High Intensity Athletes in
High Altitude Sports 264
14.5 Importance of Mental Strength: Success Metrics 265
14.6 Requirements for Athletes to Be Successful in High Altitude
Extreme Sports 265
    14.6.1 Food, Nutrition and Micronutrients for High Altitude
Extreme Sports 265
        14.6.1.1 Sodium Requirement 265
        14.6.1.2 Potassium Requirement 265
        14.6.1.3 Iron Requirement 266
        14.6.1.4 Zinc Requirement 266
        14.6.1.5 Calcium Requirement 266

    14.6.1.6   Magnesium Requirement 266
    14.6.1.7   Chromium (III) Requirement 266
    14.6.1.8   Vanadium Requirement 267
    14.6.1.9   Boron Requirement 267
    14.6.1.10 Nickel Requirement 267
    14.6.1.11 Selenium Requirement 267
  14.6.2   Vitamins and Antioxidants Requirements for High Altitude
           Extreme Sports 267
    14.6.2.1   Vitamin C 267
    14.6.2.2   Vitamin E..267
    14.6.2.3   Beta-Carotene: Vitamin A 268
    14.6.2.4   Glutamine..268
  14.6.3   Physical Requirement...268
14.7 Food Nutrients and Impacts 268
14.8 Importance of Nutraceuticals and Functional Foods for High Altitude
      Extreme Sports Athletes..269
  14.8.1   Types of Functional Food Products and Nutrition 269
  14.8.2   Disadvantages of Functional Food and Nutrition 269
14.9 Places Appropriate for High Altitude Extreme Sports.............................270
  14.9.1   Mountainous Terrain 271
  14.9.2   Water Terrain at High Altitude 272
  14.9.3   Airborne/Mid-Air...272
14.10 High Altitude Extreme Sports Statistics 273
14.11 Conclusion 273
References..274

14.1   EXTREME SPORTS AND EVOLUTION OF HIGH ALTITUDE EXTREME SPORTS

In order to understand the intricate aspects of high altitude extreme sports, we need to understand the background of high altitude sports and assess the critical aspects of high altitude living. Over the last several decades and in a number of sporting events, humans have been able to adapt. In general, high altitude regions have been defined as follows:

    a. Ultra High Altitude ≥18,000 ft
    b. Very High Altitude ≥11,001 Ft and <17,999 ft
    c. High Altitude ≥5000 Ft and <11,000 ft

Just to give context, Everest base camp has an altitude of 16,000 Ft and the summit of Mount Everest has an altitude of 29,029 Ft.

It is interesting to understand the context of altitude in terms of athletes. High altitude has different impacts based on the type of event.

    a. Explosive event: High altitude → Low atmospheric pressure → Lower resistance from atmosphere → Better performance (Examples of explosive events in sports are 100 mts sprint, 200 mts sprint, 400 mts sprint, long jump, triple jump)

b. Endurance event: High altitude → Low atmospheric pressure → Reduction in oxygen level → Reduction in performance (Examples of this type of sports include 800 mts sprint, relay race)

The above theory was well proven in the 1968 Olympics, where a number of records were created. A number of key decisions were made following the 1968 Olympics. It has been demonstrated that high altitude might lead to an increase in red blood cells, which helps in efficient training. Different training routines have been designed based on altitude – sometimes training on high altitude and sleeping at low altitude, while in other cases different trainings are conducted at different altitudes. In certain cases, the first three months of training are conducted in high altitude and the next three months are done in low altitude in a six-month training course, while elsewhere a number of permutations and combinations have been followed.

Extreme sports in high altitudes have developed from traditional sports. This chapter will cover both snow and ice as well as air based high-altitude extreme sports. [1]

14.2 BROAD CLASSIFICATION OF HIGH ALTITUDE EXTREME SPORTS [2]

High altitude extreme sports can be practiced (1) on snow and ice, and (2) in air.

Some different types of snow and ice-based games include (a) snowboarding, (b) snowblading, (c) snowmobiling, (d) skiing, (e) ice climbing, (f) snow kiting, and (g) monoskiing.

In a very strict sense, all air sports might not be high altitude sports but a number of them do fall into this category. Some examples of air sports are (1) sky diving, (2) base jumping, (3) wing suiting, (4) bungee jumping, (5) high-lining, (6) paragliding and (7) hang gliding.

14.3 SNOW AND ICE AND AIR SPORTS

14.3.1 DEEP DIVE ON SNOW AND ICE BASED SPORTS

Depending on the route, conditions and competition type, all the above sports could range from simple sports to more complicated ones. Higher degrees of complexity would turn these sports into extreme sports.

14.3.1.1 Snowboarding

In snowboarding, sportspersons are attached to the board and slide down snowy mountains and perform stunts while gliding through the snow. It is now an integral part of the Olympic games and can be done either in races or freestyle events.

The course of the expedition can often be difficult and challenging.

14.3.1.2 Snowblading

This is a combination of ski and ski skates, also known as short ski. The skis used are smaller and shorter (1 meter in length) and athletes descend the slope without the use of poles. Snowblading is limited to a comparatively shorter area and requires high agility, better movement for maneuvring around cliffs and obstacles and better control of the blade.

14.3.1.3 Snowmobiling

Snowmobiling involves motorised skiing in snow. Engine powered vehicles are used to compete in such events and/or freestyle events. In short, snowmobiling is similar to riding a motorcycle on snow. It gives a lot of rush to drive a vehicle where the athletes are whisking through the snow.

Snowmobiling is a high speed game (more than 100 miles/hr) and is generally conducted on vehicles of a small size.

14.3.1.4 Skiing

Skiing is one of most popular sports. Skis are long thin runners which can be made of wood, metal or fiberglass and are fastened to specific type of boots made for skiing. With the help of these runners, the aim of the game is to slide over the snow to move from one point to another on a downhill slope from the top of a mountain. Both slalom and freestyle options are available in skiing.

Steep falls, tough cliffs and avalanches are challenges which athletes need to overcome.

14.3.1.5 Ice Climbing

Ice climbing is accomplished by using specified tools to climb ice-covered mountains. This is one of the most difficult types of climbing. Extreme sports athletes will spend numerous days with their bodies flat on the side of glacier and frozen waterfall and use pricks and ropes to scale the difficult surface.

There is a constant danger of ice breaking, which would plunge sportsmen down a long, steep icy slope in the mountains when the ice breaks. Frostbite is a constant threat, and avalanches could appear from nowhere to derail climbers.

14.3.1.6 Snow Kiting

Snowkiting, also called kite skiing, is a sport where athletes use the power of a kite to glide down the snow. This is very similar to water-based kiteboarding. This is a very popular outdoor winter sport. Kites are used as a mode of acceleration, with both the floating power of kites and power of wind utilized in this sport. The athlete uses the pulling and floating power of a kite to glide on snow or ice, while also utilizing the power of a kite to give them extra power and the option to make large jumps.

Large jumps over high ramps are critical parts of this sport.

14.3.1.7 Monoskiing

Just as the name suggests, monoskiing involves a single wider ski where both feet face forward in the direction the athlete wants to travel. The ski has a carved shape to enable easier and faster turns.

The speed is extremely high speed and loss of control results in accidents.

14.3.2 Deep Dive on Air Based Sports

We will take a look at the following: sky diving, base jumping, wing suiting, bungee jumping, high-lining, paragliding and hang gliding

14.3.2.1 Skydiving

United States Parachuting Company (USPA) defines skydiving as 'an extreme sport' where a person or group of persons descend(s) from an aircraft to surface when the person uses a parachute during the descent. An aircraft could be any vehicle moving through the air – an airplane, helicopter, hot-air balloon, paraglider, etc.

In all modern skydiving events, skydivers have a two parachute system which has a container and two parachutes – the main and the backup. There is also a device installed which will open the reserve parachute if the skydiver is not able to open his/her parachute.

Extreme heights and continuous spins in the air, as well as higher air time means less control to maneuver which are all factors that are considered before someone completes a skydive.

14.3.2.2 Base Jumping

The word BASE stands for building, antenna, span and earth. Participants jump from various low altitude objects like cliffs or bridges and have very little time to open the parachute. There is no room for error if there is any malfunction due to the low height of the object from which the jump is initiated. Self-control is important and landing can be quite difficult.

14.3.2.3 Wing Suiting

Wing suiting involves flying in the air using a special suit which looks like a wing and is used to increase surface area of the human body to increase the lift. The jumpsuit actually consists of two arm wings and a leg wing and is supported by pressurized nylon cells allowing athletes to glide horizontal distances at lower rate of descent than in other sports like parachuting.

Coordination, speed and maneuvering are key for success.

14.3.2.4 Bungee Jumping

Bungee jumping has become very popular in the recent times and involves the act of jumping from a height towards the ground while the athlete is connected to the structure from where the jump was initiated by elastic cord. The structure has modified over the years from a tall building or a bridge but nowadays athletes do it from hot-air balloons, helicopters and even small planes. There is a steep free fall and then rebound and there is a continuous oscillation of moving up and down until all the kinetic energy is released.

14.3.2.5 High-Lining

High-lining involves moving from one point to another where the path is a narrow rope connecting the two points. Usually, a safety harness is attached to the rope. High degree of balance is required in this sport.

14.3.2.6 Paragliding

This is a sport where a parachute us attached to person's body which allows them to glide through the air after from a flight. It doesn't necessarily have to from flight but could be from any height.

Paragliding has no frames but has an elliptical shaped parachute which can fold to about the size of a backpack.

14.3.2.7   Hang Gliding

Hang gliding could be both recreation and an extreme sport. Hang gliders are mostly launched from a mountain and they are launched facing the wind. The pilot who is launched from a height holds on to the frame and shifts the body weight to have control
The objective of this game is to be airborne and stay airborne as much as possible.

14.4   DAY TO DAY ACTIVITIES FOR HIGH INTENSITY ATHLETES IN HIGH ALTITUDE SPORTS [3]

It is extremely difficult to set a regime or create a set of plans since activities are different based on the type of high altitude sports the athlete is involved in, while training would differ too. Some important factors in training activity have been determined by the following factors:

a. Duration
b. Intensity
c. Frequency

It is important to plan the workout program effectively, and a slow and steady approach is the key to success, with numerous ways to measure this. A typical routine for a high intensity workout training program is described below:

Day 1: Breakfast → High intensity workout for an hour (work interval should be above 80% of the maximum heart rate) → Mix of good protein/carbohydrate/minerals → Lunch → Evening snack → Weight lifting → Dinner → Sleep/Rest
Day 2: Breakfast → High intensity workout for an hour (work interval should be above 80% of the maximum heart rate) → Mix of good protein/carbohydrate/minerals → Lunch → Evening snack → Weight lifting → Dinner → Sleep/Rest
Day 3: Breakfast → High intensity workout for an hour (work interval should be above 80% of the maximum heart rate) → Mix of good protein/carbohydrate/minerals → Lunch → Evening snack → Swimming or other cardio → Dinner → Sleep/Rest
Day 4: Break/Day of recovery
Day 5: Breakfast → Cardio (Long distance running or jogging) → Mix of good protein/carbohydrate/minerals → Lunch → Evening snack → High intensity workout for an hour (work interval should feel that exercise is hard or very hard) → Dinner → Sleep/Rest
Day 6: Breakfast → Any form of Kickboxing → Mix of good protein/carbohydrate/minerals → Lunch → Evening snack → Light to moderate weightlifting → Dinner → Sleep/Rest
Day 7: Breakfast → Light weight lifting → Mix of good protein/carbohydrate/minerals → Lunch (could be a little out of the regular regime) → Evening snack → Easy day/could be just a small walk around the neighborhood (work interval should feel that exercise is hard or very hard) → Dinner → Sleep/Rest

Of course, the above routine needs to be changed based on the type of sport and feasibility of other external factors. It is not fit and applicable for all programs, but a basic guide to a routine/schedule for high intensity, high altitude extreme sport.

14.5 IMPORTANCE OF MENTAL STRENGTH: SUCCESS METRICS [4]

Mental strength is important for any extreme sports and is one of the most important factors to be successful in high altitude extreme sports. Mental strength is a combination of multiple factors and often the following characteristics have an important role for success in extreme sports:

- Desire
- Passion
- Drive
- Attitude
- Vitality
- Vigor
- Endurance of mind
- Mental alertness
- Promptness

It's often determined that the ideal case of an athlete would be to possess all the qualities but in all practical cases, athletes' possess a combination of multiple characteristics of the nine defined above. A good strong mentally alert athlete is believed to possess five or more of these qualities.

14.6 REQUIREMENTS FOR ATHLETES TO BE SUCCESSFUL IN HIGH ALTITUDE EXTREME SPORTS

14.6.1 FOOD, NUTRITION AND MICRONUTRIENTS FOR HIGH ALTITUDE EXTREME SPORTS

14.6.1.1 Sodium Requirement [5]

An extreme sports athlete training for high altitude games needs approximately 12 g of salt which contains approximately 4.5 g of sodium. Daily loss of sodium is approximately 150 mg (feces + urine: 50 mg/day & skin: 100 mg/day). The amount of sodium needed is 30 times from what is replaced every day (30*150 = 4.5g)

14.6.1.2 Potassium Requirement

The exact potassium requirement is about 4.7 g/day. If an athlete is running for 40 minutes at a temperature of around 65–70 degrees Fahrenheit, the loss of potassium would be around 435–440 mg/hour (approximately 200 mg/kg of weight lost while performing strenuous exercise). At the same time, it is important not to intake more than necessary since too much supplementary potassium intake could cause cardiac arrest.

14.6.1.3   Iron Requirement [6–8]

Iron requirement based on sex and age is given below:

Females 14–18 years: 15 mg
Females 19–50 years: 18 mg
Females 51+ years: 8 mg
Males 14–18 years: 11 mg
Males 19+ years: 8 mg

Iron is a very important ingredient that is required by high altitude extreme sports enthusiasts. Iron is important specifically for extreme sports athletes since iron is an important component of hemoglobin. The iron is used for hemoglobin which is used to make oxygen-carrying red blood cells.

14.6.1.4   Zinc Requirement [9]

Extreme sports athletes should take 30–60 mg of Zinc daily. Zinc is extremely important since it is used for tissue repair and helps convert food to energy.

14.6.1.5   Calcium Requirement [9]

Calcium intake for a normal human being ideally will vary from 1,000 to 1,500 mg/ day but this depends on age and gender. For an extreme sports athlete in high altitude, the calcium intake should be at least 1,200–1,500 daily.

14.6.1.6   Magnesium Requirement [9]

The recommended intake for magnesium for athletes for extreme sports should be 500–800 mg/day. A higher dose than stated above can cause diarrhea. Most athletes lose magnesium through urine and sweat.

14.6.1.7   Chromium (III) Requirement [10]

Information on trivalent chromium requirements for people who have almost no exercise or moderate exercise is not available at a very detailed level. Similarly, detailed studies on chromium requirement are not available for extreme sports athletes. It has been determined that adequate daily dietary intake of chromium for adults is 30–200 μg/d. However, there is a lack of a food composition database which makes it difficult to exactly determine the chromium requirement.

For extreme sports athletes, the chromium requirement is higher. There is no verified source of data for exact chromium intake and requirements for extreme sports, and chromium intake also varies from country to country. Reports suggest that chromium intake in sportspersons in the USA is approximately 1.2 ng Cr/MJ (5 μg/1000 kcal) to 3.6 ng Cr/MJ. The chromium requirement based on generic population for some countries is shown below:

Finland: 29 μg
England: 25 μg
Canada: 56 μg
US: 37 μg

14.6.1.8   Vanadium Requirement [10]

In terms of Estimated Average Requirement (EAR) and/or Adequate Intake (AI), there is no set requirement or limit. The upper limit for vanadium is 1.8 mg/day and it generally varies between 0.9–1.4 mg/day for extreme sports athletes.

14.6.1.9   Boron Requirement [10]

For extreme ports athletes who are into high altitude sports, boron requirement is higher than normal. The upper limit for boron is 20 mg/day.

14.6.1.10   Nickel Requirement [10]

The upper limit for nickel is 1 mg/day similar to boron requirement as mentioned above for high altitude athletes.

14.6.1.11   Selenium Requirement

Selenium helps in recovery from tissue damage and boosts immunity. Approximately 200 mcg of selenium supplement is safe for high altitude extreme sportspersons.

14.6.2   Vitamins and Antioxidants Requirements for High Altitude Extreme Sports

14.6.2.1   Vitamin C [10]

Vitamin C is extremely important for high altitude extreme sports athletes. High altitude extreme sports athletes require more Vitamin C than the general population and it has been determined that men need approximately 90 mg/day while women need approximately 75 mg/day. Depending on the level of activity and the requirements of particular sports, it has been determined that sportspersons need anywhere between 500 mg and 3000 mg/day.

Sources of vitamin C:

Vitamin C can be found in a number of fruits and vegetables.
Vegetables: Various vegetables containing vitamin C include broccoli, green pepper, red pepper, red cabbage, tomatoes, cauliflower and Brussel sprouts.

Fruits: Fruits include orange, cantaloupe, kiwi, strawberries, raspberries, blueberries, cranberries, pineapple, papaya, watermelon and mango

Overdose of vitamin C is very rare and difficult but it has been determined that taking Vitamin C on an empty stomach might cause indigestion, while taking large amounts of vitamin C from different sources might cause diarrhea.

14.6.2.2   Vitamin E

Like vitamin C, vitamin E is extremely important for high altitude extreme sports athletes. Vitamin E helps in cell repair and protects from cellular damage. It has been determined that 400–800 international units(UI)/day is required; however, at the same time, recent studies have determined too much vitamin E could be extremely harmful.

14.6.2.3   Beta-Carotene: Vitamin A

Vitamin A mainly comes from Resveratrol: grape (grape extract). Vitamin A is important for high altitude extreme sports athletes for a number of reasons – for better immune systems and helping in the regeneration of bones, soft tissues and white blood cells. Vitamin A also acts as an antioxidant which is extremely important for high altitude sports.

14.6.2.4   Glutamine

2 g/day of glutamine is necessary for extreme sports athletes.

Gold, Silver and Tungsten

Even though the importance and efficacy of gold and silver in food and the nutritional benefits are not completely understood, there are some studies that have shown the benefit of their presence and hence their importance in extreme sports activity [11].

Homeopathy has claimed the importance of gold in heart disease, arthritis and depression.

14.6.3   PHYSICAL REQUIREMENT

Since there are different types of high altitude extreme sports, it is difficult to generally categorize the physical requirements of all extreme sports. However, in general, most high altitude extreme sports athletes are immensely fit and their fitness training would cover most or all of the following:

a. Flexible joints and easy joint movements with full range of motion
b. Long distance running to improve stamina
c. Short distance/interval sprints to improve strength
d. High intensity endurance training
e. Lower back and upper back training
f. Core strength and coordination of body parts
g. Overall flexibility including hip and trunk, stability and balance

14.7   FOOD NUTRIENTS AND IMPACTS

After a detailed study of most of high altitude extreme sports athletes, it has been determined that extreme sports athletes typically have these three foods in their diet: fish containing omega-3 fatty acids, caffeine and tart cherry juice. Even though fish and caffeine were popular with other athletes, it was interesting to find tart cherry juice as one of the foods as well.

Important benefits of fish/omega 3 fatty acids are a. Decreasing inflammation; b. Increasing blood flow by 36% while exercising; c. Decreasing morning stiffness, joint pains and swollen joints (rheumatoid arthritis)

Important benefits of caffeine are a. Increased mental alertness if given in doses of 4 mg/kg; b. Increased ability in logical reasoning; c. Increased memory strength; d. Immense helpfulness in increasing the time to exhaustion for multiple extreme sports that are extremely strenuous (a category which includes high altitude extreme sports); e. Decreased exhaustion in high endurance extreme sports; f. Improved mental alertness and physical endurance during stages of sleep deprivation; g. Helpfulness in recovery from muscle pain.

The important benefits of tart cherry juice are a. High level of antioxidant and anti-inflammatory effect; b. Provides strength during high intensity and high endurance sports; c. Reduces pain.

14.8   IMPORTANCE OF NUTRACEUTICALS AND FUNCTIONAL FOODS FOR HIGH ALTITUDE EXTREME SPORTS ATHLETES

In order to understand the importance of nutraceutical and functional foods for extreme sports athletes, we should first define "functional foods". Functional foods are the types of foods that provide *"added physiological benefits above the naturally occurring benefits"*.

Functional food [12] is simply food that provides something extra. Out of a number of various important advantages, the following are the most important provided by functional foods that are highly beneficial for extreme sports athletes:

a. Helps in weight loss
b. Increases both muscle and bone strength
c. Increases joint strength
d. Decreases cardiovascular diseases
e. Decreases chance of diabetes
f. Decreases skin deformation and wrinkles
g. Helps digestion

14.8.1   TYPES OF FUNCTIONAL FOOD PRODUCTS AND NUTRITION [13, 14]

One of the most significant drawbacks of nutritional supplements is the inability to prove or support their benefits in all cases. Nutritional supplements are unique in that the effect produced by a nutritional supplement on one athlete could be different from another athlete. Supplements also have a brand loyalty [13] among athletes and athletes don't like to change supplements and brands very often, especially if certain supplements have worked well in the past.

The largest category of nutritional supplements is protein powder. Protein powder is taken by at least two thirds of extreme sportsmen/sportswomen. Most protein products help in building muscle mass and providing strength and hence are used in more strenuous trainings and workouts.

The second category of nutritional supplements contains some combination of caffeine and sugar, while other ingredients could be present such as additives like carbohydrates and plant extracts. This category is used for 'increasing energy and endurance' [14].

The third category contains combinations of protein and carbohydrates. This category of supplements is used for repairing muscles and "recovery".

Apart from the top three products, there are others that are plant based, but these have less penetration in the market and generally account for 3–5% market share.

14.8.2   DISADVANTAGES OF FUNCTIONAL FOOD AND NUTRITION [13]

Just like any other product, there are some disadvantages of functional food products for extreme sports. These might not be necessarily disadvantages but could be defined as factors that might need more understanding and analysis before claiming success for all functional foods.

There are less scientific evidence, clinical studies and results regarding the effects of functional foods:

a. More time and analysis have been spent on regular foods since they were available for a longer time, while less time has been spent on functional foods, meaning there have been fewer results on the effects of these foods on high altitude extreme sports produced. This illustrates how it is sometimes difficult to prove the impact of functional food and nutrition on extreme sports.

b. The effect of functional food and nutrition might be unique to every extreme sports athlete and might not produce the same results for everyone.

c. Too many different kinds of products are available in the market. Often times, less is better. Due to the number of products available in the market, it is sometimes extremely confusing as to which product should be purchased. In addition, there is a chance that one product is chosen over another incorrectly without an understanding of the actual difference between them.

d. The costs of functional and nutraceutical products are often very high as compared to regular food products, which might be a reason not to buy functional foods.

e. Skepticism about nutritional and functional food: oftentimes there is skepticism from athletes and coaches about the efficacy of functional food, which has hindered its growth in popularity. This is connected to point 1 above and in this case, there have been contradictory conclusions when a large number of clinical trials have been done on the same product

f. Product success is dependent on a high degree of loyalty; the success of functional food is dependent on the degree of loyalty by the sports fraternity. If product users think there is a difference in performance due to the use of functional food then athletes will definitely continue using the product. But this loyalty also has a negative impact since the product success often depends on the 'feel factor' of the athletes.

g. Extremely short time span for success: functional food and nutritional products are judged in weeks and months, not years, and sometimes in days. The extremely short span in determining the success of the product often makes it difficult for it to be successful.

h. Oftentimes the efficacy of functional food is proved through a small number of participants: in most cases, the efficacy of functional food is proved by a small athlete pool but once the product is launched it doesn't keep up to its promise.

14.9   PLACES APPROPRIATE FOR HIGH
ALTITUDE EXTREME SPORTS [15]

Even though most extreme sports don't have specific locations, a number are more popular in particular regions and locations and quite a number of high altitude extreme sports are highly popular in particular places. A few are described below (the following examples are considered due to high popularity) along with their popular location.

Based on the terrain, these popular sports could be divided into the following:

14.9.1 MOUNTAINOUS TERRAIN

(a) Ice climbing

Ouray Ice Park (Colorado, USA) was the first park used for this sport. Val David (Quebec, Canada) is another park used for ice climbing.

Other related sports involve any form of climbing exercise, often in high altitudes (could be bare rocks or snow-capped mountains)

(b) Snowmobiling

Snowmobiling involves transportation and racing on snow.

Upper Peninsula (Michigan, USA) and Alpine resorts (Canada as well as the USA) are used for snowmobiling.

Other related sports involve any form of transportation and racing across snow, e.g. using a sled on the snow-covered surfaces.

(c) Bouldering

Bouldering involves climbing but without any protective gear and backup.

Bouldering is generally held in indoor locations and it is extremely popular in the USA, UK and Germany. This is also popular in outdoor locations such as in California, USA, and Rocklands, South Africa.

(d) Zip-lining at High Altitude

Zip-lining involves holding a pulley attached to a cable and moving from point A to point B.

Zip-lining is quite popular in Zip 2000 (Sun City, South Africa) and in Selvatura Park (Costa Rica).

Other related sports involve traversing between two points (the path between could be extremely difficult).

(e) Slacklining at High Altitude

This involves walking on a thin rope which is the path between two points.

Slacklining is popular in multiple locations including Vancouver (Canada), a very popular and famous spot.

Other related sports involve tight rope walking and slacklining yoga.

(f) Downhill mountain biking

Bikes are used in downhill mountain biking to go down a steep hill, often crossing multiple obstacles on the way.

Downhill mountain biking is held in Death Road, in Bolivia, and in Whistler Bike Park in Canada.

Other related sports include other racing events.

(g) Zorbing

This involves rolling down the hill in a transparent ball.

Rotorua, USA and Guam are popular locations for zorbing.

Other related sports also involve participants moving down a steep hill.

(h) Extreme Ironing [16]

Extreme ironing is one of the comparatively new events/games, started in 1997 in Leicester, UK, where people take ironing boards to remote locations and iron items of clothing. It began as and is still usually considered a game for fun.

This sport is popular in Germany, Austria, Croatia, Chile and Australia.

14.9.2 Water Terrain at High Altitude

(a) Freshwater cave diving

Freshwater cave diving refers to underwater diving in water-filled caves. The purpose is to explore flooded caves for scientific investigation. It could also refer to activities similar to scuba divers practicing oceanic cave exploration.

Freshwater cave diving is very popular in the Yucatán Peninsula in Mexico.

Other related sports include ocean scuba diving.

(b) Ice swimming

This involves swimming for one mile where the water temperature is below 5 degrees centigrade.

This is very popular in Finland.

Another form of this sport is extremely popular in northern Europe where participants take dips in the ice-cold water between sauna sessions.

(c) Canyoning

Canyoning in short could be described as a form of white-water rafting but without the boat. It's called gorge walking where canyoners navigate through the gorges by swimming, walking, moving over the rocks and sliding down chutes.Some of the best places to go canyoning are Dundonell or Inchree Falls in Scotland, How Stean Gorge in Yorkshire, Brecon Beacons or Snowdonia National Park in Wales.

Utah and Grand Canyon treks in Arizona, US are also famous.

(d) Coasteering

Coasteering involves moving through a rocky coastline without any water vehicle. Walking, running and/or swimming are allowed.

The coastline of Pembrokeshire, Wales, UK, is the most popular place for coasteering.

Other related sports involve swimming in difficult terrain, especially rocky terrain.

(e) White water rafting

White water rafting involves moving across rapids or using rafts to create a path to move across rapids. White water rafting is rated for difficulty between one and five levels, where the fifth is most difficult.

Zambezi River, Zambia, Suarez River, Colombia and Sun Kosi River, Nepal, are the most popular spots for white water rafting.

Other related sports involve "Levels", where Level 1 is the easiest and Level 5 is the most difficult.

14.9.3 Airborne/Mid-Air

(a) Bungee Jumping

Bungee jumping involves jumping from mid-air and landing safely on the ground. A safety cord is attached by a guide/instructor and height can vary.

Queenstown, Victoria Falls, Zambia and Macau Tower are the most popular spots.

Other related sports involve base jumping and sky surfing
(b) Sky diving

Sky diving involves jumping from .mid-air and landing safely on the ground. The height of the jump can vary.

The Swiss Alps, Switzerland, and Byron Bay, Australia, are the most popular spots for sky diving.

Other related sports include base jumping, sky surfing and wingsuit surfing.

(c) Kite surfing

Kite surfing includes wakeboarding, surfing, windsurfing, paragliding, and certain gymnastics.

O'ahu, Hawaii, USA, El Gouna, Egypt, and Camber Sands, UK, are the most popular spots for kite surfing.

Other related sports include paragliding, windsurfing and surfing.

(d) Boarding, also called Heli-skiing

This involves jumping from a helicopter and using a ski, snowboard and poles to traverse the trail.

Chugach Mountain, Alaska, USA, is the most popular spot for this sport.

Other related sports include snowboarding and skiing.

We will end airborne sports with a fun game which could become extreme based on the level of competition and terrain but which is still considered a low risk sport.

(e) Cheese rolling [17]

Cheese rolling started in the 15th century and involves participants running down the hill behind cheese. Just as name suggests, a nine pound of Double Gloucester cheese is rolled from top of hill and competitors chase behind the cheese. Even though the goal of the game is to catch the cheese but often times, the cheese gains speed and it becomes difficult to catch and the first person to cross the finish line is the winner.

Cooper's Hill, Gloucester, UK, is the most notable place for this event. Other related sports include zorbing.

14.10   HIGH ALTITUDE EXTREME SPORTS STATISTICS [18]

Extreme sports have become immensely popular in the 20th century and continue to gain popularity. In terms of sales, extreme sports generate over 12 billion dollars per year of which one-third comes from high altitude sports. Over 100 million dollars is spent every year on close to 300 high intensity or extreme sports around the world; it is estimated that over 25 million athletes participate in extreme sports.

14.11   CONCLUSION

Overall, mountain and high-altitude sports are very exciting and thrilling. Strong determination, focus, enthusiasm and utmost desire are required to participate in these activities. In general, high altitude extreme sports are extremely popular among people between the ages of 20 and 35, though recently high altitude sports are becoming popular with people above the age of 40. Just like land based extreme sports, high altitude sports are also popular and current and retired army and navy veterans are also responsible for increasing the popularity of these sports. They have done similar sports during their active duty and would like to continue an active life both for themselves and to make these sports popular among their groups of friends, and also influence other people outside the army to take up extreme sports. Often times, high altitude extreme sports are commercialized by army and navy veterans. With the advent of such exercise, food and nutrition also become extremely important and there is a need for appropriate food and nutrition which can provide the motivation, strength and desire to take part in these sports. We provided a detailed review of the various activities and the nutritional requirements for the athletes involved in these mountain and high-altitude events.

REFERENCES

1. Hlodan O. Evolution in Extreme Environments. *BioScience*. 2010, 60 (6): 414–441. https://academic.oup.com/bioscience/article/60/6/414/242037 (Date accessed: May 20, 2018)
2. EXTREME. Types of Extreme Sports. 2017. https://www.extremesportscompany.com/list-of-extreme-sports (Date accessed: February 08, 2018)
3. High Intensity Interval Training. ACSM Information, American College of Sports Medicine. https://www.acsm.org/docs/brochures/high-intensity-interval-training.pdf (Date accessed: May 23, 2018)
4. Uliaszek AA, Zinbarg RE, Mineka S, Craske MG, Sutton JM, Griffith JW, Rose R, Waters A, Hammen C. The Role of Neuroticism and Extraversion in the Stress-Anxiety and Stress-Depression Relationships. *Anxiety Stress Coping*. 2010, 23 (4): 363–368
5. Kenney L. Dietary Water and Sodium Requirements for Active Adults. *Sports Science Exchange*. 2004, 92 (17). http://www.gssiweb.org/sports-science-exchange/article/sse-92-dietary-water-and-sodium-requirements-for-active-adults (Date accessed May 23, 2018)
6. Kealey S. The Iron Needs of Athletes: Who Needs More, and How to Get it Through Your Diet. http://www.sheilakealey.com/sports-nutrition/iron/ (Date accessed May 23, 2018)
7. Sly B. What Athletes Need to Know About Iron Deficiency (Breaking Muscle Newsletter). https://breakingmuscle.com/healthy-eating/what-athletes-need-to-know-about-iron-deficiency (Date accessed May 23, 2018)
8. Weinstein J. Iron and the Endurance Athlete. https://www.trainingpeaks.com/blog/iron-and-the-endurance-athlete/ (Date accessed May 23, 2018)
9. Lukaski HC. Magnesium, Zinc, and Chromium Nutriture and Physical Activity. *Am J Clin Nutr*. 2000, 72 (2 Suppl): 585S–593S
10. Institute of Medicine (US) Panel on Micronutrients. Washington (DC). Dietary Reference Intakes for Vitamin A, Vitamin K, Arsenic, Boron, Chromium, Copper, Iodine, Iron, Manganese, Molybdenum, Nickel, Silicon, Vanadium, and Zinc. National Academies Press (US); 2001 ISBN-10: 0-309-07279. https://www.ncbi.nlm.nih.gov/books/NBK222310/ (Date accessed: May 23, 2018)

11. Anderson LV. Conspicuous Consumption. How Much Gold Can You Safely Eat? http://www.slate.com/articles/technology/2012/07/the_666_gold_wrapped_douche_burger_is_it_safe_to_eat_gold_.html (Date accessed May 23, 2018)

12. Spano M. Functional Foods, Beverages, and Ingredients in Athletics. *Spano Sports Nutrition Consulting*. https://pdfs.semanticscholar.org/0c98/834914c198c854f6b57bce4068f68f0639a1.pdf (Date accessed May 23, 2018)

13. Bomgardner M. Athletes Look to Sports Nutrition Products to Improve Performance. *Chem Eng News*. 2016, 94 (6): 10–15. https://cen.acs.org/articles/94/i6/Athletes-Look-Sports-Nutrition-Products.html (Date accessed: May 23, 2018)

14. Ghose T. Extreme Workouts: The Nutritional Needs of Elite Athletes. https://www.livescience.com/55503-nutritional-needs-of-athletes.html (Date accessed: May 22, 2018)

15. Lonely Planet Writer. 20 Unmissable Extreme Sports (and Where to Try Them). https://www.lonelyplanet.com/travel-tips-and-articles/20-unmissable-extreme-sports-and-where-to-try-them/40625c8c-8a11-5710-a052-1479d277bd61 (Date accessed: May 22, 2018)

16. Shaw P. *Extreme Ironing*. 2005. London: New Holland Publishers.

17. Earley C. A Quick Guide to Cheese Rolling, England's Strangest Sport. https://theculturetrip.com/europe/united-kingdom/england/articles/a-quick-guide-to-cheese-rolling-englands-strangest-sport/ (Date accessed: May 23, 2018)

18. Perlman A. Lead Adventurer at Nerve Rush. Nerve Rush Extreme Sports. http://www.nerverush.com/extreme-sports-list/ (Date accessed: May 20, 2018)

15 Structurally Diverse Water Sports in Extreme Conditions

Sourya Datta and Debasis Bagchi

CONTENTS

15.1 What are Extreme Water Sports and Categories of Extreme Sports 278
    15.1.1 Based on Elements 278
    15.1.2 Based on Risk... 278
    15.1.3 Based on Location (Country) 279
    15.1.4 Based on Difficulty... 279
15.2 Extreme Sports and Evolution of Water Related Extreme Sports.............. 279
    15.2.1 Basic Definition of Water Sports and Types of Water Sports........ 279
15.3 Evolution of Water Sports and Extreme Water Sports 280
15.4 Deep Dive on Each of the Water Sports.. 281
15.5 Deep Dive on Popular Extreme Water Sports 288
    15.5.1 Surfing.. 288
    15.5.2 Water Skiing... 288
    15.5.3 Bodyboarding... 288
    15.5.4 Wakeboarding... 289
    15.5.5 Kiteboarding/Kitesurfing.. 289
    15.5.6 Windsurfing.. 289
    15.5.7 Cavediving.. 289
    15.5.8 Paddle Surfing.. 289
    15.5.9 Flowboarding 290
    15.5.10 Kayaking 290
    15.5.11 Cliff Diving 290
    15.5.12 Canoeing 290
    15.5.13 Scuba Diving 290
    15.5.14 Whitewater Rafting 290
    15.5.15 Kneeboarding 291
    15.5.16 Skimboarding 291
    15.5.17 Jet Skiing.. 291
    15.5.18 Flyboarding 291
15.6 Food and Nutritional Requirements to Be Successful in Extreme
    Water Sports.. 291
15.7 Future of Extreme Water Sports.. 292
15.8 Conclusion 293
References.. 294

15.1   WHAT ARE EXTREME WATER SPORTS AND CATEGORIES OF EXTREME SPORTS [1]

'Extreme Sports' is a type of activity that gives an adrenaline rush to individuals who take part in sports that are different from the generic norm. Extreme water sports are extreme sports that take place in water. Structurally, water sports are different from land and snow/ice and thus by default water extreme sports are also different from the extreme land and high altitude sports discussed in Chapters 13 and 14.

As far as the categories of extreme sports are concerned, they have been mainly divided into the following: [2]

Based on elements (water, snow, air, earth)
Based on risk, enthusiasm and zeal
Based on location (country)
Based on difficulty

15.1.1   BASED ON ELEMENTS

Although we will cover water sports in this chapter, below are some popular examples of extreme sports to show the difference.

Examples of activities/sports on water include surfing, bodyboarding, water skiing, wakeboarding, kite surfing, windsurfing, cave diving, paddle surfing, cliff jumping, scuba diving, whitewater rafting and skim boarding jet skiing.

Examples of activities/sports on snow include snowboarding, snow skiing, ice climbing and snowmobiling.

Examples of activities/sports on air include skydiving, base jumping, bungee jumping, high-lining, paragliding and slacklining.

Examples of activities/sports on earth include skateboarding, mountain boarding, sandboarding, frifting, BMX, motocross, inline skating, mountaineering, caving, slacklining, rock climbing, free climbing, bouldering, mountaineering, sand kiting and zorbing.

15.1.2   BASED ON RISK

Extreme Sports can be categorized based on risk [3, 4].

Shane Murphy, a distinguished professor at Western Connecticut State University and also a sports psychologist, sums up the personal appetite of athletes, "I can enjoy hitting the tennis ball around, because that's my skill level... But others might need the challenge of Olympic competition In most sports, risk is directly proportional to the complexity of sports. For example, if we take the above quote, Olympic games would have more risks compared to a friendly tennis match.

Risk is defined based on a number of important factors: skill, experience, zeal, enthusiasm and environment. Often times an experienced extreme sports person knows how to mitigate risks and handle difficult situations. Professor Murphy gave an excellent example of a group who were climbing Everest and wanted to do so without oxygen. For most people this is extremely risky but to the group it was just one part of a larger activity they had worked towards for years; they believed that had minimized the risks due to their extensive preparation. Most of the time, an athlete has things under control and he/she knows how to avoid the risk instead of getting into a risky/dangerous situation.

15.1.3 BASED ON LOCATION (COUNTRY)

Based on location, extreme sports can vary greatly. Each and every type of extreme sport is unique in its own way and often time the location makes it more challenging. The same type of sport could become more difficult or much easier based on the location; even within the country, depending on the location, the same type of sport could vary, such as the difficulty of the Spartan race which will vary depending on various locations in US. Even in California, based on the city (every city has its own unique features and terrains), the difficulty of Spartan race will vary.

15.1.4 BASED ON DIFFICULTY

Difficulty is often subjective and not always objective. A very well-trained athlete could find one sport moderately easier in comparison to a semi-trained athlete for whom the same sport could be much more difficult. In addition, the athlete could be a master in one type of sport and he/she could be mediocre in another type of sport. A good example is short distance running versus long distance running. An Olympic level [1] pro-athlete in short distance running might not even be able to perform in a state level competition in long distance running.

15.2 EXTREME SPORTS AND EVOLUTION OF WATER RELATED EXTREME SPORTS

Just like any other terrains, in order to understand water related extreme sports, we need to understand water sports, their evolution and different types and then the evolution of extreme water sports.

15.2.1 BASIC DEFINITION OF WATER SPORTS AND TYPES OF WATER SPORTS

Any type of sport that takes place in water could be defined as a water sport. Broadly speaking, water sports can be classified as (a) in water, (b) under water, and (c) over water.

Another way of defining water sports could be (a) individual or (b) group, while, similarly, a third method would be (a) recreational or (b) competitive.

If we combine the above two, we can also classify water sports as the following:

a. Individual recreational
b. Individual competitive
c. Group recreational
d. Group competitive

We could also apply the categories of in water, under water and over water in the sections mentioned above.

Popular games in the 'In Water' category include:

  (i) Scuba diving
 (ii) Springboard diving
(iii) Snorkeling
 (iv) Triathlon
  (v) Water Polo

Popular games in the 'Under Water' category include:

  (i) Cave diving
 (ii) Ice diving
(iii) Free diving

Popular games in the 'Over Water' category include:

   (i)   Boat racing
  (ii)   Barefoot skiing
 (iii)   Canoeing
  (iv)   Fly boarding
   (v)   Jet skiing
  (vi)   Kayaking
 (vii)   Kiteboarding
(viii)   Kneeboarding
  (ix)   Kitesurfing
   (x)   Parasailing
  (xi)   Rafting
 (xii)   Rowing
(xiii)   Surfing
 (xiv)   Wakeboarding
  (xv)   Windsurfing

15.3 EVOLUTION OF WATER SPORTS AND EXTREME WATER SPORTS [5, 6]

In general, the category of water sports is so vast that each of the sports need to be categorized and understood individually.

Broadly we can classify water sports under following heads:

  1. Aquatics
       Aquatics or Aquatic Sports are a number of sports that are played both in Olympic and other international competitions.
       a. Diving
       b. Swimming
       c. Water Polo

2. Boating
   a. Canoeing
   b. Kayaking
   c. Rafting
   d. Yachting
3. Sailing
4. Skimboarding
5. Surfing
6. Underwater
   a. Underwater diving
   b. Underwater sports
7. Windsurfing
8. Jetskiing
9. Kitesurfing
10. Packrafting
11. Paddle sports
12. Rowing
13. Sea Jousting
14. Tubing
15. Wakeboarding
16. Water basketball
17. Water Aerobics
18. Water ball
19. Water motor sports
20. Water skiing

15.4 DEEP DIVE ON EACH OF THE WATER SPORTS

Let's look at each of the sports mentioned above in detail.

1. Aquatics:
   In general, aquatics can be divided into groups. All sports described below started as regular sports and they were simpler and easier to begin with. They don't fall under the category of extreme, but all the sports described below in detail could be transformed to extreme by increasing the complexity of the sports and changing the rules.
   a. Diving
   There are different types of diving in the Olympic Games, with generally two types of diving most popular: regular diving and synchronized diving. The difference between regular and synchronized diving is that in synchronized diving, the two divers are required to perform the exact same dive simultaneously and are rated based on the diving. Synchronized diving is very similar to synchronized swimming where the total rating is given based on both the participants but in synchronized diving, additional rules are also added since there are points for synchronization between the divers. Regular diving doesn't need any

synchronization and points are awarded based on the dive of individual participants. There are other formats of diving, described below:

   i. Pool diving

   Not as popular as outdoor diving and in general competitions takes place at pools which are approximately 33 feet high. Competition takes different formats and higher points are awarded for more somersaults but, most of the time, competitors prefer less somersaults and more accurate entry into the water (more somersaults makes the dives more complex).

   ii. Outdoor diving

   Outdoor diving takes different formats but most often takes place from a cliff. Cliff diving is challenging due to extreme height as well unknown terrain (the depth of water being entered into is unknown). This is where diving can become more complex and enter the category of extreme sports.

   b. Swimming

   a. Open water swimming

   Types: ice swimming, long distance swimming, marathon swimming, winter swimming

   b. Swimming styles: freestyle, breaststroke, butterfly, backstroke

   c. Synchronized swimming: combination of swimming, dance and gymnastics

   Can take different formations: solo, duet, team, mixed duet, combination and highlight

The category of open water swimming can be made more complex and ice water swimming will be an extreme sport depending on factors like temperature and length of the event.

   c. Water polo

   Seven member team game with one member being the goalie. Just like the above types of games, the game of water polo falls under the regular sports category but can be made complex by changing the rules like how many players per side, lowering the criteria for fouls and allowing more contact in the game.

2. Boating:

   Boating is very wide, including a number of sports. Not all of these fall under the category of extreme sports but some do; of these we will cover canoeing, kayaking, rafting and yachting, since these could fall under the category of extreme sports depending on their difficulty level.

   a. Canoeing:

   The main difference between canoeing and kayaking is the position of the rider and the number of blades. Canoeing generally uses a single-bladed paddle while kayaking uses a paddle with two blades. Just like kayaking, canoeing becomes dangerous depending on the path of the course and in such situations can be considered part of extreme sports.

b. Kayaking:

   Kayaking in general sounds a non-invasive and low danger sport but could become extremely dangerous depending on the course, such as in extreme whitewater with an increased number of rapids and rocks.

c. Rafting:

   Rafting initially started as a leisure sport but over time has developed from low action to medium and finally to high action extreme sports depending on the course of the water. The International Rafting Federation looks over rafting competitions around the world and depending on the course rafting can view them as easy or extremely dangerous, with the latter entering into the category of extreme sports. There are six main types of courses depending on the size of the wave and the water movement.

   Class 1: Very basic rapids, easy flow of water

   Class 2: A small number of rocks, may need some skillful movement along the water

   Class 3: A couple of drops might be in the course, low danger

   Class 4: White water, requires medium to high experience in rafting, also needs skilled movement of the rafts

   Class 5: Larger waves, presence of medium to larger rocks, high skillful movement of rafts required

   Class 6: Extremely dangerous and requires trained rafters. High waves, large rocks and a number of large drops could be in the path, meaning safety is a big factor and that this is considered extreme sport

d. Yachting:

   Yachting most likely started in the Netherlands as early as the seventeenth century. Initially it wasn't the sport that it has evolved into now but rather it started with small sailing boats which later gave way to more powerful custom-built boats or yachts in England for competitions. Skiff racing is one variety of yachting that falls into the category of extreme sports, with the unpredictability pf the weather playing a very important role here. Different types of races are common and vary from short distance (or dinghy racing) races to longer point races.

3. Sailing:

   Sailing was the main from of transportation in early ages which has given way to competitions today. Ships are still a significant part of transportation but different forms of sailing have been adopted for various forms of competition. Two popular classes of sailing competitions are based on:

   A. Disciplines:

      a. Match Racing: Two boats race against each other
      b. Team Racing: Two team race against reach other
      c. Fleet Racing: Pre-defined course for racing
      d. Wave Riding: Boats need to ride waves to complete a course

   B. Gender: A number of formats are available – both mixed races as well as male only and female only

4. Skimboarding:

Skimboarding, also known as skimming, is used to ride along the water and then meet an incoming wave so as to return to the shore with the wave.

5. Surfing:

One of the most popular sports in water is surfing. Here the surfer rides towards the shores, forward off a wave which helps their movement in this direction.

There are a number of types of surfing with the most common types listed below:

a. Stand-up surfing: surfer stands up and rides the wave
    i.   Short boarding
    ii. Long boarding
    iii. Stand up paddling
b. Body boarding: Surfer uses a body board and most of the time either lies on their front or sits down with their knee in front, or can stand on the board
c. Knee boarding: using drop knee
d. Surf matting : inflatable mats are used for surfing
e. Foil boarding: using foils
f. Body surfing: surfer uses his/her own body and doesn't use a board
    Surfing is being introduced in the Summer Olympics in 2020.

    Surfing takes place mostly in the ocean but often in lakes, rivers and even using artificial waves.

    Different moves at surfing include hanging ten and hanging five, as well as the cutback, floater and airs. Just like different moves, there are different rotations as well. Different types of rotations include:

a. 180 degrees: surfer does a 180 and lands backwards first before returning to their original position
b. 360 degrees: a full 360 where the surfer lands at the exact same position where they started
c. 540 degrees: the surfer does a full/complete rotation and then a 180
d. Backflip: highly skilled surfers perform this move, which involves a flip
e. Rodeo flip: a backflip with a 180 rotation
f. Grabs: a movement completed by grabbing the surfboard, of which there are different variations

6. Underwater: [7]

There are a number of underwater games and the most popular underwater games are shown below. Most of the games are regular but just like a number of water games, each of the sports could be made more complex by changing a few rules.

(i)   Finswimming
(ii)   Freediving
(iii) Spearfishing
(iv)   Sport diving
(v)   Underwater football
(vi)   Underwater hockey

(vii)   Underwater ice hockey
(viii)   Underwater orienteering
  (ix)   Underwater photography
   (x)   Underwater rugby
  (xi)   Underwater target shooting
7. Windsurfing: Combination of Surfing and Sailing
    Both surfing and sailing use wind to propel forward. There are two main types of competitions, freestyle and wave, with these based on both technique and diversity. Most windsurfers call themselves sailors due to the close proximity of their sport with sailing style and the rules. Officially, windsurfing for men began in 1984 and for women in 1992. Currently there are two events, RS:X for men and women.
8. Jet skiing:
    Jet skiing refers to the use of jet ski to travel through the water. The jet ski was originally manufactured by Kawasaki but this term now refers to all watercrafts used for either recreational or any extreme sport. A number of manufacturers have started making jet skis, with Yamaha one well known company that makes jet skis.
9. Kitesurfing:
    Kitesurfing is extremely interesting; it combines snowboarding, surfing, windsurfing, skateboarding and paragliding. The reasons behind the combination of so many sports are the location and the manner in which the sports are taking place. In general, kiteboarding uses a power kite and uses the strength of wind for the movement.
Water: Kiteboard is used (very similar to surfboard)
Land: Foot-steered buggy is used
Snow: Skis or snowboards are used
        Types of Kitesurfing:
        Freeride: The most fun and simple type of kitesurfing –designed to have the most fun
        Waveriding: Directional board is used, and this involves a combination of kiteboarding and surfing
        Freestyle: Perform multiple tricks on the air, with smaller sized boards are used
        Airstyle: The name air refers to how the kitesurfer jumps in the air and performs various tricks
        Wakestyle: Tricks are often performed in the air with jumps also are performed, generally on flat water
        Wakeskate: Very similar to skateboarding and mostly done on flat water
        Course racing: As the name suggests, this involves some kind of race and thus involves speed. Main goal is to compete against other kitesurfers
        Park riding: More intense/difficult version of wakestyle and kite-surfers need to cross obstacles and/or perform tricks on the obstacles
        Speed racing: Speed is the key, with the goal to achieve maximum speed when the distance is greater than 500 meters

10. Packrafting:

Packrafting refers to the use of inflatable boats in whitewater. There are certain features in packrafts which are extremely important such as their being extremely lightweight and generally having paddles and oars that can be collapsed so these can be used over a longer distance. Most packrafts can only carry a single passenger and weigh less than nine pounds, with modern packrafts sturdier and can carry more weight than earlier ones. It is believed that packrafting started in US (probably in Alaska) but slowly gained popularity in parts of Asia, Australia, New Zealand and South America. Even though packrafts were used in Class II level or below the sport is slowly becoming popular at Class V levels which used to allow kayaks or much larger rafts initially. Packrafts at present are used for multiple purposes: whitewater rafting, adventure racing, remote fishing, and mountain climbing access points.

11. Paddle boarding/Paddle sports:

Paddle boarding is a sport where a person uses a surf board and long paddles to move in the water. There are different types of paddle boarding with the most common being (a) standing paddle boarding (b) lying paddle boarding (c) kneeling paddle boarding. In the future, paddle boarding could become an Olympic sport.

12. Rowing:

This goal here is to move the boat forward using oars. Rowing was planned to debut in the Olympic Games in 1896 but couldn't start due to bad weather, instead beginning in 1900 for men, with women's rowing starting in 1976. The Olympics has a total boat class of 14 while the World Rowing Championship involves 22 boat classes. Some popular domestic competitions include the Harvard-Yale Regatta and Head of the Charles Regatta in the US.

The two main types of rowing are: (a) sweep, where each rower has one oar (b) sculling, where each rower has two oars.

Types of rowing races/competitions:

a. Side by side : Boats competing with each other and starting the race at the same time, with the fastest finisher the winner, also known as regatta. The standard distance for Olympic versions of this is 1.24miles (2 KM).

b. Head races: Instead of competing side by side, boats start at intervals of 10–20 seconds between them, with the length generally the same as regatta (1.24 miles); some races, however, could be up to 7.46 miles.

c. Bumps races: As the name suggests, this race involves bumping by boats. This is a multi-day race where the goal is to bump a boat in the front and avoid getting bumped by a boat from behind. The boat that has bumped another boat will start at the beginning the next day.

d. Stake races: Competitors start at the same time, travel to a certain point, complete a 180 turn and then return to their starting point. In most cases, competition takes place between two boats.

13. Sea Jousting:

Sea jousting or water jousting is mainly a European sport and probably started in Egypt and later became popular in Ancient Greece and Rome. At present it is a very popular European sport and widely practiced in France and Germany. The aim is to knock the other boat off balance while maintaining one's own balance.

14. Tubing:

   The rider sits on a tube and has either ropes or strings attached with the boat. The main goal is to maintain balance and ride with the waves while being pulled forward on the water by the boat. Tubing can be towed (by a motor boat in most cases) or free floating (use hands to paddle).

   Another popular form of tubing is snow tubing, which takes place in colder regions of the world where there is abundance of snow.

   Another form of high-speed water tubing is kite tubing, when the tube becomes air borne and takes off due to high speed.

15. Wakeboarding:

   Like most other water extreme sports, wakeboarding is a combination of sports, here water skiing, snowboarding and surfing. After a number of modifications in recent years, the current wakeboard is small and rectangular, with two places for the feet. Wakeboards usually travel between 20–25 miles/hour and are tied behind a boat.

16. Water basketball:

   Water basketball is a combination of basketball and water polo. It is a team game with five people per side with the player in possession of the ball having to shoot within a specific time of receiving possession. This game is a recent phenomenon and, unlike other games, started in Australia and then became popular in other European nations such as Italy and Netherlands.

17. Water aerobics:

   Like water basketball, water aerobics is a recent phenomenon which involves aerobic exercises in the water. In its simplest form, water aerobics includes aerobic exercises which are forms of resistance training. Different forms of water aerobics include Zumba in water, yoga in water, jogging (standing in one place and trying to move the legs one at a time just like walking), and resistance training.

18. Water ball:

   A giant ball approximately two meters in diameter holds a person inside and allows them to walk across water. Safety is often a significant concern here and in a few cases some people have been hurt using water balls.

19. Water motor sports:

   Water motor sports are extremely popular and began more than 100 years back in the 1908 Olympics. However, after the 1908 Olympics, it was announced that there motor sports would no longer feature. There were three main races: (a) open class/Class A (b) 60 feet/Class B and (c) up to eight meters/Class C.

   Even though they were stopped after just one Olympic Games, motor sports are extremely popular at present.

20. Water skiing:

   Water skiing is a surface water sport where the sportsperson is pulled by the boat and the rider moves through the water or just taps on the water surface. Different formats are available, with either one ski or two skis used. The most important requirements for sportspersons performing water skiing is to have strength and endurance. Even though water skiing is popular across all parts of the world it is extremely popular in US, where there are around eleven million water skiers, while Australia has around 1.3 Million water skiers. There are a number of water skiing events, with some of most popular listed above:

a. Barefoot water skiing
b. Show skiing
c. Ski racing
d. Freestyle jumping
e. Marathon
f. 3 events:
   i. Slalom
   ii. Jump
   iii. Trick

15.5 DEEP DIVE ON POPULAR EXTREME WATER SPORTS [8, 9]

15.5.1 SURFING

Surfing is the sport of riding water waves in an upright position. The aim of surfing is to glide or move across the water surface until the waves lose their momentum. Surfing could be done in the ocean, a river or even man-made water.

There are different types of surfing waves:

a. Spilling waves
b. Plunging waves
c. Surging waves
d. Collapsing waves

Balance and timing are the key to be successful in this sport.

15.5.2 WATER SKIING

This is a game where athletes use rope to hold oneself to a boat and move along the water in great speed. An athlete is tied to the boat with a rope and then pulled behind.

Great balance is needed.

15.5.3 BODYBOARDING

Bodyboarders use surf boards to ride the waves. The bodyboard is actually hydrodynamic foam and athletes also use swim fins for greater stability and control. The bodyboarder rides the board towards the wave and the wave carries the bodyboarders back towards the shore.

Timing is key in this sport so that the surfers ride the wave accurately at the right time.

15.5.4   WAKEBOARDING

In wakeboarding, the athlete stand on a board and is given a rope to hold with the other end tied to a powerboat boat which zooms across the water. The athlete jumps and flips in the air before landing on the water again.

Wakeboarding is the fastest growing water sport in the world and needs great balance and measurement and timing of spin in the air.

15.5.5   KITEBOARDING/KITESURFING

Kiteboarding refers to a game where an athlete attaches himself/herself to a surf board, holds a massive kite and then performs a number of stunts like spins in the air. The kiteboarder holds the handles of the large powerkite which moves in the wind which makes the athlete move across the water.

Kiteboarding combines wakeboarding, snowboarding, windsurfing, surfing, paragliding and skateboarding.

This sport needs careful attention to the direction of wind and strength of waves.

15.5.6   WINDSURFING

Windsurfing is an interesting game which combines some aspects of surfing and some aspects of sailing. It is a form of sailing where the athlete is on a surfboard-like board and the wind moves this board across the water. There is a basic difference with regular surfing – surfing uses wave force while windsurfing uses wind to move forward and this makes this sport enjoyable in rivers, lakes, seas and oceans.

Windsurfers need to be aware of high waves and high winds.

15.5.7   CAVEDIVING

Cavediving is a form of underwater diving taking place in water-filled caves. Cavedivers use scuba gear and go under the water until they find an entrance to a cave deep underwater. As the divers go deeper and deeper into the caves, different types of plants and fishes could appear, and the rock formations change. The deeper it is the more challenging it is, and it is an extremely dangerous sport due to complete darkness and unknown areas.

Apart from numerous other dangerous, losing the way has been very common in this sport.

15.5.8   PADDLE SURFING

Paddle surfing, as the name would suggest, is regular surfing with the help of a paddle. This sport could have originated in Hawaii and it follows the same principle as surfing, but the paddle surfer uses their paddles to go through the water and the board is used for balance and control to move through water.

15.5.9 Flowboarding

Flowboarding is a very interesting sport, where athletes surf on water but are stationary. Flowboarding takes ideas from surfing, bodyboarding, wakeboarding and other related sports. Powerful pumps are used to create artificial waves at a speed of ~30mile/hour and flowboarders ride along the waves. These are stationary waves and there is no movement of water. Often times there are artificial rock formations to make changes in the course of the water gushing out at high speed from the pumps.

15.5.10 Kayaking

Kayaking involves moving across water in a small boat with a double bladed oar for paddling. This type of activity is benign on the surface, but competitions bring in requirements of high speed, presence of rocks, also deep crevices and high drops, making it extremely challenging.

15.5.11 Cliff Diving

Just as the name suggests, cliff diving is a sport where the divers jump from a high cliff/rock. This game is one of the least complicated – there are no special clothes and no equipment is needed. The extreme nature of this sport is due the height of landing, often times the height is 85 feet.

Risks include the position of the jump and the position of landing.

15.5.12 Canoeing

Movement across a number of different obstacles along a course using a canoe with single blade paddle. Canoeing is made extreme by choosing the course and the path.

15.5.13 Scuba Diving

Scuba diving is a type of underwater diving. Since the diver is going under water, the diver needs underwater breathing system, usually in the form of tanks of compressed air. Scuba diving could be lot of fun but there is always an issue of dangerous animals in the water.

15.5.14 Whitewater Rafting

Whitewater rafting is a game where riders ride boats or rafts down a stream of whitewater. Whitewater rafting is an extremely fast paced sport, and the riders have to manuover through the water and have to watch out for rocks which could derail them from their course and high and dangerous waterfalls makes the route more complex. There are many levels of rapids which determine the difficulty level of rafting.

Class I : Flat moving water with almost no obstacles.
Class II : Water has some waves and rocks.
Class III : Water has moderate waves and a fast current, some rocks that may need to be avoided.
Class IV : Turbulent water, extremely fast currents, and drops are higher.

Class V : Intense water, extremely fast cross currents, drops are longer and larger. Extremely difficult to ride.

Class VI : Impossible to navigate.

An extreme form of rafting is riverboarding where riders surf rapids without any rafts.

15.5.15 KNEEBOARDING

Kneeboarding is a combination of surfing, water skiing and wake boarding. The surfers get towed on a board behind a motorboat. The riders first kneel on the boards and are secured with a strap over the thighs. Once the motorboat starts, the rider is pulled, and the rider needs to shift their weight effectively to avoid a fall.

15.5.16 SKIMBOARDING

Very similar to surfing but a freestyle version of the extreme sport. The surf board is smaller and more compact which helps for an easy ride for this type of sport. The smaller surf board is used by skimboarders to move across the water and meet an incoming wave and reach the shore. The smaller boards have no fins and are easy to maneuver and move. However, while that gives flexibility, faster movements are required in order to be successful.

15.5.17 JET SKIING

Riders use a self-propelled vehicle or scooter and used to skim across the water; control and steering are done with handlebars. The more extreme games are competitions where riders compete against each other at extremely high speeds and the first to reach the end is declared the winner.

15.5.18 FLYBOARDING

A flyboard is a hoverboard that can be used on water. Once the flyboard is attached to the personal watercraft, water will propel the device upward and it can take the flyboarders as high as 49 feet. It has the capability of diving through the water down to 8 feet. Championships and competitions started from 2012 and are gaining in popularity every year. Balance is the key to be successful in this game.

15.6 FOOD AND NUTRITIONAL REQUIREMENTS TO BE SUCCESSFUL IN EXTREME WATER SPORTS [10–12]

Six different types of food are extremely important - proteins, amino acid supplements, vitamins, herbal extracts, glutamine, probiotics and fish oil

Proteins and amino acid supplements: used for muscle repair
When to take: both before and after workout

Which types of food provide necessary nutrition: meat (red meat), beans, green vegetables
Food product extensions: protein powder
Ingredients: soy protein, whey protein

Vitamins: used for improving bone health, better immunity and muscle function
When to take: part of regular diet
Which types of food provide necessary nutrition: apart from food, sunlight is a great source
Food product extensions: supplements
Ingredients: Vitamins C, D and E

Herbal extracts: used for reducing inflammation and provides oxidation
When to take: part of regular diet
Which types of food provide necessary nutrition: dark color vegetables and fruits
Food product extensions: supplements
Ingredients: green tea extract, quercetin, anthocyanins, oligomeric proanthocyanidins

Glutamine: used for improving immunity and gut health
When to take: part of a regular diet and also important after workout
Which types of food provide necessary nutrition: protein rich foods, spinach, parsley
Food product extensions: supplements
Ingredients: L-glutamine, creatine, L-carnitine, etc.

Probiotics: used for improving immunity and gut health
When to take: part of a regular diet and also important after workout
Which types of food provide necessary nutrition: yogurt, curd, fermented foods
Food product extensions: supplements
Ingredients: live friendly bacteria probiotics.

Fish oil: used for improving immunity and also reduces inflammation
When to take: part of regular diet
Which types of food provide necessary nutrition: fish
Food product extensions: supplements
Ingredients: Omega-3

15.7 FUTURE OF EXTREME WATER SPORTS [13]

The future of water extreme sports is very interesting. On one hand, the existing sports are becoming more and more popular and people who were not previously a part of the extreme sports community are taking part while, on the other hand, existing sports are becoming more complex which is attracting new sets of people and also opening up new revenue streams for companies/individuals who are creating new sports or modifying an existing sport to make it extreme or adding further complexities.

Location:

In the future, more regions will become new destinations for extreme sports. At present, the most popular locations for extreme sports are the United States, Canada, the United Kingdom, as well as other places in Europe such as Germany, France and Italy. Australia and New Zealand are also very popular places for extreme water sports, as is Scandinavia. However, future projections for locations show both current locations becoming more popular and new locations such as South America (especially Brazil) along with countries such as Hungary, Poland, Croatia and Czech Republic becoming more popular.

In addition, competition is heating up to host extreme sports among the most popular countries for these, such as United States, United Kingdom, Canada, Australia, New Zealand, France, Norway and Switzerland. This is not an all-inclusive list but some major countries where extreme water sports are extremely popular as well as those that want to be seen as current and future spots for water extreme sports.

Age group:

Overall, considering most of the extreme water sports, the age group of 20 to 35 has been identified as the age group that most enjoys taking part in extreme water sports. But over time, the age profile is broadening and more people of different age groups are participating in extreme water sports. More students are taking part in more extreme sports as well as new young entrepreneurs, with new water sports especially popular.

Growth potential:

Even though extreme water sports have gained a lot of popularity in the recent past and continue to gain popularity, in terms of actual numbers, it is extremely small. In the future that number should rise but the most important factor at present is the perception of the sports and popularity of extreme eater sports, which is determined by the popularity of the sport at that current time. More recently, extreme water sports are becoming popular with two sets of people: 1. middle aged and retired people who are taking on more water sports such as rafting and 2. students who are taking time off and traveling either before or after college.

15.8   CONCLUSION

Lots of attention are being observed in these challenging sports and activities, especially in young and middle-aged athletes and the para-military and military forces. Appropriate technological strategies and nutritional supports are also being designed by health professionals, sports nutritionists, dieticians and nutritionists. Innovation strategies are in progress to support these athletes.

REFERENCES

1. EXTREME. Types of extreme sports by Brand EXTREME (an iconic lifestyle brand fueled by the passion, creativity and freedom of action); 2017. https://www.extremesportscompany.com/ (Date accessed: May 22, 2018)
2. EXTREME. Types of extreme sports by Brand EXTREME (an iconic lifestyle brand fueled by the passion, creativity and freedom of action); 2017. http://www.extremetime.com/exploring-information-types.html (Date accessed: February 8, 2018)
3. Brody J.E. Taking sports to the extreme. *New York Times*; 2016. https://well.blogs.nytimes.com/2016/08/15/taking-sports-to-the-extreme/ (Date accessed: July 2018)
4. Glor J. Are extreme sports too dangerous? *CBS News*; 2012. https://www.cbsnews.com/news/are-extreme-sports-too-dangerous/ (Date accessed: July 2018)
5. Fry K. Water sports. *Ask About Sports*; 2009. http://www.askaboutsports.com/about/water-sports.htm (Date accessed: July 2018)
6. Different types of water sports: Enjoyed by people. *Sports x Fitness*; 2014. http://sportsxfitness.com/ (Date accessed: July 2018)
7. Underwater sports. https://www.underwatersports.com/ (Date accessed: July 2018)
8. Brymer E. Risk taking in extreme sports: A phenomenological perspective. *Annals of Leisure Research*, 2010. 13 (1); 218–238.
9. Risks in sport/8 of the most dangerous adventure sports. *Business Insider*; 2016. https://www.businessinsider.com/adventure-extreme-sports-injury-concussion-rates-2016-9 (Date accessed: July 2018)
10. Deakin University. Sporting performance and food. *Better Health Channel*. https://www.betterhealth.vic.gov.au/health/healthyliving/sporting-performance-and-food (Date accessed: July 2018)
11. Quinn E. An overview of nutrition for athletes; 2018. https://www.verywellfit.com/sports-nutrition-4157011 (Date accessed: July 2018)
12. Swearingen D. Eating before competition. https://www.cwu.edu/sports-nutrition/eating-competition (Date accessed: July 2018)
13. Extreme sports (current and future growth); 2018. https://www.onecaribbean.org/content/files/ExtremeSportCaribbeanNicheMarkets.pdf (Date accessed: July 2018)

Section V

Importance of Hydration
and Use of Gelatin

16 An Overview on the Beneficial Effects of Hydration

Douglas S. Kalman

CONTENTS

16.1 Introduction 297
16.2 Water and Its Diverse Biochemical and Physiological Functions 298
16.3 Salient Beneficial Features of Water 299
16.4 Hydration and Thirst 299
16.5 State of Hydration: Optimal Health 300
16.6 Athletic Performance and Hydration Status 301
16.7 Hydration and Measurement 303
16.8 Diverse Rehydration Techniques 304
16.9 Fluid Intake and Replacement 307
16.10 Summary and Conclusions 308
References 308

16.1 INTRODUCTION

A human body contains approximately 60% or greater water, the largest constituent of the human body. Water/hydration is important for vital physiological and biochemical functions including body temperature, heart rate and blood pressure, as well as for maintaining optimal health, especially for dermal health, hair and nails. In 2004, the Institute of Medicine (IOM) announced the official recommendation related to water/hydration needs. Simultaneously, the Food and Nutrition Board of the National Academies of Sciences, Engineering, and Medicine established the nutrient recommendations on water, salt and potassium to maintain health and reduce chronic disease risk. It was emphasized that an adult woman should consume 2.7 L of water, while an adult man should consume 3.7 L of water per day. Approximately 80% of this water comes from drinking water and beverages, while 20% is derived from food and nutrients.

A significant question arises on how a human body utilizes the processes of hydration and thermogenesis because the volume of water regulates nutrition, physical and physiological activities. For example, an increase in core body temperature during physical performance and exercise is coupled with heat dissipation. Heat dissipation will result in cutaneous vasodilation and change in heat transfer and exchange in conjunction with fluid/water. If heat transfer via radiation and convection is not adequate in reducing the heat load, sweating will occur and heat will be lost by evaporation along with fluid loss. If the water loss exceeds fluid intake, hypohydration leading to dehydration will occur, which will cause lethargy.

Water is a vital macronutrient and hydrating agent which is merely neglected and ignored. The IOM has created a level of water intake deemed to describe the "Adequate Intake" (AI). The AI is meant to "to prevent deleterious, primary acute, effects of dehydration, which include metabolic and functional abnormalities."[1] It is very challenging to establish a specific level of water intake/hydration in sportspersons involved in diverse sports activities. However, awareness that optimal hydration status/fluid balance is extremely essential for individuals involved in diverse sports activities, exercise or regular household or office work is important. The ultimate aim is to maintain adequate hydration and optimal health under all potential conditions.

An intricate relationship exists between hydration states and optimal health along with disease relationships, which allows for the belief that a strong correlation exists between hydration and disease/dysfunction. Furthermore, it has been repeatedly demonstrated that hydration plays a key role in the prevention of prolonged labor, urolithiasis, urinary tract infections, bladder cancer, constipation, pulmonary/bronchial disorders, heart disease, hypertension, venous thrombosis and diverse degenerative diseases.[2,3]

This review provides important information as related to the aspects that affect hydration needs and fluid balance. The provision of fluid guidelines for the physically active adult and the non-active adult are included. However, the total lifecycle hydration aspect is not covered herein, but can be read elsewhere.[4]

16.2   WATER AND ITS DIVERSE BIOCHEMICAL AND PHYSIOLOGICAL FUNCTIONS

Water is a fluid that acts as a solvent and a mode of transportation system within the human body. Water is the human body's most important nutrient, rather an overlooked macronutrient. It is utilized in each and every intricate function of the body, including the maintenance of body temperature, body fat metabolism, digestion, lubricating and cushioning organs, transporting nutrients and flushing toxins. Overall, water plays a central role in thermoregulation and maintenance of optimal health. Water can modulate multiple metabolic processes as well as physical performance and mental acuity.

Although nutrition-oriented research studies are primarily focused on obesity, diabetes, metabolic syndrome, arthritis and cancer, hydration has been totally neglected or ignored. As a result, the relationship between fluid intake and human health is not very clearly understood.

It is important to know that a reduction in total body water stores by as little as 2% can adversely impact aerobic performance, orthostatic tolerance and cognitive function. The body is comprised of approximately 60% water and the water/fluid is stored or circulating. It is interesting to know that muscle contains about 73% water, blood 93% and fat mass 10%. Approximately 5–10% of total body water is turned over daily through obligatory losses through respiratory functions, urinary excretion and sweating. Respiratory water losses are typically replenished through the production of metabolic water formed by substrate oxidation. Fluid losses during and post-exercise also affect overall fluid balance. Thus, fluid balance is easiest thought of as wanting to achieve a balance between fluid output and intake. It has been reported that physically active adults living in warmer climates have daily water needs of 6 L, with highly active populations needing even more to remain euhydrated.[5]

In the USA, average fluid intake is currently 1,440 mL per day, with 19% of the fluid intake coming from foods.[6] Thus, Americans are typically under-hydrated based on IOM guidelines where it is generally recommended that men aged 19 to 70+ consume 3.7 L/day and women aged 19 to 70+ consume 2.7 L/day.

16.3 SALIENT BENEFICIAL FEATURES OF WATER

As indicated earlier, water is a multifunctional macronutrient and its most vital function is body heat regulation. Water acts as a buffer; if there is high specific heat (the specific heat of water equals one when one kg of water is heated one degree Celsius between 15 and 16°C). The body is about 60% fluid, therefore a 70 kg man will contain ~42 kg of water throughout the body.[7] For every one degree rise in temperature in a 70 kg person, ~58 calories (kilo-calories, termed herein as calories) will be oxidized, thus the heat buffering effect of water also results in an increased metabolic rate.

Exercise physiology and physical activity are closely associated with physical activity, as evidenced by the evaporation of sweat; for every gram of sweat evaporated (liquid to vapor) from the skin, the body expends 0.58 calories (or 2.43 kjoules).[7,8] Thus, it is quite obvious that water not only has high specific heat, but also assists in the transfer of heat from areas of production to dissipation. Heat transport occurs with minimal change in actual blood temperature.

Water readily transverses through all cell membranes in the body. Osmotic and hydrostatic gradients and force dictate the movement and direction of water. Movement of water is also guided by the activity of adenosine triphosphatase (ATPase) sodium–potassium pump (Na-K pump). When exercise is accompanied on a regular basis by a person who previously did not engage in activity, fluid shifts occur and plasma volume will expand. However, the body regulates fluid balance tightly.

16.4 HYDRATION AND THIRST

Thirst, a sensation of dryness in the mouth, is subjective. It is basically the craving for fluids, resulting in the basic instinct to drink to quench the thirst. Thirst initiates a unique mechanism involved in fluid balance. The perception of being thirsty is a subjective motivator to quench thirst in animals and humans.[9] Circulatory systems maintain body fluid levels essential for long-term healthy survival. Factors influencing fluid needs and urge to drink include cultural and societal habits combined with internal psychogenic drive and the regulatory controls to maintain fluid homeostasis. Regulatory control includes maintaining the fluid content of various bodily compartments, the osmotic gradient of the extracellular fluids or working with specific hormones to assist in the regulation.

During the physiological process when a human body loses water, it is usually depleted from both the extracellular and intracellular spaces. These losses might not be equal in volume. Water and sodium chloride, the major solute of the extracellular fluid, results in proportionately more extracellular fluid depletion than if water alone is lost. If fluid losses come from the gastrointestinal tract (i.e., diarrhea) and are of normal osmotic load (isotonic) then the depletion will be entirely from the extracellular fluid. On the contrary, if hypertonic fluid is added to the extracellular compartment, there will be an osmotic depletion of water from the intracellular compartment into the extracellular fluid, and this latter compartment will be expanded.

A series of compensatory responses occur as a consequence of the fluid losses from either the intra- or extra-cellular space. Considering the effects of vasopressin secretion, stimulation of the renin–angiotensin–aldosterone system, sympathetic activation and reduced renal solute and water excretion is important when addressing hydration in athletes. However, hormonal responses to fluid losses are not solutions to returning the athlete to a euhydrated state. The only means to do this is by hydrating the individual to the tune of 600 mL per 0.46 kg weight lost (~1320 mL per kg weight lost). Thirst can be thought of as one component, the "vocal" component of the body's response to fluid shifts or losses.

Osmoregulation is considered a vital part of thirst regulation. The osmotic pressure of the fluid (plasma osmolality) typically lies between 280–295 mosmol/kg/H_2O. Losses as small as 1–2% of body weight stimulate thirst. Increased thirst is directly proportional to the osmotic gradient. Changes in NaCl and/or glucose induce this response by not crossing cell membranes so easily. The osmotic differences between the intracellular and extracellular spaces are what dictate the flow of fluids (higher to lower concentration occurring typically by osmosis). Osmosis is partially regulated by osmoreceptors (relative to vasopressin) in the brain and in the liver. The hypothalamus, an integral component of the brain, initiates thirst regulation and control.

Thirst regulation is multifactorial. Within the central nervous system (CNS) osmotic, ionic, hormonal and nervous signals are integrated and impact the perception of thirst. Overcoming hypo or dehydration following the ingestion of water or fluid involves additional pathways and factors that are beyond the scope of this chapter. The fact that disease or metabolic disorder states can impact hydration status cannot be overlooked even in the apparently healthy athlete.

16.5 STATE OF HYDRATION: OPTIMAL HEALTH

Fluid loss from the human body occurs from both the intra- and extracellular compartments, while the loss of sodium chloride occurs from the extracellular space. During sweating, sodium chloride is lost at a rate of 7:1 compared to potassium.[9] Thus, fluid losses of 1–2% of body weight or greater induce the need for fluid and electrolyte replacement. Although these facts are known, the importance of hydration state and health or disease prevention is often ignored. Moreover, advancing age may also serve as a potential risk factor for dehydration.

Although many diseases/dysfunctions have multifactorial origins, lifestyle, genetics, environment and other factors including the state of hydration are worthy of investigation. Moderate dehydration plays a factor in the development of various diseases and disorders. Conditions associated with the negative impacts of hypohydration or dehydration include alterations in amniotic fluids, prolonged labor, cystic fibrosis, and renal toxicity secondary to dehydration altering how contrast agents are metabolized. The effects of chronic hypohydration or dehydration (systemic effects) include associations with (ranging from weak to mild) urinary tract infections, gallstones, constipation, hypertension, bladder and colon cancer, venous thromboembolism, cerebral infarcts, dental diseases, kidney stones, mitral valve prolapse, glaucoma and diabetic ketoacidosis.[3] Rehydration and proper hydration improve the pathophysiological conditions, disease prevention and improvement of health. Multiple factors which may affect the state of hydration include high ambient temperature, the relative humidity, rate of sweating, increased body temperature, exercise duration, training status of the individual, exercise intensity, high body fat percentage, underwater exercise, use of diuretic medications and uncontrolled diabetes. The assessment of an athlete for hydration status should include a review of all of these factors.

The ultimate goal with each individual, whether athletic or not, is euhydration or appropriate state of hydration. IOM has clearly outlined the necessity of hydration for both genders. However, the practicality of application is hard for the everyday consumer. It is important to have convenient "rule of thumb" hydration guidelines for general health. Many dietitians recommend their clients to shoot for a goal, such as drinking the equivalent in ounces to half their body weight. If one weighs 68 kg (150 pounds), then the goal of hydration per day with normal activities should be 1500–2250 mL (50–75 oz) of non-alcoholic fluid.

16.6   ATHLETIC PERFORMANCE AND HYDRATION STATUS

A large body of evidence from diverse research studies and athletic associations shows that dehydration can significantly impact performance, especially in warm, hot, dry or humid climatic conditions. Therefore, hydration status and fluid replacement guidelines have been well established in order to minimize exertional dehydration. Dehydration is defined by a 2% loss of euhydrated body weight,[10] which negatively impacts and affects athletic performance and physiological well-being. Dehydration is associated with a reduction or an adverse effect on muscle strength, endurance, coordination, mental acuity and the thermoregulatory processes.

As stated earlier, water loss takes place during exercise and athletic performance. Furthermore, large inter-individual variations in sweat rates are so wide that no universal recommendations are used. The closest universal rule is that one replaces 600 mL of water per ~1/5 kg of body weight (20 oz [1.25 pints] per pound of body weight) lost between the initiation of exercise and its cessation (L Armstrong, personal communication).

Both fluid and sodium losses take place during prolonged exercise. It is important to know that human sweat contains 40–50 mmol sodium per liter.[10] In a healthy person, large fluid losses are followed by large sodium losses. The typical sodium to potassium ratio is 7:1. On average, an athlete engaged in prolonged exercise can lose 5 L of fluid per day with a range of 4,600 to 5,750 mg sodium and much smaller amounts of potassium. It has been demonstrated that heat acclimated athletes benefit from enhanced sodium reabsorption which results in better protection of plasma volume by reducing the sodium losses. Also, the training state of the athlete and their physico-chemical characteristics are very important when contemplating fluid needs. Salt losses do not directly impact physical performance; however, using salts in fluid replacement is proven to enhance the thirst response and aid in rehydration.

Hypohydration (1% body weight loss) has been shown to decrease the ability of the athletes to perform. As a routine practice, athletes do not replace sweat/sodium losses enough during the event. On average, a marathon runner will lose up to 3% body weight and if the run is in an elevated temperate climate the losses could be 5%. Generally, Maughan elite marathoners tend to lose or sweat at a rate of 2 L/hour. Surprisingly, this sweat rate exceeds the intestinal absorption capability of the gut.[11,12]

Studies have demonstrated a negative impact of hypohydration and dehydration on athletic performance (ranging from 1% to 8% fluid losses). Sports performance or situations designed to mimic a sport have noted a decrement in performance for soccer, basketball, running/racing, cycling and other sports. In addition, better hydration is associated with lower esophageal temperature, heart rate and ratings of perceived exertion – all factors that may impact performance.[13]

Sports performance or exercise increases the metabolic rate and since energy is converted into heat, water losses will occur. In cold climates (winter sports or outdoor sports in mild or cold climates), heat is lost via radiation and convection, while as the temperature increases the losses are noticeable as sweat. The physiological response to exercise is to expand the blood volume and to increase the sensitivity for sweating to occur. Athletes and their coaches, trainers and nutritionists must be cognizant of changes in osmolarity. Body temperature and the volume of the liquid being ingested, as well as the osmolarity, can affect performance.

Hypohydration or dehydration has a potential impact on the athlete's cognitive functions. The mental aspect of sports coupled with neuromuscular integration shouldn't be ignored as dehydration has significant impact. Molecular and behavioral aspects of the neuropsychological impact of hydration are relatively new areas of research. Brain behavior and cognitive assessment are comparatively new to the exercise physiology field since a significant number of novel cognitive assessment tools have become available, despite research from the 1940s on fluid and salt intake.[14,15] Lieberman et al. (2006) demonstrated that hypohydration and dehydration were associated with increased fatigue, impaired discrimination, impaired tracking, impaired short-term memory, impaired recall and attention, while arithmetic ability also decreased and a faster response time to peripheral visual stimuli was noted.[14,15] The applications have been tested in both academic and military settings. Interestingly enough, dehydration induced by heat as compared to dehydration caused by exercise cause the same changes in cognitive performance yielding that dehydration is the cause, not exercise. Under dehydrated cognition, cognitive performance significantly declines with increased fatigue, tracking errors (visual-brain connection) and a decrease in short-term memory. Ironically, when a person is hyperhydrated, short-term memory is increased while most of the other parameters mentioned remain neutral with no negative impacts.[16,17,18]

16.7   HYDRATION AND MEASUREMENT

There is no universal technique for assessing hydration status, with at least 13 techniques suggested to assess hydration. As indicated earlier, water is the body's currency as it is an integral part of circulatory functions, biochemical reactions, temperature regulation and other physiological processes. Moreover, fluid turnover occurs as water is lost from fluid-electrolyte balance, as well as fluid loss from the lungs, skin and kidneys. Water/hydration is gained via the diet as well as fluid intake.

The types of hydration assessment methods (in the field and lab) include:

1. stable isotope dilution
2. neutron activation analysis
3. bioelectrical impedance (BIA)
4. body mass change
5. plasma osmolality
6. plasma volume change
7. urine osmolality
8. urine specific gravity
9. urine conductivity
10. urine color
11. 24-hour urine volume
12. salivary flow rate (osmolality, flow rate, protein content)
13. rating of thirst

A convenient tool which is clinically used is the Hydration Assessment (HA) Checklist. However, the HA Checklist is a lengthy, in-depth assessment designed to screen for hydration problems.[17] In older populations, HA is most often used in clinical conditions. As it is obvious that older adults both in the community as well as in the nursing home are grossly under-hydrated, ingesting on average less than about 0.26 gallons (1 L) daily, which is substantially lower than recommended. Of the ~half-gallon of fluid, few take in water, an essential element supporting cellular and organ health, electrolyte balance, medication absorption and distribution as well as kidney, bladder and integumentary functioning.

It has been extensively outlined in the literature why one gold standard technique is not available for measuring hydration:[19]

1. Water turnover or physiological regulations of total body water volume, as well as fluid concentrations, are complex and dynamic. Renal, thirst and sweat gland responses are involved to varying degrees, depending on the prevailing activities. Also, renal regulation of water balance (i.e., arginine, vasopressin) is distinct from the regulation of tonicity.
2. The 24-hour fluid deficit varies greatly amongst sedentary individuals and athletes primarily due to the exercise and morphology. However, this deficit can be matched by food and fluid intake.
3. It has been well demonstrated that sodium and osmolyte consumption affects the daily water requirement and consumption. Regional customs impact the

"Standard Value" used within biochemical assessment of hydration. For example, the mean 24-hour urine osmolality in Germany is 860 mOsm/kg while in Poland it is 392 mOsm/kg and in the United States it is in the range of 280–295 mOsm/kg. It is very important to establish an International Standard.

4. Measurement of hydration depends on two prime factors, (i) volume and (ii) time of fluid intake. Pure water or hypotonic solutions ingested rapidly can cause dilute urine prior to cellular equilibrium taking place.

5. Urine samples (spot) do not represent the true 24-hour void (all urine losses over a 24 hour period).

6. Diverse experimental designs differ in assessment techniques (blood versus urine).

7. A number of stable isotopes are used to assess hydration. However, it is not known if the isotopes are uniformly distributed throughout the body, thus the assumption used in these techniques is faulty.

8. It has been well documented that exercise and physical labor (as well as pregnancy labor) increases blood volume, while decreasing renal blood flow and altering the glomerular filtration rate affecting hydration.

9. Significant changes in osmolarity and osmolality can affect the readings for hydration on certain devices (i.e., BIA).

Moreover, many questions exist to consider plasma osmolality as a biomarker for hydration. Incidentally, plasma osmolality varies extensively depending upon the conditions being tested, the environment of the test, the pre-exercise hydration status and the intervention being evaluated.

The biggest question remains: is there a way to extrapolate laboratory techniques with those in the field so that athletes, coaches and related personnel can better help athletes?

The first item to explore is the intervention and educational sessions that athletes should receive from appropriate professionals (i.e., exercise physiologist, registered dietitian, Sports Nutritionist-CISSN, athletic trainer, etc.). Education, learning and appropriate training are the key parameters to prevent dehydration. Combining the learning experience with fluid stations on the field or in the general area of training, available to the athletes at specific intervals with or without *ad libitum* intake available, may make euhydration an easier goal to maintain.

Using the routine field technique of incorporating the combination of weighing the athlete before and after the training or competition and using the weight change as the guide for rehydration may just be the best standard when controlling for applicability, financial impact and easy of education. The rehydration is 600 mL per 0.5 kg body weight lost. Other techniques that may be able to be used in combination with monitoring weight changes include using blood and urine testing if available. Testing for osmolality (both), sodium (both) and hematocrit levels (blood) are typical and inexpensive.

16.8 DIVERSE REHYDRATION TECHNIQUES

Humans consume a wide range of fluids and beverages to quench their thirsts as well as for hydration during their entire lifespan. As demonstrated earlier, fluid homeostasis and retention can be challenging to maintain during physical work and heat stress. As emphasized, an average human body weight comprises 60% water, and during the normal physiological process and regular activities about 5–10% of total body water undergoes obligatory loss. The greater the fluid losses (from non-emergent situations, not medical or surgical), the longer the time it will take for rehydration and replenishment (4% weight loss may take up to 24 hours to rehydrate), thus prevention and use of foods or fluids that may aid in more expedient rehydration is of importance.[20]

Human body water is counterbalanced and maintained by matching daily water loss with fluid intake. Metabolic water production also contributes to a small degree hydration (metabolic hydration yields ~250 mL/day). The Food and Nutrition Board has established an adequate intake level of 3.7 L/day and 2.7 L/day for men and women, respectively.[1] The Continuing Survey of Food Intakes by Individuals (CSFII) arrived at a conclusion that adults receive about 25% of their daily fluid intake from foods.[21]

Maintaining fluid and electrolyte balance in the body means that active individuals need to replenish the water and electrolytes lost during physiological processes, routine physical activities and sweating. Overall, active individuals, regardless of age, strive to hydrate well before exercise, drink fluids throughout exercise and rehydrate once exercise is over. As outlined by the American College of Sports Medicine (ACSM) and the National Athletic Trainer's Association (NATA), generous amounts of fluids should be consumed 24 hours before exercise and 400–600 mL of fluid should be consumed two hours before exercise (this is ~6–10 oz).[22]

During exercise, active individuals should attempt to drink ~150–350 mL (6–12 oz) of fluid every 15–20 minutes. If the exercise or athletic performance is continued for a longer duration (usually >1 hour or 75 minutes) or occurs in a hot environment, sports drinks containing carbohydrate and sodium could be consumed. Following completion of the exercise, the most active individuals have some level of dehydration. Drinking enough fluids to cover ~150% of the weight lost during exercise may be required to replenish fluids lost in sweat and urine. This fluid can be part of the post-exercise drink or meal, which should also contain sodium, either in the food or beverages, since diuresis occurs (fluid losses) when only plain water is ingested. Sodium helps the rehydration process by maintaining plasma osmolality and the desire to drink.

Fluid content of foods should not be underestimated or underappreciated by sports nutritionists or health professionals. High water content foods include (water content in percentages): iceberg lettuce (96%), cooked squash (94%), pickle (92%), cantaloupe (90%), orange (87%), apple (86%) and pear (84%), as compared to steak (50%), cheddar cheese (37%), white bread (36%), cookies (4%) and nuts (about 2%). Therefore including the national recommendation of five to nine fruits and vegetables in the daily diet also assists with hydration.

In pre-exercise some athletes use beverages that contain >100 mmol/l NaCl, temporarily inducing hyper-hydration and thus aiding in rehydration. Adding glycerol to the typical sports beverage or oral rehydration solution at a dose of 1.0 to 1.5 gm/kg/ BW also assists in inducing hyperhydration.[22]

Non-water sources of hydration include caffeinated beverages. Caffeine is stated to be a mild diuretic, however, the vast evidence indicates that caffeinated beverages help to hydrate over a 24-hour period. Fiala et al. (2004) have demonstrated that caffeine is oft rumored to be a mild diuretic, while noting that caffeine itself can enhance exercise performance (typical dose at 5 mg/kg). This study utilized 10 athletes who completed two-a-day practices (2 hour/practice = 4 hours/day) for three consecutive days at 23°C. The study utilized a randomized double blind design offering of caffeine rehydration agent versus no caffeine (Coca-Cola® vs. caffeine-free version). No scientific data exhibited that caffeine intake impairs rehydration. Furthermore, no differential effects on urine or plasma osmolality, plasma volume, hematocrit, hemoglobin or body weight were observed. The caffeine (cola) intake was about 244 mg caffeine/day served in ~7 cans/day of soda (~35 mg caffeine/360 mL).[23] (24). Grandjean et al. (2000) conducted a study using a randomized crossover design using 18 volunteers with a free-living 24-hour capture design. Four beverages (carbonated, caffeine caloric cola, non-caloric caffeinated cola and coffee) were evaluated along with their respective effects on 24-hour hydration status. Urine samples were collected over a period of 24 hours and analyzed for electrolytes, body weight, osmolality, hemoglobin, hematocrit, blood urea nitrogen, creatinine and other biomarkers. No differences were observed. Thus, it can be concluded that caffeine-containing beverages significantly contribute to hydration.[24]

Recent investigation supports the inclusion of small amounts of protein with carbohydrates for hydration recovery. In an investigation in 2001, 10 endurance trained males were employed to investigate the ergogenic effects of isocaloric carbohydrate (CHO, 152.7 g) and carbohydrate–protein (CHO-PRO, 112 g CHO with 40.7 g PRO) drinks ingested after a glycogen lowering diet and exercise bout. The study was conducted in a double-blind and counterbalanced fashion. Following the completion of a glycogen lowering diet and run, two dosages of a drink were administered with a 60 minute interval between dosages. The CHO-PRO trial resulted in higher serum insulin levels (60.84 vs 30.1 mU/mL) 90 minutes into recovery than the CHO only trail ($p < 0.05$). Moreover, the time to run to exhaustion was longer during the CHO-PRO trial (540.7 ± 91.56 sec) than the CHO only trial (446.1 ± 97.09 sec, $p < 0.05$). It was concluded that a CHO-PRO drink following glycogen depleting exercise may facilitate a greater rate of muscle glycogen resynthesis than a CHO only beverage, hasten the recovery process and improve exercise endurance during a second bout of exercise performed on the same day.[25] Later studies have confirmed that adding protein in the ratio of one part protein to every four parts carbohydrate has been found to induce exercise hydration on the magnitude of 15% better than the typical carbohydrate beverage and 40% more than water alone.[26,27]

Subsequently, Seifert's study[28] concluded "contrary to popular misconception, adding protein to a carbohydrate-based sports drink … led to improved water retention by 15% over [a carbohydrate-only sports drink] and 40% over plain water."[27] In this investigation, cyclists exercised until they lost 2% of their body weight (through sweating) and then drank either a carbohydrate–protein sports drink (Accelerade™), a carbohydrate-only sports drink (Gatorade®), or water. Over the next three hours, measurements were continued to determine how much of each beverage was retained in the body (versus the amount lost through urination). The carbohydrate–protein sports drink was found to rehydrate the athletes 15% better than the carbohydrate-only sports beverage and 40% better than water. Furthermore, all three drinks emptied from the stomach and were absorbed through the intestine at the same rate. In addition, there was no difference between the carbohydrate–protein drink and the carbohydrate-only drink in terms of effects on blood plasma volume. This concludes that the carbohydrate–protein drink resulted in increased water retention in the body within and between cells. Thus, a carbohydrate–protein sports drink may be a preferable choice, over plain water and a carbohydrate–electrolyte sports drink, when rehydration and fluid retention are a concern.

Another interesting investigation by Seifert found that "consumption of a carbohydrate-protein beverage minimized muscle damage indices during skiing compared to placebo and no fluid." A total of 31 recreational skiers were divided into three groups. All three groups skied 12 runs, which took about three hours. One group drank nothing. A second group drank 6 oz (0.18 L) of a placebo (flavored water) after every second run. A third group drank an equal amount of the carbohydrate–protein sports drink (Accelerade). After the 12th run, blood samples were taken from each skier and analyzed for two biomarkers of muscle stress (myoglobin and creatine kinase). Subjects that received the carbohydrate–protein sports drink exhibited no signs of muscle damage, while indicators of muscle damage increased by 49% in subjects consuming only water.[28] Therefore, it is concluded that in skiing, a carbohydrate–protein drink is more beneficial as compared to water alone for maintaining skeletal integrity and hydration.

In general, hydration and rehydration for athletes are done with a 6–8% glucose–electrolyte solution. Newer innovation and research exhibit that adding just a small amount of protein to this type of sports beverage not only enhances hydration and rehydration (or hydration maintenance) but also promotes muscle protein synthesis (which does not happen with CHO alone) and glycogen reaccumulation while reducing markers of muscle damage. These beverages are gaining popularity for their multiple benefits that seem to make them superior to the typical sports beverage during exercise or post-exercise nutrition.

16.9 FLUID INTAKE AND REPLACEMENT

This review demonstrates the importance of fluid replacement and how research shows that the volume of fluid intake generally increases when water or the beverage is flavored.[29] In general the following fluid recommendations are used by sports nutritionists:[30,31]

- 480–600 mL. Fluid: 1–2 hours pre-exercise
- 300–480 mL. Fluid: 15 minutes pre-exercise
- 120–180 mL. Fluid: every 10–15 minutes during exercise
- In general start fluid intake 24 hours prior to exercise event.

Additionally, fluid derived from food must also be considered, however, in the post-exercise recovery period, hydration is best achieved by the ingestion of either the typical glucose–electrolyte solution or a carbohydrate–protein mixture. However, if the exercise has a duration of less than 60–75 minutes, then water (which can be flavored) is recommended. There are no proven ergogenic effects or benefits from vitamin or mineral enriched waters except that they provide absorbable nutrients at lower caloric costs than some foods.

The athletes must consider keeping the consumption record of the volume of his or her beverage in order to become more familiar with how the body responds to proper rehydration.[32] Moreover, the athlete should personalize his or her fluid intake based upon what types of beverages result in improved recovery as measured by hydration, return to normal body weight, subsequent exercise performance and effects on mental abilities/cognition.

16.10   SUMMARY AND CONCLUSIONS

Exercise increases the metabolic rate. Energy production leads to heat loss and fluid status is affected. The climate has an underappreciated effect on hydration status. In cold climates, the thermoregulatory response includes enhanced heat production by a variety of means; all result in increased fluid losses. Exercising in temperate climates is actually a little easier, as the body's accommodation response is to increase blood volume and sweating mechanism sensitivity. Athletes, along with their trainers and coaches, must be cognizant about the physiological impacts of exercise, such as changes in body temperature and blood volume, in their surrounding climate. Elevated temperature is related to blood volume reduction and performance. Maintaining fluid balance reduces the effects of climate and or blood volume on hydration status. For exercise lasting less than an hour, water or non-caloric fluid is recommended. It is not well known if "non-intensive" exercise requires that the rehydration solution include carbohydrate and electrolytes; most data notes no need for the calories and salts with short-term exercise bouts. If the exercise is longer in duration, maintaining hydration and rehydration is much more important. Beverages beneficial for enhancing rehydration include carbohydrate–electrolyte solutions and carbohydrate–protein beverages. Caffeinated beverages with and without calories also add to hydration and rehydration, although in the immediate post-exercise period, data are mounting for carbohydrate–protein to be the superior post-exercise rehydration and recovery beverage. Future research will focus on the multiple applications of this admixture beverage along with other potentially beneficial effects. Taste acceptance is very important for any of these beverages to actually be used by athletes; therefore, overcoming taste issues for beverages that contain protein remains an issue for researchers and food scientists to overcome. In conclusion, maintaining euhydration and understanding how to rehydrate after exercise is an important aspect of sports nutrition that is under-discussed or under-appreciated.

REFERENCES

1. Institute of Medicine and Food and Nutrition Board. *Dietary Reference Intakes for Water, Potassium, Sodium, Chloride and Sulfate.* Washington DC: National Academies Press, 2004. Available from: http://www.nationalacademies.org/hmd/Reports/2004/Dietary-Reference-Intakes-Water-Potassium-Sodium-Chloride-and-Sulfate.aspx.
2. Health effects of mild dehydration. 2nd international conference on hydration throughout life. Dortmund, Germany, October 8–9 2001. *Eur J Clin Nutr* 2003;57(Supplement 2).

3. Manz F. Hydration and disease. *J Amer Coll Nutr* 2007;26(Supplement 5):535s–541s.
4. Hydration and health promotion. ILSI North America conference on hydration and health promotion. November 29–30, 2006. *J Amer Coll Nutr* 2007;26(Supplement 5): 529s–532s.
5. Welch BE, Bursick ER, Iampietro PF. Relation of climate and temperature to food and water intake in man. *Metabolism* 1958;7:141–158.
6. Bullers AC. *Bottled Water: Better than Tap?* Rockville, MD: FDA, 2002. Available from: www.fda.gov/fdac/features/2002/402_h2o.html.
7. Senay LC. Water and electrolytes during physical activity. In: Wolinsky I (ed.), *Nutrition in Exercise and Sport*, 3rd edition. Boca Raton, FL: CRC Press, 1998, pp. 258–273.
8. Guyton AC. *Textbook of Medical Physiology*, 8th edition. Philadelphia, PA: WB Saunders, 1991, p 799.
9. McKinley MJ, Johnson AK. The physiological regulation of thirst and fluid intake. *News Physiol Sci* 2004;19(1):1–6.
10. Sharp RL. Role of sodium in fluid homeostasis with exercise. *J Amer Coll Nutr* 2006;25(Supplement 33):231s–239s.
11. Whiting PH, Maughan RL, Miller JDB. Dehydration and serum biochemical changes in marathon runners. *Eur J Appl Physiol* 1984;52(2):183–187.
12. Maughan RJ. Fluid and electrolyte loss and replacement in exercise. *J Sports Sci* 1991;9(Supplement 1):117–142.
13. Murray B. Hydration and physical performance. *J Amer Coll Nutr* 2006;26(Supplement 5):542s–548s.
14. Grandjean AC. Dehydration and cognitive performance. *J Amer Coll Nutr* 2006;26(Supplement 5):549s–554s.
15. Lieberman HR. Hydration and cognition: A critical review and recommendations for future research. *J Amer Coll Nutr* 2006;26(Supplement 5):555s–561s.
16. Cian C, Koulmann N, Barraud P, Raphel C, Jimeniz C, Meli B. Influence of variations on body hydration on cognitive function: Effect of hyperhydration, heat stress, and exercise-induced dehydration. *J Psychophysiol* 2000;14(1):29–36.
17. Posner BM, Jette AM, Smith KW, Miller DR. Nutrition and health risks in the elderly: The nutritional screening initiative. *Amer J Publ Health* 1993;83(7):972–978.
18. Zembrzuski CD. A three-dimensional approach to hydration of elders: Administration, clinical staff, and in-service education. *Geriatr Nurs* 1997;18(1):2.
19. Armstrong LE. Assessing hydration status: The elusive gold standard. *J Amer Coll Nutr* 2006;26(Supplement 5):575s–584s.
20. Kenefick RW, Sawka M. Hydration at the work site. *J Amer Coll Nutr* 2006;26(Supplement 5):597s–603s.
21. Heller KE, Sohn W, Burt BA, Eklund SA. Water consumption in the United States in 1995–1996 and implications for water fluoridation policy. *J Publ Health Dent* 1999;59(1):3–11.
22. Shirreffs SM, Armstrong LE, Cheuvront SN. Fluid and electrolyte needs for preparation and recovery from training and competition. *J Sports Sci* 2004;22(1):57–63.
23. Fiala KA, Casa DJ, Roti MW. Rehydration with a caffeinated beverage during the non-exercise periods of 3 consecutive days of 2-a-day practices. *Int J Sport Nutr Exerc Metab* 2004;14(4):419–429.
24. Grandjean AC, Reimers KJ, Bannick KE, Haven MC. The effect of caffeinated, non-caffeinated, caloric and non-caloric beverages on hydration. *J Amer Coll Nutr* 2000;19(5):591–600.
25. Niles ES, Lachowetz T, Garfi J. Carbohydrate-protein drink improves time to exhaustion after recovery from endurance exercise. *J Exer Physiol Online* 2001;4(1):45–52.
26. Ivy JL, Goforth HW Jr, Damon BM, McCauley TR, Parsons EC, Price TB. Early postexercise muscle glycogen recovery is enhanced with a carbohydrate-protein supplement. *J Appl Physiol* 2002;93(4):1337–1344.

27. Seifert JG, Harmon J, DeClercq P. Protein added to a sports drink improves fluid retention. *Int J Sports Nutr Exerc Metab* 2006;16(4):420–429.

28. Seifert JG, Kipp RW, Amann M, Gazal O. Muscle damage, fluid ingestion, and energy supplementation during recreational alpine skiing. *Int J Sports Nutr Exerc Metab* 2005;15(5):528–536.

29. Minehan MR, Riley MD, Burke LM. Effect of flavor and awareness of kilojoule content of drinks on preference and fluid balance in team sports. *Int J Sports Nutr Exerc Metab* 2002;12(1):81–92.

30. Pivarnik JM. Water and Electrolytes during Exercise. In: Hickson JF, Wolinsky I (eds.), *Nutrition in Exercise and Sports*, 1st edition. Boca Raton, FL: CRC Press, 1989, pp 185–200.

31. McArdle WD, Katch FI, Katch VL. *Sports & Exercise Nutrition*. Philadelphia, PA: Lippincott Williams and Wilkens, 1999, pp. 275–276.

32. Zembrzuski CD. Hydration assessment checklist. *Geriatr Nurs* 1997;18(1):20–26.

17 Versatile Use of Gelatin in Functional Food and Nutraceuticals

Douglas S. Kalman

CONTENTS

17.1   Introduction 311
17.2   Evolution of Gelatin Manufacturing 312
17.3   Human Consumption: Trend 313
17.4   Economics and Worldwide Trend 314
17.5   Uses in the Food and Pharmaceutical Industry 314
17.6   Clinical Trials in Bone and Joint Diseases 315
17.7   Gelatin and Anaphylactic Reaction 316
17.8   Application in Sports Nutrition and Athletic Performance 317
17.9   Gelatin and Delivery Modules 317
17.10 Summary 318
References 318

17.1   INTRODUCTION

Gelatin is a colorless, flavorless and opaque protein derived from collagen, which is obtained from various animal body parts. Commercially, gelatin is manufactured from skin and bone from slaughtered animals that have been approved for human consumption. The collagen contained in these raw materials, viz. bone and skin, is the actual starting material used in the manufacturing of gelatin. It is widely used as a gelling agent in food, pharmaceuticals, capsules and cosmetic manufacturing. It is a unique functional food ingredient which has extensive applications in the functional food and nutraceutical industries. It is widely available in many prepared foods, especially in diverse sport foods, gummy-bears and snack bars. The type of gelatin used in these bars is collagen or hydrolyzed collagen. Athletes are mainly exposed to gelatin or hydrolyzed collagen as a protein source.

Gelatin is derived from collagen, an insoluble fibrous protein which is the principal constituent of connective tissues and bones. Collagen is distinctive in that it contains an unusually high level of the cyclic amino acids proline and hydroxyproline. Collagen consists of three helical polypeptide chains around each other and connected by intermolecular cross-links.

Structurally, gelatin is primarily composed of the amino acid glycine (about 33%) and proline/hydroxyproline (22%), with the remaining 45% made up by 17 amino

311

acids (18 in total). Of these 17 remaining acids, alanine is the most abundant in gelatin, followed by glutamic acid, arginine and aspartic acid. It should be noted that gelatin does not have any cysteine or cystine, but does have trace amounts of methionine (<1% by weight). Gelatin does not contain all of the essential amino acids, as it lacks tryptophan. Gelatin is the soluble form (via hydrolysis) of collagen. Commercially edible gelatins are 84–90% protein, 8–12% water and 2–4% minerals salts. Gelatin in and of itself contains no fat or carbohydrates.[1] However, the caloric value of gelatin is 3.6 calories/gram.

17.2 EVOLUTION OF GELATIN MANUFACTURING

Gelatin is mainly manufactured from pig skin, although it can also be produced from cattle skin and bones. However, it is very important that all of the raw materials used in the production of gelatin come from registered slaughterhouses. These slaughterhouses test all animals aged above 30 months for the presence of bovine spongiform encephalopathy (BSE). Under the auspices of the European Commission, multisite studies were carried out in Scotland (Institute for Animal Health in Edinburgh), the Netherlands (ID-Lelystad) and in the United States (Baltimore Research and Education Foundation) in order to determine if BSE or related pathogens could survive. The studies found that no harmful organisms survived the manufacturing process for gelatin. Thus, safety or toxicity should not be a potential concern.[2]

Gelatin is derived from collagen by hydrolysis. Several varieties of gelatin are available. The composition of gelatin depends on the source and nature of collagen and the hydrolytic treatment used for its manufacturing. Gelatin, as it is typically made, is not Kosher; however, if made from cattle slaughtered under Kashruth law and strict supervision, the gelatin can be certified as Kosher. In North America, cattle hides are the least used gelatin raw material.[2] In particular, gelatin extracted from bone is used primarily in photographic applications, while some is used in pharmaceuticals.

The so-called green bone from the slaughter of cattle is cleaned, degreased, dried, sorted and crushed to a particle size of about 1–2 cm. The pieces of bone are then treated with dilute hydrochloric acid to remove mineral salts. The resulting sponge-like material is called ossein. From this point on in the manufacture of Type B gelatin, both cattle hides and bone tissues receive similar treatment.

Cattle hides are available from trimming operations in leather production. They are usually dehaired chemically using a lime/sulfide solution followed by mechanical loosening. For the production of Type B gelatin, both bone tissues (or ossein) and cattle hide pieces are subjected to lengthy treatment with an alkali (usually lime) and water at ambient temperature. Depending on previous treatment, the nature of the material, the size of the pieces and the exact temperature, liming can take between 5 and 20 weeks, though the usual timeframe is 8–12 weeks. The process is controlled by the degree of alkalinity of the lime liquor as determined by titration with acid, or by making test extractions.

Pork skin is currently the most abundant raw material for the production of edible gelatin in North America. Pork skins, free from flesh and fat, are obtained either fresh or frozen from slaughterhouses and meat processing plants. Pork skin hairs are removed by scalding with a hot dilute caustic soda solution.

For Type A gelatin, pork skins are washed with cold water and then soaked in cold dilute mineral acid for several hours until maximum swelling has occurred. The most commonly used acids are hydrochloric acid and sulfuric acid. Following the processing, the remaining acid is drained off and the material is again washed several times with cold water. Subsequently, the pork skins are prepared for the extraction using hot water.

Reaction time, temperature, pH and number of extractions vary from processor to processor depending on product needs, type of equipment employed, time of operations and economics. For both type A and type B gelatins, extraction procedures are closely controlled to optimize both quality and quantity. Although continuous extraction is used by some processors, most methods still employ discrete batch fractions. Stainless steel vessels equipped with the provisions for heating and temperature control are used for extraction. The number of extractions varies, with 3–6 typical. The grade, type and quality of gelatin produced is dependent upon the needs of the customer.

Gelatin is gaining increasing popularity in diverse food products. It is extensively used in functional food and confectionary products (jubes, gums, marshmallows, toffies, lozenges, licorice, etc.), dairy products (for its fat-like mouthfeel), desserts (i.e., jello), meat products (as a coating, extender, glazing or emulsifier), bakery products (i.e., icing) and in the pharmaceutical industry (i.e., gel-caps, binding agents, emulsifiers). However, in each industry that gelatin is used, there are quality controls for handling and processing, thus providing one or multiple steps of protection from contamination.

17.3 HUMAN CONSUMPTION: TREND

The first process for gelatin was started by Papin as early as 1682 with a slow cooking extraction technique using a bone mixture. Following its invention, the word gelatin (Latin gelatinus, meaning stiff or frozen) was coined in 1700. The first patent was granted in 1754 in England for the use of gelatin as an adhesive (joiner's glue). In 1871, Dr. Richard Leach Maddox provided a new direction by using gelatin to further process pictures in photography and painting. Visualizing the versatile applications of gelatin, a new revolution was started in the manufacturing of gelatin and full-scale factory processing began. The processing of gelatin slowly evolved from 1875 to 1950 while later, in 1974, the first professional association dedicated to the art and science of gelatin was established (Gelatin Manufacturers of Europe; GME).[3]

Gelatin is consumed extensively by humans in diverse food and dairy products, frozen foods, desserts, gummi bears, marshmallows, circus peanuts, lozenges, wafers, bakery fillings and icings, meat products and alcohol. Gelatin is also used to fortify reduced-calorie foods. Gelatin hydrolysates are mostly used in soups, shakes and fruit drinks.

Overall, it is quite obvious that over the past 400 or more years, the use and consumption of gelatin and/or collagen have been a part of the human diet.

17.4 ECONOMICS AND WORLDWIDE TREND

Basically, gelatin has become a big commodity item with widespread applications. In 2001, 110,400 metric tons of pig skin was used for the manufacturing of gelatin. Usage has only increased since 2001, especially with the increased production of higher protein bars and foods, whereas gelatin is used in part for a protein source. About 77,200 metric tons of bovine hides are used in gelatin production, while 80,800 metric tons of bones and 1,000 metric tons of other animal parts are utilized in the production of edible and pharmaceutical gelatin. In worldwide sales, gelatin business generated $1.2 billion.

North and South America consume 60,500 and 39,500 metric tons of gelatin per year, respectively, while Western Europe and Eastern Europe consume 117,000 and 5,000 metric tons, respectively. Germany, France and Belgium are the largest gelatin consumers, while Switzerland consumes only 300 metric tons per year. The annual sales of gelatin worldwide are estimated to grow approximately 2–3% per annum.[2,3]

17.5 USES IN THE FOOD AND PHARMACEUTICAL INDUSTRY

Gelatin has a number of functional properties and, thus, a number of food and pharmaceutical products can be fortified. These include

1. As a gel and a number of gelatin-based products can be designed to prepare desserts, lunch meats, pâté and consommé
2. In whipping agents including nougats, mousses, soufflés, marshmallows, chiffons and whipped cream
3. Being used to develop protective colloid-based products such as meat rolls, canned meat, confectionary, cheeses and dairy products
4. Being used as a clarifying agent in diverse products including wine, beer, fruit juices and vinegar
5. Being applied as a film coating ingredient, as for example coating for meats, fruits or deli items
6. As a thickener in powdered drinks, bouillon etc.
7. In gravies, sauces, puddings and allied confectionary products
8. As a process aid for microencapsulation of colors, flavors, oils and vitamins
9. As an emulsifier viz., cream soups, fat-replacer, flavorings, etc.
10. As a stabilizer in cream cheese, chocolate milk, yogurt and icings
11. Acting as an adhesive to affix nonpareils, coconut-layered confections, bind frosting, etc.
12. Use in the pharmaceutical industries for two-piece hard capsules, soft elastic gelatin capsules, tablets, tablet coating and as a gelatin emulsifier/filler.
13. For microencapsulation (of oil or hydrophobic compounds)
14. As a water insoluble sponge during surgical procedures (Gelfoam™)
15. As a film (GelFilm™ for laboratory printing of specific types of analysis (i.e., DNA)
16. Use in medical troches and pastilles (lozenge like products)
17. In research laboratories, where gelatin is also used in bacterial culture media

Moreover, gelatin is used in the fabrics industry (to coat yarn), in the manufacture of paper (coating and surface sizing), printing (lithography) and as a cleansing agent. Gelatin is used as a binder for the material in matches, coating adhesives, as a filter, in cosmetics (creams and lotions) and in the chemical industries.[2]

17.6   CLINICAL TRIALS IN BONE AND JOINT DISEASES

The safety and efficacy of a gelatin-based dietary supplement in 175 adults with mild symptoms of knee-based osteoarthritis for symptomatic relief of osteoarthritis was investigated in a randomized, double-blind, placebo-controlled clinical trial over a period of 14 weeks. A total of 80 subjects received the supplement (Knox NutraJoint™ manufactured by Nabisco, which contains 10 grams of hydrolyzed gelatin derived from collagen source plus amino acids as well as vitamins C, D and K, plus calcium, copper, manganese and zinc), while 95 subjects received the placebo.[4,5] To assess joint strength and work performance, a series of isokinetic and isometric leg strength tests were performed using the Biodex Multi-Joint System B2000. Subjects also filled out questionnaires regarding perceived effects on the ability to carry out daily living events (pain, stiffness and mobility). Gelatin-based products did show an improvement in knee function and strength compared with those in the placebo group. The Principal Investigator stated in a press release, "These results suggest that gelatine supplementation has the potential to improve knee function during activities which place a high amount of stress on the joint, like walking or jogging. They also encourage further research to evaluate the long-term benefits of this type of treatment."[6] However, this study was never published in a peer-reviewed journal.

Another meta-analysis of studies utilizing collagen hydrolysate in the treatment of osteoarthritis (OA) and osteoporosis was recently published.[7] Hydrolyzed gelatin products are Generally Regarded as Safe (GRAS) and have a long history of use in the food and pharmaceutical industries. Pharmaceutical-grade collagen hydrolysate use is associated with reduced pain in those with OA of the knee or hip. Pharmacokinetic data indicates an associated increase in serum concentrations of hydroxyproline, along with preferential uptake by cartilage suggesting a beneficial effect of the collagen hydrolysate. In ranking pain severity relief of those who achieved perceived benefit when using the collagen hydrolysate, those patients with the most severe symptomology appear to experience the greatest relief. A typical dose of 10 grams of collagen hydrolysate was used for clinical benefit in OA.

Clinical efficacy of collagen hydrolysate supplementation on bone metabolism was investigated. The investigation was to confirm the potential use of collagen hydrolysate in osteoporosis because the collagen matrix is vital for bone integrity. Furthermore, since collagen hydrolysate has been shown to exert a positive impact on cartilage uptake and synthesis, it may also have an effect on the osteoclast and osteoblast activity. Delivering calcitonin with the collagen hydrolysate appears to slow the destruction of collagen as evidenced by reduced urinary pyridinoline cross-links, a novel marker of bone turnover.

Thus, collagen hydrolysate may serve as a promising nutraceutical supplement in osteoporosis prevention. The effective daily dose of collagen hydrolysate for osteoporosis was observed to be 10 grams.[7]

OA, a degenerative joint disease accompanied by joint pain, swelling and stiffness, impairs activities of daily living, reduces the quality of life and is the most common form of arthritis worldwide. Dietary supplements exhibited significant promise in the treatment of osteoarthritis. Clinical investigations using soluble undenatured type II collagen supplements from bovine and avian sources have yielded equivocal results in rheumatoid and osteoarthritis. A recent investigation examined if a Hydrolyzed Type II Collagen product (avian source: Biocell™) would have any positive effects in adults with OA when compared to placebo.[8]

Another randomized, double-blind placebo-controlled study was conducted over a period of two months in 16 subjects who are suffering from OA of the knee and hand. During recruitment, subjects were balanced for age, race, gender and location of osteoarthritis. In addition, subjects taking cyclo-oxygenase-2 inhibitor (COX-2 inhibitor) or non-steroidal anti-inflammatory drugs (NSAID) therapies were allowed to continue their therapy during this investigation. However, subjects who were taking nutraceuticals or dietary supplements were excluded. Also, subjects who had clinically significant medical conditions were excluded. Subjects with allergies to dietary collagen, who were pregnant or lactating or who had recently participated in a clinical trial were also excluded. Subjects were randomized and treated with either active Biocell™ (1000 mg BID; n = 8) or placebo (PLA, cellulose; n = 8) treatment over a period of eight weeks. Measurements included changes in the Western Ontario and McMaster Universities Osteoarthritis Index (WOMAC), Quality of Life short form (QoL), sleep quality ratings (via visual analog scale) as well as clinical markers of safety (i.e., liver function tests, renal function, white blood counts, blood pressure, heart rate, etc.). Following the completion of the study and statistical assessment, it was observed that Hydrolyzed Type II Collagen experienced a significant improvement in their WOMAC score, as well as stiffness and activities of daily living scores when compared to the placebo ($p < 0.05$ for all subsets and for total WOMAC scores). Additionally, the Biocell™ group achieved a significant improvement in QoL scores ($p < 0.05$) compared to baseline values. Adverse events were not different between the groups, while the study compliance was 93–94% as determined by returned capsule counts. Investigators concluded that Hydrolyzed Type II Collagen appeared to be a safe and effective dietary supplement for the adjunctive treatment of OA.[8]

17.7   GELATIN AND ANAPHYLACTIC REACTION

As a preventive measure, infants are given a series of immunizations shots throughout the first few years of life. Following immunization, some infants develop anaphylaxis. It is a serious and potentially life-threatening condition. As a routine practice, gelatin is used in the production and delivery of vaccines for measles, mumps, rubella (MMR), varicella, diphtheria-tetanus-acellular pertussis (DTP) and Japanese encephalitis. People who receive any of these vaccines develop a sensitization to the gelatin as evidenced by elevated immunoglobin E (IgE) antibodies (anti-gelatin antibodies). It is quite obvious that someone who is given a DTP vaccine and develops a sensitization to the gelatin may develop an anaphylactic reaction when given a subsequent vaccine (i.e., MMR). Mayo Clinic (Minneapolis, MN, USA) conducted a retrospective case control study and reported that 27% of the sample tested had anti-gelatin antibodies (anti-gelatin IgE) whereas none of the control subjects had.[9] Simultaneously, the Centers for Disease Control and Prevention (CDC) reported that since the introduction of DTP there has not been a substantial increase in the number of allergic responses reported. Furthermore, CDC stated that anaphylactic reactions to MMR are rare and the incidence is unchanged. Based on the observations, it was estimated that 25% of all people who have a reaction to MMR are hypersensitive to gelatin in the vaccine. Accordingly, CDC announced that allergy testing or evaluation should be conducted on infants who exhibit any symptoms of hypersensitivity to gelatin. Overall, gelatin seems to be non-toxic, tolerable and healthy as a food ingredient and GRAS; however, it may induce an adverse effect in a small population of unsuspecting infants/toddlers.[9]

17.8   APPLICATION IN SPORTS NUTRITION AND ATHLETIC PERFORMANCE

Scientific research or clinical studies haven't yet demonstrated any evidence of athletic performance enhancement following the use of gelatin or hydrolyzed collagen. However, hydrolyzed collagen or gelatin exerted potential benefit for the relief of osteoarthritis and pain alleviation; thus, athletes, those who engage in athletic performances, muscle building and exercise may consider the adjunctive use of hydrolyzed collagen or gelatin.

Sports nutritionists and athletes always prefer to consume a protein enriched diet, which significantly contributes to their sports and athletic performances. As demonstrated earlier, gelatin is derived from collagen, while collagen is a protein source in many foods.

However, gelatin is an incomplete protein of low biological value when compared to egg, milk, whey, etc., and, thus, it should not play a major role as the primary dietary protein constituent in athletes.

17.9   GELATIN AND DELIVERY MODULES

As discussed earlier, gelatin is used in many food ingredients, and widely used in paper and pharmaceutical industries, as well as in photographic processing. In the nutraceutical and functional food industries, gelatin is used in tablets and capsules (as a binder or for the capsule itself). Use of gelatin has grown significantly as a pharmaceutical delivery molecule. The remarkable area of interest is twofold: oral-muco delivery (gel films that melt on the tongue or in the mouth which deliver a nutritional or pharmaceutical agent) and as part of a microsphere used in the parenteral treatment of specific disease states.

Particularly, for the controlled release of a medication, microspheres allow for the delivery of novel bioactive proteins to the target tissue. Thus, this novel delivery system is particularly suitable in osteoarthritis which affects one joint (monoarthritis).[10]

17.10 SUMMARY

Taken together, gelatin is a protein derived from collagen which has diverse applications in the nutrition, functional food, nutraceuticals, chemical and pharmaceutical industries. Sports nutritionists and athletes who consume protein bars and protein shakes or consume gel caps are exposed to gelatin. A significant amount of clinical evidence has proven that hydrolyzed gelatin and hydrolyzed collagen are safe and efficacious for the symptomatic relief of osteoarthritis. Furthermore, research studies have shown that hydrolyzed collagen can help in pain alleviation and possibly the enhancement/repair of cartilage tissue.

In particular, athletes involved in sports and weightlifting exhibiting the signs of osteoarthritis or joint pain/stiffness might benefit from the prophylactic use of hydrolyzed gelatin. Additional research investigations are required in order to determine if gelatin or hydrolyzed collagen has protective or recovery properties for joint pain or cartilage-based disorders. However, gelatin and/or collagen supplementation as a potential protein source is not recommended.

REFERENCES

1. www.gelita.com/dgf-english/gelatine/gelatine_was.html. Accessed December 13, 2002.
2. www.gelatin-gmia.com/html/rawmaterials_app.html. Accessed June 18, 2003.
3. www.gelatine.org. Accessed December 13, 2002.
4. http://www.nutrajoint.com/aboutus/article11-22.shtml. Accessed November 11, 2002.
5. McCarthy SM, Carpenter MR, Barrell M, Morrissey D, Jacobson E, Kline G, Rowinski M, Freedson P, Gootman JP, O'Brien D, Knipe SJ, Rippe JM. The effectiveness of gelatine supplementation treatment in individuals with symptoms of mild osteoarthritis. Annual Meeting of the American Academy of Family Physicians. Dallas, Texas, September 22, 2000.
6. Rippe JM., McCarthy S., Abbott Waite M. *The Joint Health Prescription: 8 Weeks to Stronger, Healthier, Younger Joints.* New York: Balantine Books, 2001.
7. Moskowitz RW. Role of collagen hydrolysate in bone and joint disease. *Seminars in Arthritis and Rheumatism* 2000;30(2):87–99.
8. Kalman D, Almada AL, Schwartz, Prachon J, Sheldon E. A randomized double blind clinical trial evaluating the safety and efficacy of hydrolyzed collagen type II in adults with osteoarthritis. Annual Meeting of the American College of Rheumatology. Orlando, FL, 2003.
9. Pool V, Braun MM, Kelso JM, Mootrey G, Chen RT, Yunginger JW, Jacobson RM, Gargiullo PM. Prevalence of anti-gelatin IgE antibodies in people with anaphylaxis after measles-mumps rubella vaccine in the United States. *Pediatrics* 2002;110(6):e71.
10. Brown KE, Leong K, Huang CH, Dalal R, Green GD, Haimes HB, Jiminez PA, Bathon J. Gelatin/chrondroitin 6-sulfate microspheres for the delivery of therapeutic proteins to the joint. *Arthritis and Rheumatism* 1998;41(12):2185–2194.

Section VI

*Impact of Eccentric Exercise
on Muscle and Adaption
of Body and Muscles*

18 Skeletal Muscle Damage and Recovery from Eccentric Contractions

Eisuke Ochi and Yosuke Tsuchiya

CONTENTS

18.1 General Introduction 321
18.2 Damage from Eccentric Contractions 322
    18.2.1 Muscle Function 322
    18.2.2 Delayed-Onset Muscle Soreness 324
    18.2.3 Joint Flexibility and Muscle Stiffness 325
    18.2.4 Swelling and Edema 326
    18.2.5 Blood Proteins (Creatine Kinase and Myoglobin) 327
    18.2.6 Nerve Function 328
18.3 Protection and Recovery from Muscle Damage 329
    18.3.1 Pre-Exercise Intervention (Prevention) 329
    18.3.2 Post-Exercise Intervention (Post-Intervention) 331
18.4 Summary and Future Directions 331
References 333

18.1 GENERAL INTRODUCTION

The contraction modalities of skeletal muscle are classified into "isometric contractions", which generate strength during muscle contraction with unchanged muscle length; "concentric contractions", which generate strength during muscle contraction while muscles are contracting; and "eccentric contractions (ECCs)", which generates strength while muscles are stretched in the opposite direction of the muscle contraction. All of these contraction modalities occur in exercise, sports, or resistance training. A typical example of ECCs is forcibly stretching the muscle with loads that exceed the maximum muscle strength generated. Examples of such movements are the gradual lowering of a dumbbell and off-loading an item. Thus, if the muscle is to be stretched when the level of muscle strength generated is intentionally smaller than the load, the muscle will be accidentally stretched to absorb the shock. As such, submaximal ECCs occasionally occur even in daily activities. Fewer motor units may be recruited for a given submaximal load during eccentric versus concentric contractions, which implies that there will be a greater force per active motor unit (Bigland-Ritchie and Woods 1976; Isner-Horobeti et al. 2013; Ochi, Tsuchiya, and Nosaka 2016). Therefore, exercise-induced muscle damage (EIMD), such

321

as persistent decrease in muscle strength and muscle soreness lasting a few days, occurs after ECCs (Guilhem, Cornu, and Guevel 2010). The EIMD from the ECCs appears to be greater with higher loads (McHugh and Tetro 2003), faster contraction velocities (Chapman et al. 2006), longer muscle lengths during exercise (Nosaka et al. 2005; Proske and Allen 2005), and in untrained subjects (Newton et al. 2008). Several review articles have described the mechanism of muscle damage due to ECCs (Clarkson and Hubal 2002; Douglas et al. 2017; Hyldahl and Hubal 2014; Peake et al. 2017; Proske and Allen 2005). Since EIMD is caused by extreme and rare sports, the prevention of EIMD must be crucial. In this chapter, the exercise conditions (repetition of contractions, patterns of exercise movement, contraction velocity, etc.), differences in subject characteristics (individual differences, genetic background, etc.), and the relationship between the respective muscle damage markers in the ECCs model are reviewed. In addition, we introduce factors involved in the early recovery from muscle damage.

18.2 DAMAGE FROM ECCENTRIC CONTRACTIONS

18.2.1 MUSCLE FUNCTION

The decline in muscle strength capabilities in the days following ECCs is considered one of the most reliable indirect markers of EIMD (Paulsen et al. 2012; Warren, Lowe, and Armstrong 1999). Loss in muscle strength is generally representative of the severity of histological damage (Clarkson and Hubal 2002). Reductions of 10–60% of muscle strength have been reported for up to a week following ECCs (Guilhem, Cornu, and Guevel 2010; Murayama et al. 2000; Ochi, Tsuchiya, and Nosaka 2016; Ochi, Tsuchiya, and Yanagimoto 2017; Tsuchiya et al. 2015, 2016). The magnitude of muscle strength impairment appears to be directly associated with the number of muscle fibers with myofibrillar disruption and excitation–contraction coupling dysfunction (Peake et al. 2017; Raastad et al. 2010). In addition, the reduced neuromuscular performance with EIMD may, at least partly, be underpinned by impaired sarcolemmal activity, potential alteration of conduction velocity (Piitulainen et al. 2010), and transient changes (e.g. 24 h) in central nervous system activity (Isner-Horobeti et al. 2013).

The extent of muscle strength loss and the time to full recovery is typically dependent on several factors including the mode, muscle parts, contractions times, intensity, contraction velocity, training status, and age. For example, paradigms using the quadriceps, such as downhill running, typically generate 10–30% loss of force following exercise when compared to maximal ECCs of the biceps, which typically results in 50–60% loss of strength post-exercise (Eston et al. 1996; Newham, Jones, and Clarkson 1987). Isolated ECCs of the quadriceps on a dynamometer or using weights can generate higher strength losses than downhill running. Chen et al. (2011) tested these changes by measuring indirect markers of muscle damage following 30 maximal isokinetic (90°/sec) ECCs for the knee extensors and flexors and compared them with the elbow flexors and extensors of the same subjects. The results showed that the muscle strength decreased significantly immediately following exercise for the elbow flexors ($33 \pm 4\%$), elbow extensors ($30 \pm 3\%$), knee flexors ($17 \pm 2\%$), and knee extensors (5 ± 2%). The magnitude of the decrease was significantly greater for the elbow extensors and elbow flexors than for the knee extensors and knee flexors. However, while there was no significant difference between the elbow flexors and elbow extensors, a significant difference between knee flexors and knee extensors was observed. In addition, it became clear that the degree of the decrease in muscle strength differs according to the repetitions of isokinetic contractions. Nosaka, Newton, and Sacco (2002) compared the extent of the decrease in muscle strength after 12 and 24 maximal ECCs of the elbow flexors. They reported that a decrease in muscle strength was significantly higher with 24 contractions (58.1% decrease) than with 12 contractions (47.1% decrease). Even in ECCs by knee extension, muscle strength decreased by 5% (Chen et al. 2011) in a study where 30 contractions were performed and by approximately 40% in a study where 100 contractions were performed (Xin et al. 2014). Furthermore, the decrease in muscle strength was shown to vary according to the contraction velocity. Chapman et al. (2006) performed ECCs of the elbow flexors at contraction velocities of 30°/sec and 210°/sec and reported that the decrease in muscle strength was large at the contraction velocity of 210°/sec. Conversely, the results of animal studies are controversial. In our previous study, muscle strength was greatly decreased after fast contraction velocity (180°/sec) than with a slow contraction velocity (30°/sec). Moreover, the increase in Forkhead transcription factors of the O class (FOXOs) was reported to be high (Ochi et al. 2010). In the investigation by Warren et al. (1993), where differing contraction velocities (0.5, 1.0, and 1.5 L0 (resting length)/sec) during elongation contraction were examined using rat soleus muscle *in vitro*, the authors concluded that the decrease in the tension generated subsequently was not affected. Therefore, the effect of contraction velocities on muscle function following s may differ depending on assessment made *in vitro* or *in vivo*. In addition, the decrease in muscle strength has also been reported to be affected by the range of motion (ROM). Nosaka et al. (2001) demonstrated that the magnitude of the decrease in muscle strength after s of the elbow flexors was greater at the elbow joint ROM of 50–130° than at 100–180° (complete extension; 50–130°: 45% decrease, 100–180°: 69% decrease). Moreover, a study comparing the magnitude of muscle damage after isotonic ECCs of the elbow flexors using a dumbbell at 40% maximal voluntary isometric contraction (MVC) in young and elderly men demonstrated that the decrease in muscle strength of young men (70% decrease) was greater than that of elderly men (50% decrease) (Lavender and Nosaka 2006). In addition, the magnitude of the decrease in muscle strength is considered to be greater after isotonic ECCs than after isokinetic ECCs. In a study where 30 ECCs were performed using a dumbbell at 100% MVC, muscle strength decreased by approximately 50–55% post-exercise (Chen et al. 2010; Chen, Nosaka, and Sacco 2007). Meanwhile, in the previous studies where 30 isokinetic ECCs were performed similarly, muscle strength decreased by approximately 30–40% (Chen et al. 2010; Ochi, Tsuchiya, and Nosaka 2016; Tsuchiya et al. 2016; Tsuchiya, Nakazato, and Ochi 2018). Conversely, in our previous study, 60 ECCs were performed using a dumbbell at 40% MVC and the magnitude of decrease in muscle strength post-exercise was 23.2% (Ochi, Tsuchiya, and Yanagimoto 2017). This suggests that isotonic ECCs induce a decrease in muscle strength in an intensity-dependent manner. In addition, the magnitude of decrease in muscle strength after ECCs was reported to be small in subjects who performed regular training (trained) as compared with those who did not (untrained) (Newton et al. 2008). A "repeated bout effect (RBE)," described below, is likely a related cause.

18.2.2 Delayed-Onset Muscle Soreness

Although delayed-onset muscle soreness (DOMS) is also a common symptom of muscle damage, the mechanisms responsible for DOMS remain somewhat uncertain. DOMS refers to the dull, aching pain felt during movement or upon palpation of the affected tissue and often accompanies EIMD (Clarkson, Nosaka, and Braun 1992). It is commonly believed that micro-trauma of myofibers and subsequent inflammation causes DOMS. However, mechanical hyperalgesia occurs 1–3 days after ECCs in rats, without any apparent microscopic damage of the muscle or signs of inflammation (Hayashi et al. 2017). Indeed, muscle soreness in humans appears in the hours following ECCs, peaking 1–3 days after ECCs, and disappearing after 7–10 days (Cheung, Hume, and Maxwell 2003).

Two pathways are involved in inducing mechanical hyperalgesia after ECCs: (1) activation of the B2-bradykinin receptor-nerve growth factor pathway and (2) activation of the COX-2-glial cell line-derived neurotrophic factor pathway. It appears that these neurotrophic factors are produced by muscle fibers and/or satellite cells (Mizumura and Taguchi 2016). These agents may induce DOMS directly by stimulating muscle nociceptors. Alternatively, they may act indirectly by binding to the extracellular receptor and inducing secretion of neurotrophins from muscle fibers, which results in nociceptor stimulation and DOMS (Hyldahl and Hubal 2014). It is likely that DOMS is associated with inflammation in the extracellular matrix, rather than with myofiber damage and inflammation (Damas et al. 2016).

Interestingly, DOMS appears to be independent of other markers (e.g. MVC, ROM and plasma creatinine kinase [CK]) of EIMD (Nosaka, Newton, and Sacco 2002). The study by Warren, Lowe, and Armstrong (1999) also reported that DOMS after ECCs correlated poorly with other muscle damage markers. In addition, Nosaka, Newton, and Sacco (2002) compared the magnitude of the decrease in muscle strength after 12 and 24 maximal ECCs of the elbow flexors and reported that no significant difference was observed in peak DOMS (12 contractions: 40.8 mm, 24 contractions: 40.9 mm). Furthermore, a study that compared trained and untrained subjects also demonstrated no notable differences in the level of DOMS after ECCs of the elbow flexors (Newton et al. 2008). Moreover, no difference was observed even in isotonic and isokinetic ECCs. In a previous study where dumbbells were used with 30–60 ECCs of the elbow flexors at 40–100% MVC, the DOMS after the exercise was reported to be approximately 35–57 mm (Chen et al. 2010; Chen, Nosaka, and Sacco 2007; Lavender and Nosaka 2006; Ochi, Tsuchiya, and Yanagimoto 2017), and that after 12–60 maximal isokinetic ECCs of the elbow flexors was 20–60 mm (Chen et al. 2009; Chen et al. 2011; Muthalib et al. 2011; Newton et al. 2013; Nosaka and Clarkson 1996a; Nosaka, Newton and Sacco 2002; Ochi, Tsuchiya, and Nosaka 2016; Tsuchiya et al. 2016; Tsuchiya, Nakazato, and Ochi 2018). Meanwhile, the level of DOMS following ECCs was reported to be influenced by the contraction velocity. Chapman et al. (2006) examined ECCs of the elbow flexors at contraction velocities of 30° or 210°/sec and reported that the level of DOMS was higher at a contraction velocity of 210°/sec (20.6 vs 42.0 mm). Moreover, in a study comparing the magnitude of muscle damage after 30 maximal isokinetic ECCs of the elbow and knee flexors and extensors, the level of DOMS was shown to be lower with the knee flexors (15 mm) and extensors (20 mm) than with the elbow flexors (50 mm) and extensors (40 mm) (Chen et al. 2011). However, the DOMS after 100 maximal isokinetic ECCs of the knee extensors was reported to be 40 mm (Xin et al. 2014), which suggests that the difference in the level of DOMS due to the site is likely dependent on the repetitions of contraction. Furthermore, DOMS is also affected by the joint angle associated with ECCs. Nosaka et al. (2001) demonstrated that the level of DOMS after ECCs of the elbow flexors was higher at an elbow joint ROM of 100°–180° (complete extension) than at 50°–130° (50°–130°: 20 mm, 100°–180°: 40 mm). Moreover, a study comparing the magnitude of muscle damage after ECCs of the elbow flexors in young and elderly men demonstrated that peak DOMS following exercise was greater in young (35 mm) than in the elderly men (15 mm) (Lavender and Nosaka 2006).

18.2.3   Joint Flexibility and Muscle Stiffness

Passive tension, muscle swelling, and an increase in muscle hardness (Murayama et al. 2000) may all contribute to the reduced range of joint motion often observed following ECCs (Clarkson, Nosaka, and Braun 1992). A sense of force and position can both be negatively affected by ECCs (Proske and Allen 2005), which may have implications on the performance of various sports. In fact, we confirmed that joint passive resistive torque increased transiently after ECCs of the ankle dorsiflexors (Ochi, Ishii, and Nakazato 2007). It has been demonstrated that the decrease in relaxed elbow joint angle is also associated with increased muscle stiffness (Chleboun et al. 1998; Howell, Chleboun, and Conatser 1993; Jones, Newham, and Clarkson 1987). Jones, Newham, and Clarkson (1987) measured the force required to extend the flexed elbow joint after ECCs of the elbow flexor muscles, showing that muscle stiffness increased after exercise. Howell, Chleboun, and Conatser (1993) and Chleboun et al. (1998) have also reported an increase in muscle stiffness after ECCs of the elbow flexor muscles. They used a device that extended the elbow joint and recorded the torque required to hold the forearm at successive angles. More recently, elastographic techniques have been used to assess the shear elastic modulus (i.e., elasticity) of a localized area in the muscle at rest (Debernard et al. 2011; Gennisson et al. 2010; Lacourpaille et al. 2014; Shinohara et al. 2010), during isometric contraction (Dresner et al. 2001; Shinohara et al. 2010), and during passive stretching (Koo et al. 2014; Maisetti et al. 2012). Lacourpaille et al. (2014) showed that the shear elastic modulus of the biceps brachii and brachialis increased at 1 h after ECCs using elastographic techniques. The increase in the shear elastic modulus after ECCs was associated with both Ca^{2+} release, due to cell membrane damage, and with sarcomere disruption during ECCs (Lacourpaille et al. 2014).

In many studies, the joint ROM from the extension position to that of flexion of the elbow joint has been used to evaluate joint flexibility. Nosaka, Newton, and Sacco (2002) compared change in the ROM after 12 and 60 maximal isokinetic

ECCs of the elbow flexors and reported that the ROM limitation was significantly larger with 60 contractions (extension position: −14.4°, flexion position: −9.6°) than with 12 contractions (extension position: −10.4°, flexion position: −5.6°). Moreover, in a study comparing the magnitude of muscle damage after 30 maximal isokinetic ECCs of the elbow and knee flexors and extensors, limitation of the ROM was smaller with the knee flexors (−4°) and extensors (−2°) than with the elbow flexors (−10°) and extensors (−10°) (Chen et al. 2011). Furthermore, the limitation of ROM was reported to be larger after fast-velocity (210°/sec) ECCs than after slow-velocity (30°/sec) ECCs (30°/sec: −10.2°, 210°/sec: −23.9°) (Chapman et al. 2006). Similar to DOMS, the limitation of the ROM is also affected by the joint angle associated with ECCs (Nosaka and Sakamoto 2001). The limitation of ROM following the ECCs of the elbow flexors was greater in an elbow joint ROM of 100–180° (complete extension) than in an elbow joint ROM of 50–130° (50–130°: −14°, 100–180°: −28°) (Nosaka and Sakamoto 2001). Moreover, a study that compared the magnitude of muscle damage after ECCs of the elbow flexors in young and elderly men demonstrated that the limitation of the ROM after exercise was greater in young (−35°) than in elderly men (−25°) (Lavender and Nosaka 2006). Even in our study using rat models, passive resistive torque after ECCs increased greatly in young rats as compared to older rats (Ochi et al. 2008). With regard to the status of training, unlike DOMS, limitation of the ROM was reported to be larger in untrained (−18°) than in trained (−8°) subjects after ECCs (Newton et al. 2008). Conversely, limitation of the ROM after ECCs showed no notable differences for isokinetic or isotonic contractions (Chen et al. 2010; Chen, Nosaka, and Sacco 2007; Ochi, Tsuchiya, and Nosaka 2016; Ochi, Tsuchiya, and Yanagimoto 2017; Tsuchiya, Nakazato, and Ochi 2018). Moreover, in a study that evaluated shear elastic modulus using elastographic techniques, the shear elastic modulus of the upper arm increased by 70–150% in 30 min after 30 or 60 maximal ECCs of the elbow flexors (Lacourpaille et al. 2014). In other words, one can consider limitation of the ROM after ECCs to be associated with increased muscle stiffness. In the latter study, an increase in muscle stiffness and a decrease in muscle strength after exercise were also shown to be significantly correlated ($r = -0.80$) (Lacourpaille et al. 2017).

18.2.4 Swelling and Edema

The delayed onset of swelling (2–4 days) has been documented previously (Clarkson and Dedrick 1988; Hill and Richardson 1989; Howell et al. 1985), although no study has documented the time course of the swelling lasting as long as 9 days. As with soreness and tenderness, considerable individual variation in swelling was observed. The muscle swelling and edema after ECCs appear to be associated with inflammatory swelling (Nosaka and Clarkson 1996a) due to an accumulation of fluid in the area. When fluid accumulation exceeds the capability of the lymphatic drainage system, the result is edema (Nosaka and Clarkson 1996).

Swelling and edema after ECCs are evaluated by measuring the circumference of the limbs using a measuring tape or measuring the cross-sectional area of the limb with an ultrasound device or magnetic resonance imaging (MRI). To date, upper arm circumference after isokinetic or isotonic ECCs of the elbow flexors has been confirmed to increase by approximately 4–20 mm (Chapman et al. 2006; Lavender and Nosaka 2006; Newton et al. 2008; Newton et al. 2013; Nosaka, Newton, and Sacco 2002), while the cross-sectional area of the upper arm muscles (biceps brachii and brachialis) increases by approximately 19–40 mm^2 (Ochi, Tsuchiya, and Nosaka 2016; Ochi, Tsuchiya, and Yanagimoto 2017; Tsuchiya, Nakazato, and Ochi 2018). Similar to other muscle damage markers, changes in limb circumference after ECCs have been shown to differ according to repetitions and site of contractions (Nosaka, Newton, and Sacco 2002). Specifically, upper arm circumference has been reported to increase by 12 and 20 mm after 12 and 60 isokinetic ECCs of the elbow flexors, respectively (Nosaka, Newton, and Sacco 2002). Moreover, in a study where the ECCs of the elbow and knee flexors and extensors were evaluated, limb circumference was shown to increase less in the knee flexors (5-mm increase) and extensors (3-mm increase) than in the elbow flexors (10-mm increase) and extensors (8-mm increase) (Chen et al. 2011). Similarly, swelling and edema have been reported to be affected by contraction velocity and range of the joint angle. The increase in upper arm circumference post-exercise has been reported to be greater in ECCs at a slow contraction velocity (30°/sec) than at a fast contraction velocity (210°/sec) (Chapman et al. 2006). Moreover, the increase in upper arm circumference has been reported to be greater in ECCs where the elbow joint ROM was 100°–180° than in ECCs where the elbow joint ROM was 50°–130° (50–130°: no change, 100°–180°: 15-mm increase) (Nosaka and Sakamoto 2001). In addition, the increase in upper arm circumference after ECCs of the elbow flexors was greater in young (15-mm increase) than in elderly men (5-mm increase), which is similar to the findings associated with muscle strength and joint ROM (Lavender and Nosaka 2006). Even in the comparison of trained and untrained subjects, the increase in upper arm circumference after ECCs of the elbow flexors was significantly greater in untrained (15-mm increase) than in trained subjects (5-mm increase) (Newton et al. 2008). Moreover, changes in the cross-sectional area of muscles on MRI showed that the elbow flexor muscle group (biceps brachii and brachialis) after 30 isokinetic ECCs of the elbow flexors increased by 19–22 mm^2 (Ochi, Tsuchiya, and Nosaka 2016; Tsuchiya, Nakazato, and Ochi 2018). Furthermore, in isotonic ECCs, the cross-sectional area of the elbow flexor muscles, measured using an ultrasound device after 60 ECCs of 40% MVC using a dumbbell, was shown to increase by 40 mm^2 (Ochi, Tsuchiya, and Yanagimoto 2017).

18.2.5 Blood Proteins (Creatine Kinase and Myoglobin)

When muscle tissue is damaged due to ECCs, oxygen transport in the muscle; plasma levels of myoglobin (Mb), which is an oxygen storage protein; and CK activity, which plays a primary role in the production of ATP, lactate dehydrogenase (LDH), aldolase (ALD; a glycolytic enzyme catalyst), aspartate transferase (AST; an enzyme in the liver and skeletal muscle cells), and alanine amino transferase (ALT; predominant in the liver) are increased. Of these, CK and Mb, which are abundantly contained in skeletal muscles, are commonly used as muscle damage markers in many studies. Many reports have indicated that peak CK and Mb levels are reached in 3–5 days after exercise and have been shown to be linked with delayed-onset inflammatory reactions (Manfredi et al. 1991). In addition, the correlation of CK and Mb with other muscle damage markers has also been investigated. Nosaka and Clarkson (1996b) investigated the correlation between the increase in CK and muscle damage markers levels after 24 ECCs of the elbow flexors. They reported that an increase in CK level correlated significantly with a decrease in muscle strength ($r = 0.73$), limitation of the ROM ($r = 0.69$), and an increase in upper arm circumference ($r = 0.91$). Meanwhile, the increase in CK level did not correlate significantly with DOMS (Nosaka and Kuramata 1991). Although increased plasma levels of CK after ECCs correlated with muscle damage markers, the inter-subject variation in the levels was high. The inter-subject range of peak CK levels after ECCs has been reported to be 236–25,244 IU/l (Nosaka and Clarkson 1996b) and 93–10,528 IU/l (Tsuchiya et al. 2016). Therefore, careful attention is required when using CK levels as an index for evaluating muscle damage.

The increase in CK and Mb levels after ECCs are similar to the decrease in muscle strength, limitation of the ROM, and swelling. Peak CK levels after 12 and 24 isokinetic ECCs of the elbow flexors have been reported to be 5,549 IU/l after 12 contractions and 15,284 IU/l after 60 contractions (Nosaka, Newton, and Sacco 2002). Moreover, in a study were ECCs of the elbow and one flexor and extensor were performed, both peak CK and Mb levels were lower for the knee flexors (CK: 1,000, Mb: 200) and extensors (no change) than for the elbow flexors (CK: 2,500 IU/l, Mb: 400 IU/l) and extensors (CK: 2,000 IU/l, Mb: 400 IU/l) (Chen et al. 2011). In addition, similar to other muscle damage markers, these are also affected by contraction velocity and range of joint angle. In addition, the peak CK level was reported to be higher after fast velocity (210°/sec) ECCs than after slow-velocity (30°/sec) ECCs (30°/sec: no change, 210°/sec: 1,298.2 IU/l) (Chapman et al. 2006). Similarly, the peak CK level after ECCs was shown to be higher at the elbow joint ROM of 100–180° than when it was 50°–130° (50°–130°: 2,891 IU/l, 100°–180°: 10,640 IU/l) (Nosaka and Sakamoto 2001). Moreover, in a study comparing young and elderly men, peak CK and Mb levels after isotonic ECCs of the elbow flexors increased significantly in the elderly men, where the peak CK level was approximately 6,000 IU/l and the Mb level was 1,000 IU/l (Nosaka and Sakamoto 2001). Similar results were demonstrated even in a study that compared trained and untrained subjects. The peak CK level after 60 isokinetic ECCs of the elbow flexors increased to approximately 2,000 IU/l in the untrained subjects, whereas it did not increase significantly in the trained subjects (Newton et al. 2008).

18.2.6 Nerve Function

It has been shown that ECCs cause histological damage in rats, not only in the myofibrils, the extracellular matrix, and the triads of the cytoplasmic membrane system (Piitulainen et al. 2008; Proske and Morgan 2001), but also in nerve fibers and cause thinning of myelin sheaths (Kouzaki et al. 2016). Kouzaki et al. (2016) reported that M-wave latency was delayed by 12% at 24 h and 24% at 48 h after 60 ECCs of the elbow flexors in women, which suggests musculocutaneous nerve impairment. However, a significant correlation was not observed between the delay in nerve conduction velocity and the decrease in muscle strength. Moreover, a study in which 60 isotonic ECCs were performed using a 40% MVC dumbbell demonstrated that the M-wave latency was delayed by 32% immediately after completion of the exercise (Ochi, Tsuchiya, and Yanagimoto 2017). However, in this study, the relationship between nerve conduction velocity and other muscle damage markers was not investigated. Thus, there are still several issues that need to be clarified with regard to the relationship between decreased nerve function due to ECCs and muscle damage. The studies on the effect of ECCs on nerve function are extremely limited and detailed studies using human subjects to investigate motor nerve conduction velocity are warranted. Moreover, investigations on sensory nerve function are necessary in the future.

18.3 PROTECTION AND RECOVERY FROM MUSCLE DAMAGE

The number of muscle fibers showing a disruption of normal myofibrillar band patterns is increased immediately after ECCs (Gibala et al. 1995). Disruption of Z disks and sarcomeres appears to peak between 1–3 days after exercise (Crameri et al. 2007; Friden, Sjostrom, and Ekblom 1983; Newham et al. 1983; Yu, Carlsson, and Thornell 2004), but may remain elevated up to 6–8 days after exercise (Friden, Sjostrom, and Ekblom 1983; Jones et al. 1986; Yu, Carlsson, and Thornell 2004). There is a temporal association between the extent of the loss of muscle strength after exercise and the time required to restore muscle strength to normal levels. When muscle strength decreases by ~20% immediately after exercise, it is usually restored within 2 days after exercise (Crameri et al. 2007; Malm et al. 2004). In contrast, when muscle strength decreases by ~50% immediately after exercise, especially on initial exposure to ECCs, it remains below pre-exercise values at 7 days after exercise (Lauritzen et al. 2009; Paulsen et al. 2010a; Paulsen et al. 2010b). As shown in Figure 18.1, a previous review article (Peake et al. 2017), reported that the time course of changes in muscle strength, ROM, DOMS, limb circumference (i.e., swelling), and blood CK activity in the days after intense ECCs varies. Even when recovery of muscle strength is prolonged, DOMS is resolved by 4 days after exercise (Damas et al. 2016). Muscle swelling peaks 4–5 days after exercise and increases in serum biomarkers of muscle damage, such as CK activity, are also delayed (Damas et al. 2016). Changes in muscle strength appear to influence the magnitude and time course of changes of other EIMD markers.

18.3.1 PRE-EXERCISE INTERVENTION (PREVENTION)

A range of physiotherapeutic, nutritional, and pharmacological strategies has been evaluated to investigate their effectiveness in restoring muscle function, relieving muscle soreness, and reducing intramuscular inflammation after exercise. Some individual studies have reported benefits of these strategies for recovery from EIMD. In particular, several reports have stated that the ingestion of amino acids, proteins, vitamins, polyphenols, omega 3 fatty acids, etc., inhibits muscle damage after ECCs (Foure and Bendahan 2017; Nakazato, Ochi, and Waga 2010; Ochi, Tsuchiya, and Yanagimoto 2017; Owens et al. 2018; Rahimi et al. 2017; Tsuchiya et al. 2016). In our recent study, subjects ingested omega 3 fatty acids in the form of

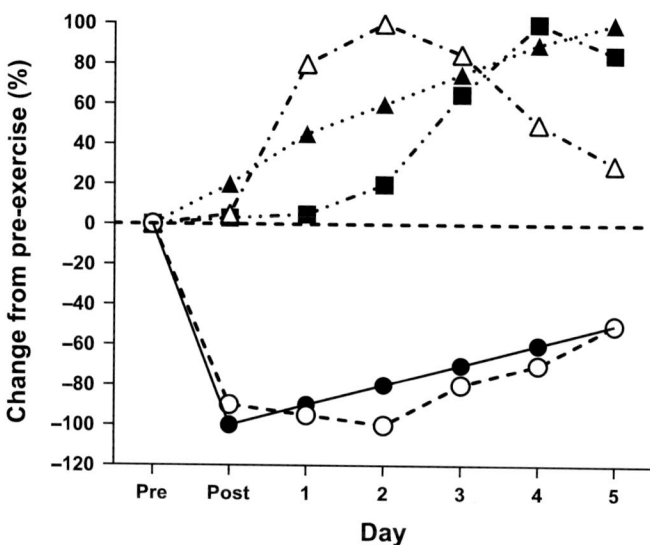

FIGURE 18.1 Schematic illustration displaying model data for the typical magnitude and time course of changes in maximal voluntary contraction torque of the elbow flexors (maximum voluntary contraction), range of motion at the elbow joint, swelling measured by upper arm circumference, delayed-onset muscle soreness assessed by a visual analog scale, and creatine kinase activity in the blood before (Pre), immediately after (Post), and 1–5 days after 30 maximal eccentric muscle contractions of the elbow flexors performed by healthy young men who were unaccustomed to the exercise. Data are derived from separate analysis published elsewhere (Damas et al. 2016; Peake et al. 2017). ●, strength; ▲, swelling; △, soreness; ○, range of motion; ■, creatine kinase.

eicosapentaenoic acid (EPA) (600 mg/day) and docosahexaenoic acid (DHA) (240 mg/day) for 8 weeks prior to exercise. Muscle damage after 30 ECCs of the elbow flexors was significantly inhibited (Tsuchiya et al. 2016). Furthermore, ingestion of EPA and DHA also inhibited the delay in nerve conduction velocity that occurs after ECCs (Ochi, Tsuchiya, and Yanagimoto 2017). Moreover, a study that investigated the effect of apple polyphenols in rats confirmed that the decrease in muscle strength and the increase in oxidative stress that occurred after ECCs was inhibited when apple polyphenols were ingested for 3 weeks prior to the exercise (Nakazato, Ochi, and Waga 2010).

The most well-known intervention which is able to promote recovery from EIMD is previous muscle damage (Peake et al. 2017). After an initial bout of muscle-damaging exercise, the muscle learns to adapt and is protected, such that the signs and symptoms of EIMD are less severe and exhibit a more rapid return to normal after subsequent bouts of exercise (Nosaka et al. 2001; Paulsen et al. 2009; Stupka et al. 2001). This phenomenon is known as the RBE. The protective effect is provided by low-intensity ECCs or maximal isometric contractions at a long muscle length (Chen et al. 2012; Lin et al. 2015). Interestingly, the RBE is also conferred to the contralateral muscles, such that a second bout of ECCs performed by the contralateral arm induces less EIMD than the initial bout of the opposite arm (Chen et al. 2016; Tsuchiya, Nakazato, and Ochi 2018).

18.3.2 POST-EXERCISE INTERVENTION (POST-INTERVENTION)

Recent results from systematic reviews and meta-analyses combining all of these studies revealed no major or consistent advantages from applying any of these strategies (Peake et al. 2017). However, massage, wearing compression garments, and cold-water immersion somewhat inhibit DOMS (Hohenauer et al. 2015; Marques-Jimenez et al. 2016; Poppendieck et al. 2016). Compression garments and cold-water immersion also enhanced recovery of muscle strength (Leeder et al. 2012; Marques-Jimenez et al. 2016). With respect to ingestion of supplements immediately after exercising, Wilson et al. (2009) reported that when 3 g of the leucine metabolite, beta-hydroxy-beta-methylbutyrate (HMB), was ingested immediately after ECCs of the knee flexors and extensors, muscle damage was not inhibited. Future studies on post-exercise interventions that alleviate muscle damage are anticipated.

18.4 SUMMARY AND FUTURE DIRECTIONS

The details of the effects of different conditions of ECCs and the characteristics of subjects in terms of muscle damage markers are shown in Table 18.1.

TABLE 18.1

Effects of the Conditions of Eccentric Contractions and Subject Characteristics Relative to Muscle Damage Markers

	Condition of Eccentric Contractions				Characteristics of Subjects		
	Repetitions	Parts of the Muscle	Contraction Velocity	Range of Motion	Training Status	Age	Genetics
Muscle strength	affected	affected	affected	affected	affected	affected	affected
Delayed onset muscle soreness	unaffected	affected	affected	affected	unaffected	affected	unaffected
Range of motion and muscle stiffness	affected	affected	affected	affected	affected	affected	affected
Swelling and edema	affected	affected	affected	affected	affected	affected	–
Serum creatine kinase and myoglobin	affected	affected	affected	affected	affected	affected	–

–: No data

1. In individuals who performed high repetitions of ECCs, the magnitude of the decreases in muscle strength, the limitation of the joint ROM, swelling, and the increases in plasma CK and Mb levels was high, while DOMS was not affected by the repetitions of contractions.

2. With isokinetic ECCs, the magnitude of the decreases in muscle strength, DOMS, limitation of the ROM, swelling, and the increases in plasma CK and Mb levels was larger in the elbow flexors and extensors compared to those observed when the knee flexors and extensors were exercised.

3. In ECCs performed with a fast contraction velocity, the magnitude of the decreases in muscle strength, DOMS, limitation of the joint ROM, swelling and increases in plasma CK and Mb levels after exercise was greater when compared to the magnitude of those observed after slow ECCs.

4. When ECCs were performed with muscles in the elongated position, the magnitude of the decreases in muscle strength, DOMS, limitation of the joint ROM, swelling and increases in plasma CK and Mb levels after exercise was greater than the magnitude of those observed after ECCs with muscles in the shortened position.

5. In ECCs with conditions of relatively similar intensity, the magnitude of the decreases in muscle strength, DOMS, limitation of the joint ROM, swelling and increases in plasma CK and Mb levels after exercise were greater in the young than those observed in elderly men.

6. The magnitude of the decreases in muscle strength, limitation of the joint ROM, swelling and increase in plasma CK and Mb levels after ECCs was greater in untrained subjects compared to those observed in trained subjects. Moreover, DOMS was not affected by training status.

Furthermore, the correlation with muscle damage markers is shown in Table 18.2. Previous studies have demonstrated that plasma CK is significantly correlated with decreases in muscle strength, DOMS, and limitations in the joint ROM (Nosaka and Clarkson 1996b). In addition, increases in the shear elastic modulus (as measured by elastographic techniques) after ECCs have been reported to be significantly correlated with decreases in muscle strength (Lacourpaille et al. 2017). Since there was no significant correlation with the other muscle damage markers, we suggest that these muscle damage markers were independent. Many factors relating to the correlation between nerve damage and muscle damage remain unclear and will need to be investigated in detailed studies in the future.

Importantly, the correlation between ECC-induced muscle damage and genes is being investigated. Although the mechanism(s) responsible for the reported discrepancies in loss of strength among individuals following ECCs is still poorly understood, there is evidence that genetic variability may play a role (Hubal et al. 2010; Hubal, Rubinstein, and Clarkson 2007). Recently we have examined the effect of the *ACTN3 R577X* gene polymorphism on the decreases in muscle strength, limitation of the ROM, and DOMS after ECCs. We found that limitation of the ROM after ECCs was significantly smaller in individuals with the *RR* allele compared to those possessing either the *RX* or *XX* allele (Kikuchi et al. 2018). Conversely, there was

TABLE 18.2

Matrix of the Correlation of Muscle Damage Markers Induced by Eccentric Contractions

	Muscle Strength	Delayed Onset Muscle Soreness	Range of Motion and Muscle Stiffness	Swelling and Edema	Serum Creatine Kinase	Nerve
Muscle strength		×	○	×	×	–
Delayed onset muscle soreness	×		×	×	×	–
Range of motion and muscle stiffness	○	×		×	○	–
Swelling and edema	×	×	×		×	–
Serum creatine kinase	○	○	○			–
Nerve function	×	–	–	–	–	

○: Correlation Present, ×: No Correlation, –: No Data

no significant difference between the groups with respect to the decrease in muscle strength (Kikuchi et al. 2018). In the future, detailed studies examining the role of genetic factors in determining the magnitude of muscle damage are necessary.

While it is clear that ECCs cause a transient decrease in muscle function and an increase in muscle soreness, it is also evident that increases in blood pressure, heart rate, and subjective exercise intensity were limited during the exercise (Okamoto, Masuhara, and Ikuta 2006; Penaililo et al. 2013). Moreover, in our previous study, we confirmed that ECCs cause an increase in blood levels of bone metabolic markers (Tsuchiya, Sakuraba, and Ochi 2014). This demonstrates that insulin-like growth factor-1 (IGF-1) induced by ECCs is involved in this increase in bone formation and bone absorption. Although the long-term benefits are unclear, one can predict that ECCs have a positive effect on bone health. As detailed above, when ECCs are incorporated appropriately in training and exercise programs, these can improve health and competitive performance.

REFERENCES

Bigland-Ritchie, B., and J. J. Woods. 1976. Integrated electromyogram and oxygen uptake during positive and negative work. *J Physiol* 260 (2):267–77.

Chapman, D., M. Newton, P. Sacco, and K. Nosaka. 2006. Greater muscle damage induced by fast versus slow velocity eccentric exercise. *Int J Sports Med* 27 (8):591–8.

Chen, T. C., H. L. Chen, M. J. Lin, C. J. Wu, and K. Nosaka. 2009. Muscle damage responses of the elbow flexors to four maximal eccentric exercise bouts performed every 4 weeks. *Eur J Appl Physiol* 106 (2):267–75.

Chen, T. C., H. L. Chen, M. J. Lin, C. J. Wu, and K. Nosaka. 2010. Potent protective effect conferred by four bouts of low-intensity eccentric exercise. *Med Sci Sports Exerc* 42 (5):1004–12.

Chen, T. C., H. L. Chen, M. J. Lin, H. I. Yu, and K. Nosaka. 2016. Contralateral repeated bout effect of eccentric exercise of the elbow flexors. *Med Sci Sports Exerc* 48 (10):2030–9.

Chen, T. C., H. L. Chen, A. J. Pearce, and K. Nosaka. 2012. Attenuation of eccentric exercise-induced muscle damage by preconditioning exercises. *Med Sci Sports Exerc* 44 (11):2090–8.

Chen, T. C., K. Y. Lin, H. L. Chen, M. J. Lin, and K. Nosaka. 2011. Comparison in eccentric exercise-induced muscle damage among four limb muscles. *Eur J Appl Physiol* 111 (2):211–23.

Chen, T. C., K. Nosaka, and P. Sacco. 2007. Intensity of eccentric exercise, shift of optimum angle, and the magnitude of repeated-bout effect. *J Appl Physiol 1985* 102 (3):992–9.

Cheung, K., P. Hume, and L. Maxwell. 2003. Delayed onset muscle soreness: Treatment strategies and performance factors. *Sports Med* 33 (2):145–64.

Chleboun, G. S., J. N. Howell, R. R. Conatser, and J. J. Giesey. 1998. Relationship between muscle swelling and stiffness after eccentric exercise. *Med Sci Sports Exerc* 30 (4):529–35.

Clarkson, P. M., and M. E. Dedrick. 1988. Exercise-induced muscle damage, repair, and adaptation in old and young subjects. *J Gerontol* 43 (4):M91–6.

Clarkson, P. M., and M. J. Hubal. 2002. Exercise-induced muscle damage in humans. *Am J Phys Med Rehabil* 81 (11 Suppl):S52–69.

Clarkson, P. M., K. Nosaka, and B. Braun. 1992. Muscle function after exercise-induced muscle damage and rapid adaptation. *Med Sci Sports Exerc* 24 (5):512–20.

Crameri, R. M., P. Aagaard, K. Qvortrup, H. Langberg, J. Olesen, and M. Kjaer. 2007. Myofibre damage in human skeletal muscle: Effects of electrical stimulation versus voluntary contraction. *J Physiol* 583 (1):365–80.

Damas, F., K. Nosaka, C. A. Libardi, T. C. Chen, and C. Ugrinowitsch. 2016. Susceptibility to exercise-induced muscle damage: A cluster analysis with a large sample. *Int J Sports Med* 37 (8):633–40.

Debernard, L., L. Robert, F. Charleux, and S. F. Bensamoun. 2011. Characterization of muscle architecture in children and adults using magnetic resonance elastography and ultrasound techniques. *J Biomech* 44 (3):397–401.

Douglas, J., S. Pearson, A. Ross, and M. McGuigan. 2017. Eccentric exercise: Physiological characteristics and acute responses. *Sports Med* 47 (4):663–75.

Dresner, M. A., G. H. Rose, P. J. Rossman, R. Muthupillai, A. Manduca, and R. L. Ehman. 2001. Magnetic resonance elastography of skeletal muscle. *J Magn Reson Imaging* 13 (2):269–76.

Eston, R. G., S. Finney, S. Baker, and V. Baltzopoulos. 1996. Muscle tenderness and peak torque changes after downhill running following a prior bout of isokinetic eccentric exercise. *J Sports Sci* 14 (4):291–9.

Foure, A., and D. Bendahan. 2017. Is branched-chain amino acids supplementation an efficient nutritional strategy to alleviate skeletal muscle damage? A systematic review. *Nutrients* 9 (10).

Friden, J., M. Sjostrom, and B. Ekblom. 1983. Myofibrillar damage following intense eccentric exercise in man. *Int J Sports Med* 4 (3):170–6.

Gennisson, J. L., T. Deffieux, E. Mace, G. Montaldo, M. Fink, and M. Tanter. 2010. Viscoelastic and anisotropic mechanical properties of in vivo muscle tissue assessed by supersonic shear imaging. *Ultrasound Med Biol* 36 (5):789–801.

Gibala, M. J., J. D. MacDougall, M. A. Tarnopolsky, W. T. Stauber, and A. Elorriaga. 1995. Changes in human skeletal muscle ultrastructure and force production after acute resistance exercise. *J Appl Physiol* 78 (2):702–8.

Guilhem, G., C. Cornu, and A. Guevel. 2010. Neuromuscular and muscle-tendon system adaptations to isotonic and isokinetic eccentric exercise. *Ann Phys Rehabil Med* 53 (5):319–41.

Hayashi, K., K. Katanosaka, M. Abe, A. Yamanaka, K. Nosaka, K. Mizumura, and T. Taguchi. 2017. Muscular mechanical hyperalgesia after lengthening contractions in rats depends on stretch velocity and range of motion. *Eur J Pain* 21 (1):125–39.

Hill, D. W., and J. D. Richardson. 1989. Effectiveness of 10% Trolamine Salicylate cream on muscular soreness induced by a reproducible program of weight training. *J Orthop Sports Phys Ther* 11 (1):19–23.

Hohenauer, E., J. Taeymans, J. P. Baeyens, P. Clarys, and R. Clijsen. 2015. The effect of post-exercise cryotherapy on recovery characteristics: A systematic review and meta-analysis. *PLOS ONE* 10 (9):e0139028.

Howell, J. N., A. G. Chila, G. Ford, D. David, and T. Gates. 1985. An electromyographic study of elbow motion during postexercise muscle soreness. *Journal of Applied Physiology* 58 (5):1713–8.

Howell, J. N., G. Chleboun, and R. Conatser. 1993. Muscle stiffness, strength loss, swelling and soreness following exercise-induced injury in humans. *J Physiol* 464 (1):183–96.

Hubal, M. J., J. M. Devaney, E. P. Hoffman, E. J. Zambraski, H. Gordish-Dressman, A. K. Kearns, J. S. Larkin, K. Adham, R. R. Patel, and P. M. Clarkson. 2010. CCL2 and CCR2 polymorphisms are associated with markers of exercise-induced skeletal muscle damage. *J Appl Physiol* 108 (6):1651–8.

Hubal, M. J., S. R. Rubinstein, and P. M. Clarkson. 2007. Mechanisms of variability in strength loss after muscle-lengthening actions. *Med Sci Sports Exerc* 39 (3):461–8.

Hyldahl, R. D., and M. J. Hubal. 2014. Lengthening our perspective: Morphological, cellular, and molecular responses to eccentric exercise. *Muscle Nerve* 49 (2):155–70.

Isner-Horobeti, M. E., S. P. Dufour, P. Vautravers, B. Geny, E. Coudeyre, and R. Richard. 2013. Eccentric exercise training: Modalities, applications and perspectives. *Sports Med* 43 (6):483–512.

Jones, D. A., D. J. Newham, and P. M. Clarkson. 1987. Skeletal muscle stiffness and pain following eccentric exercise of the elbow flexors. *Pain* 30 (2):233–42.

Jones, D. A., D. J. Newham, J. M. Round, and S. E. Tolfree. 1986. Experimental human muscle damage: Morphological changes in relation to other indices of damage. *J Physiol* 375 (1):435–48.

Kikuchi, N., Y. Tsuchiya, K. Nakazato, N. Ishii, and E. Ochi. 2018. Effects of the ACTN3 R577X genotype on the muscular strength and range of motion before and after eccentric contractions of the elbow flexors. *Int J Sports Med* 39 (2):148–53.

Koo, T. K., J. Y. Guo, J. H. Cohen, and K. J. Parker. 2014. Quantifying the passive stretching response of human tibialis anterior muscle using shear wave elastography. *Clin Biomech* 29 (1):33–9.

Kouzaki, K., M. Kobayashi, K. I. Nakamura, K. Ohta, and K. Nakazato. 2016. Repeated bouts of fast eccentric contraction produce sciatic nerve damage in rats. *Muscle Nerve* 54 (5):936–42.

Kouzaki, K., K. Nosaka, E. Ochi, and K. Nakazato. 2016. Increases in M-wave latency of biceps brachii after elbow flexor eccentric contractions in women. *Eur J Appl Physiol* 116 (5):939–46.

Lacourpaille, L., A. Nordez, F. Hug, A. Couturier, C. Dibie, and G. Guilhem. 2014. Time-course effect of exercise-induced muscle damage on localized muscle mechanical properties assessed using elastography. *Acta Physiol* 211 (1):135–46.

Lacourpaille, L., A. Nordez, F. Hug, V. Doguet, R. Andrade, and G. Guilhem. 2017. Early detection of exercise-induced muscle damage using elastography. *Eur J Appl Physiol* 117 (10):2047–56.

Lauritzen, F., G. Paulsen, T. Raastad, L. H. Bergersen, and S. G. Owe. 2009. Gross ultra-structural changes and necrotic fiber segments in elbow flexor muscles after maximal voluntary eccentric action in humans. *J Appl Physiol 1985* 107 (6):1923–34.

Lavender, A. P., and K. Nosaka. 2006. Responses of old men to repeated bouts of eccentric exercise of the elbow flexors in comparison with young men. *Eur J Appl Physiol* 97 (5):619–26.

Leeder, J., C. Gissane, K. van Someren, W. Gregson, and G. Howatson. 2012. Cold water immersion and recovery from strenuous exercise: A meta-analysis. *Br J Sports Med* 46 (4):233–40.

Lin, M. J., T. C. Chen, H. L. Chen, B. H. Wu, and K. Nosaka. 2015. Low-intensity eccentric contractions of the knee extensors and flexors protect against muscle damage. *Appl Physiol Nutr Metab* 40 (10):1004–11.

Maisetti, O., F. Hug, K. Bouillard, and A. Nordez. 2012. Characterization of passive elastic properties of the human medial gastrocnemius muscle belly using supersonic shear imaging. *J Biomech* 45 (6):978–84.

Malm, C., T. L. Sjodin, B. Sjoberg, R. Lenkei, P. Renstrom, I. E. Lundberg, and B. Ekblom. 2004. Leukocytes, cytokines, growth factors and hormones in human skeletal muscle and blood after uphill or downhill running. *J Physiol* 556 (3):983–1000.

Manfredi, T. G., R. A. Fielding, K. P. O'Reilly, C. N. Meredith, H. Y. Lee, and W. J. Evans. 1991. Plasma creatine kinase activity and exercise-induced muscle damage in older men. *Med Sci Sports Exerc* 23 (9):1028–34.

Marques-Jimenez, D., J. Calleja-Gonzalez, I. Arratibel, A. Delextrat, and N. Terrados. 2016. Are compression garments effective for the recovery of exercise-induced muscle damage? A systematic review with meta-analysis. *Physiol Behav* 153:133–48.

McHugh, M. P., and D. T. Tetro. 2003. Changes in the relationship between joint angle and torque production associated with the repeated bout effect. *J Sports Sci* 21 (11):927–32.

Mizumura, K., and T. Taguchi. 2016. Delayed onset muscle soreness: Involvement of neurotrophic factors. *J Physiol Sci* 66 (1):43–52.

Murayama, M., K. Nosaka, T. Yoneda, and K. Minamitani. 2000. Changes in hardness of the human elbow flexor muscles after eccentric exercise. *Eur J Appl Physiol* 82 (5–6):361–7.

Muthalib, M., H. Lee, G. Y. Millet, M. Ferrari, and K. Nosaka. 2011. The repeated-bout effect: Influence on biceps brachii oxygenation and myoelectrical activity. *J Appl Physiol 1985* 110 (5):1390–9.

Nakazato, K., E. Ochi, and T. Waga. 2010. Dietary apple polyphenols have preventive effects against lengthening contraction-induced muscle injuries. *Mol Nutr Food Res* 54 (3):364–72.

Newham, D. J., D. A. Jones, and P. M. Clarkson. 1987. Repeated high-force eccentric exercise: Effects on muscle pain and damage. *J Appl Physiol 1985* 63 (4):1381–6.

Newham, D. J., G. McPhail, K. R. Mills, and R. H. Edwards. 1983. Ultrastructural changes after concentric and eccentric contractions of human muscle. *J Neurol Sci* 61 (1):109–22.

Newton, M. J., G. T. Morgan, P. Sacco, D. W. Chapman, and K. Nosaka. 2008. Comparison of responses to strenuous eccentric exercise of the elbow flexors between resistance-trained and untrained men. *J Strength Cond Res* 22 (2):597–607.

Newton, M. J., P. Sacco, D. Chapman, and K. Nosaka. 2013. Do dominant and non-dominant arms respond similarly to maximal eccentric exercise of the elbow flexors? *J Sci Med Sport* 16 (2):166–71.

Nosaka, K., and P. M. Clarkson. 1996a. Changes in indicators of inflammation after eccentric exercise of the elbow flexors. *Med Sci Sports Exerc* 28 (8):953–61.

Nosaka, K., and P. M. Clarkson. 1996b. Variability in serum creatine kinase response after eccentric exercise of the elbow flexors. *Int J Sports Med* 17 (2):120–7.

Nosaka, K., and T. Kuramata. 1991. Muscle soreness and serum enzyme activity following consecutive drop jumps. *J Sports Sci* 9 (2):213–20.

Nosaka, K., and K. Sakamoto. 2001. Effect of elbow joint angle on the magnitude of muscle damage to the elbow flexors. *Med Sci Sports Exerc* 33 (1):22–9.

Nosaka, K., M. Newton, and P. Sacco. 2002. Delayed-onset muscle soreness does not reflect the magnitude of eccentric exercise-induced muscle damage. *Scand J Med Sci Sports* 12 (6):337–46.

Nosaka, K., M. Newton, P. Sacco, D. Chapman, and A. Lavender. 2005. Partial protection against muscle damage by eccentric actions at short muscle lengths. *Med Sci Sports Exerc* 37 (5):746–53.

Nosaka, K., K. Sakamoto, M. Newton, and P. Sacco. 2001. How long does the protective effect on eccentric exercise-induced muscle damage last? *Med Sci Sports Exerc* 33 (9):1490–5.

Ochi, E., T. Hirose, K. Hiranuma, S. K. Min, N. Ishii, and K. Nakazato. 2010. Elevation of myostatin and FOXOs in prolonged muscular impairment induced by eccentric contractions in rat medial gastrocnemius muscle. *J Appl Physiol 1985* 108 (2):306–13.

Ochi, E., N. Ishii, and K. Nakazato. 2007. Effects of acute eccentric contractions on rat ankle joint stiffness. *J Sports Sci Med* 6 (4):543–8.

Ochi, E., K. Nakazato, H. Song, and H. Nakajima. 2008. Aging effects on passive resistive torque in the rat ankle joint after lengthening contractions. *J Orthop Sci* 13 (3):218–24.

Ochi, E., Y. Tsuchiya, and K. Nosaka. 2016. Differences in post-exercise T2 relaxation time changes between eccentric and concentric contractions of the elbow flexors. *Eur J Appl Physiol* 116 (11–12):2145–54.

Ochi, E., Y. Tsuchiya, and K. Yanagimoto. 2017. Effect of eicosapentaenoic acids-rich fish oil supplementation on motor nerve function after eccentric contractions. *J Int Soc Sports Nutr* 14 (1):23.

Okamoto, T., M. Masuhara, and K. Ikuta. 2006. Cardiovascular responses induced during high-intensity eccentric and concentric isokinetic muscle contraction in healthy young adults. *Clin Physiol Funct Imaging* 26 (1):39–44.

Owens, D. J., C. Twist, J. N. Cobley, G. Howatson, and G. L. Close. 2019. Exercise-induced muscle damage: What is it, what causes it and what are the nutritional solutions? *Eur J Sport Sci* 19 (1): 1–15.

Paulsen, G., R. Crameri, H. B. Benestad, J. G. Fjeld, L. Morkrid, J. Hallen, and T. Raastad. 2010a. Time course of leukocyte accumulation in human muscle after eccentric exercise. *Med Sci Sports Exerc* 42 (1):75–85.

Paulsen, G., I. M. Egner, M. Drange, H. Langberg, H. B. Benestad, J. G. Fjeld, J. Hallen, and T. Raastad. 2010b. A COX-2 inhibitor reduces muscle soreness, but does not influence recovery and adaptation after eccentric exercise. *Scand J Med Sci Sports* 20 (1):e195–207.

Paulsen, G., F. Lauritzen, M. L. Bayer, J. M. Kalhovde, I. Ugelstad, S. G. Owe, J. Hallen, L. H. Bergersen, and T. Raastad. 2009. Subcellular movement and expression of HSP27, alphaB-crystallin, and HSP70 after two bouts of eccentric exercise in humans. *J Appl Physiol 1985* 107 (2):570–82.

Paulsen, G., U. R. Mikkelsen, T. Raastad, and J. M. Peake. 2012. Leucocytes, cytokines and satellite cells: What role do they play in muscle damage and regeneration following eccentric exercise? *Exerc Immunol Rev* 18:42–97.

Peake, J. M., O. Neubauer, P. A. Della Gatta, and K. Nosaka. 2017. Muscle damage and inflammation during recovery from exercise. *J Appl Physiol 1985* 122 (3):559–70.

Penailillo, L., A. Blazevich, H. Numazawa, and K. Nosaka. 2013. Metabolic and muscle damage profiles of concentric versus repeated eccentric cycling. *Med Sci Sports Exerc* 45 (9):1773–81.

Piitulainen, H., R. Bottas, P. Komi, V. Linnamo, and J. Avela. 2010. Impaired action potential conduction at high force levels after eccentric exercise. *J Electromyogr Kinesiol* 20 (5):879–87.

Piitulainen, H., P. Komi, V. Linnamo, and J. Avela. 2008. Sarcolemmal excitability as investigated with M-waves after eccentric exercise in humans. *J Electromyogr Kinesiol* 18 (4):672–81.

Poppendieck, W., M. Wegmann, A. Ferrauti, M. Kellmann, M. Pfeiffer, and T. Meyer. 2016. Massage and performance recovery: A meta-analytical review. *Sports Med* 46 (2):183–204.

Proske, U., and T. J. Allen. 2005. Damage to skeletal muscle from eccentric exercise. *Exerc Sport Sci Rev* 33 (2):98–104.

Proske, U., and D. L. Morgan. 2001. Muscle damage from eccentric exercise: Mechanism, mechanical signs, adaptation and clinical applications. *J Physiol* 537 (2):333–45.

Raastad, T., S. G. Owe, G. Paulsen, D. Enns, K. Overgaard, R. Crameri, S. Kiil, A. Belcastro, L. Bergersen, and J. Hallen. 2010. Changes in calpain activity, muscle structure, and function after eccentric exercise. *Med Sci Sports Exerc* 42 (1):86–95.

Rahimi, M. H., S. Shab-Bidar, M. Mollahosseini, and K. Djafarian. 2017. Branched-chain amino acid supplementation and exercise-induced muscle damage in exercise recovery: A meta-analysis of randomized clinical trials. *Nutrition* 42:30–6.

Shinohara, M., K. Sabra, J. L. Gennisson, M. Fink, and M. Tanter. 2010. Real-time visualization of muscle stiffness distribution with ultrasound shear wave imaging during muscle contraction. *Muscle Nerve* 42 (3):438–41.

Stupka, N., M. A. Tarnopolsky, N. J. Yardley, and S. M. Phillips. 2001. Cellular adaptation to repeated eccentric exercise-induced muscle damage. *J Appl Physiol 1985* 91 (4):1669–78.

Tsuchiya, Y., N. Kikuchi, M. Shirato, and E. Ochi. 2015. Differences of activation pattern and damage in elbow flexor muscle after isokinetic eccentric contractions. *Isokinet Exerc Sci* 23 (3):169–75.

Tsuchiya, Y., K. Nakazato, and E. Ochi. 2018. Contralateral repeated bout effect after eccentric exercise on muscular activation. *Eur J Appl Physiol* 118 (9):1997–2005.

Tsuchiya, Y., K. Sakuraba, and E. Ochi. 2014. High force eccentric exercise enhances serum tartrate-resistant acid phosphatase-5b and osteocalcin. *J Musculoskelet Neuronal Interact* 14 (1):50–7.

Tsuchiya, Y., K. Yanagimoto, K. Nakazato, K. Hayamizu, and E. Ochi. 2016. Eicosapentaenoic and docosahexaenoic acids-rich fish oil supplementation attenuates strength loss and limited joint range of motion after eccentric contractions: A randomized, double-blind, placebo-controlled, parallel-group trial. *Eur J Appl Physiol* 116 (6):1179–88.

Warren, G. L., D. A. Hayes, D. A. Lowe, and R. B. Armstrong. 1993. Mechanical factors in the initiation of eccentric contraction-induced injury in rat soleus muscle. *J Physiol* 464 (1):457–75.

Warren, G. L., D. A. Lowe, and R. B. Armstrong. 1999. Measurement tools used in the study of eccentric contraction-induced injury. *Sports Med* 27 (1):43–59.

Wilson, J. M., J. S. Kim, S. R. Lee, J. A. Rathmacher, B. Dalmau, J. D. Kingsley, H. Koch, A. H. Manninen, R. Saadat, and L. B. Panton. 2009. Acute and timing effects of beta-hydroxy-beta-methylbutyrate (HMB) on indirect markers of skeletal muscle damage. *Nutr Metab* 6:6.

Xin, L., R. D. Hyldahl, S. R. Chipkin, and P. M. Clarkson. 2014. A contralateral repeated bout effect attenuates induction of NF-kappaB DNA binding following eccentric exercise. *J Appl Physiol 1985* 116 (11):1473–80.

Yu, J. G., L. Carlsson, and L. E. Thornell. 2004. Evidence for myofibril remodeling as opposed to myofibril damage in human muscles with DOMS: An ultrastructural and immunoelectron microscopic study. *Histochem Cell Biol* 121 (3):219–27.

Section VII

Growth, Marketing Techniques, and Future of Extreme Sports

19 Extreme Sports: Growth Prospect, Marketing Potential, and Opportunities
A Commentary

Sourya Datta and Debasis Bagchi

CONTENTS

19.1 Current Situation 342
19.2 Marketing of Extreme Sports 342
    19.2.1 Popular Offline Marketing Techniques 343
        19.2.1.1 Videos/Ads during Advertisement Breaks in TV/
                 Radio 343
        19.2.1.2 Ticket Sales/Free Giveaway/Scratch and Get Code 343
        19.2.1.3 Merchandise Sales.. 343
    19.2.2 Popular Marketing Techniques.. 343
        19.2.2.1 Blogs.. 343
        19.2.2.2 Search Engine Optimization... 343
    19.2.3 Challenges with Marketing for Extreme Sports............................. 343
19.3 Difference between Extreme Sports and Other Competitive Sports like
    the Olympic Games.. 344
19.4 Motivation Behind Extreme Sports.. 344
19.5 Popularity of Extreme Sports in Different Countries.................................. 345
19.6 Which Countries Fall Behind in the Popularity of Extreme Sports............ 346
19.7 Commercialization of Extreme Sports... 347
19.8 Some Popular Sports: Spartan Races and Tough Mudder 347
19.9 Nutraceuticals, Sports Nutrition and Food Supplements............................ 348
19.10 Future of Extreme Sports 349
19.11 Future Trends 350
    19.11.1 How Will Extreme Sports Look in the Near Future:
        (< 3 Years)?.. 350
    19.11.2 How Will Extreme Sports Look in the Longer Term:
        (> 3 Years)?.. 350
References.. 350

19.1   CURRENT SITUATION

At present, extreme sports are quite fragmented. There are professional bodies who conduct selected extreme sports involving interested athletes. For the individual, extreme sports is a combination of having thrill and fun at their own expense. The same individual could also take part in activities organized by a group/company or organization. In short, the extreme sports bodies and individual athletes are extremely scattered, unlike the Olympic structure or a World Cup structure. It is difficult to have one governing body since extreme sports are evolving all the time; a few groups like ESPN, with their Gen X sports, have tried to have a more focused approach but have had limited scope and success.

19.2   MARKETING OF EXTREME SPORTS

Marketing is a very important technique that is often used for any sport but is particularly useful for something newer and more innovative like extreme sports.

Broadly, marketing techniques have been classified under online and offline marketing.

Before going deeper into online and offline marketing, let's try to understand the difference between online and offline marketing.

Online marketing: This is a strategy in which customer traffic is attracted by using different online channels. The different online channels are (a) social media (b) blogs (c) email marketing (d) search engine (e) content marketing (f) video blogging and (g) online classifieds. This form of marketing has become extremely popular and has become one of the most efficient ways to attract millennials. Let's take the example of how a popular race company goes through the process. Once the date of the event is decided by the company, the company publishes advertisements through multiple social media channels. The advertisements could be extremely costly depending on where and when the ads are shown. Facebook ads are often bought by the organizing company who is in charge of the games. The company also pays Google for both search results and AdWords in order to populate the google search with the result of the event. A classic example would be search results between Tough Mudder and Spartan race. Someone who is searching for their next race and is not aware of the different races could choose one race over the other depending on the search result of his/her query. The organizations use multiple methods to attract new customers and have their own blogs and classifieds as well. They also send emails to customers who have signed up before and have taken part in the games.

Offline marketing: The offline marketing technique involves getting new leads by using methods other than websites. Offline marketing involves (a) television (b) radio (c) flyers (d) banners (e) newspapers (f) posters and (g) pamphlets. Even though online marketing has become more popular in recent times, at the same time traditional ads in TV, radio and newspapers are important sources to attract enthusiasts. Often times, a TV ad is carefully selected and is played, for example, during the X-games, where the organizations know that a similar set of people who are more interested in extreme sports tend to watch.

There are different costs involved in online versus offline marketing. While online marketing has web development, hosting and search engine optimization costs, offline marketing has costs for media, ads, for newspaper advertising space and television slots.

In most cases, the most effective way of marketing for any sports or extreme sports has been some kind of mixed approach between online and offline marketing [1]

Some popular offline marketing techniques for extreme sports are described below:

19.2.1   POPULAR OFFLINE MARKETING TECHNIQUES

19.2.1.1   Videos/Ads during Advertisement Breaks in TV/Radio

Most of the time extreme sports marketing teams use commercial breaks for advertising.

19.2.1.2   Ticket Sales/Free Giveaway/Scratch and Get Code

Another great way of marketing is doing a giveaway. This form of marketing has become very popular where the hosts distribute scratchcards and tickets which can be obtained by scratching and revealing a code, or where a customer buying a ticket for an extreme sports event can get another at 50% off.

19.2.1.3   Merchandise Sales

One technique that has become extremely popular is different merchandisers making their products available for sale, e.g. Spartan tee shirts are becoming more and more popular and people love the Spartan gear.

19.2.2   POPULAR MARKETING TECHNIQUES

These are based on online marketing described below.

19.2.2.1   Blogs

Most extreme sports events have a number of individual athletes signing up and often, extreme sports authorities both have their own blogs and depend on athletes' blogs for marketing.

19.2.2.2   Search Engine Optimization

A number of extreme sports bodies have a significant budget to work on search optimization and spend a lot of money to get the best results from search optimization.

19.2.3   CHALLENGES WITH MARKETING FOR EXTREME SPORTS [2]

One of the biggest challenges in the case of extreme sports marketers is how to maintain the level of excitement in the bottom marketing funnel. Assuming that excitement in the upper funnel is created by various events, blogs, shows etc., there is a huge challenge to keep the excitement going in extreme sports in the lower half of the marketing funnel. Both the optimization of great ideas and the creation of fresh ideas are important for attracting more enthusiasts.

19.3 DIFFERENCE BETWEEN EXTREME SPORTS AND OTHER COMPETITIVE SPORTS LIKE THE OLYMPIC GAMES

Within the next five years (and the process has started already), there will be a huge boom in extreme sports. A number of current sports will become more complex and new sports will emerge. It has been observed that current Olympic sports are becoming less and less popular, and people are more excited to watch and be a part of extreme sports. There are mainly two reasons behind this:

1. Unlike Olympic sports, where it is extremely difficult to be a part of the team representing a country (as competition is very high), everyone is welcome to join extreme sports since most are not team games, and it is easier to participate. Of course, we are not talking about the level of difficulty of extreme sports and whether anyone and everyone can be successful, but the barrier to enter or participate in an extreme sport is much lower than a sport at the Olympics.
2. The goal of an extreme sport is to complete the sport and not necessarily win, unlike Olympic games. Completing extreme sports is the goal here, and is a major achievement in itself.
3. Extreme sports are less stressful than Olympic sports. People taking part in extreme sports want to have fun and are not necessarily looking to win the competition, whereas there is immense pressure in representing one's country in the Olympics.

However, along with the advantages, there are a number of disadvantages as well:

1. Since extreme sports are more focused on the individual, both the planning and preparation of extreme sports is undertaken by an individual, while it is more of an undertaking to train without the supervision or guidance of a coach and other team players.
2. There is no set structure: e.g. a Spartan racer running the race in extreme conditions might be performing snowboarding the next year. This lack of specific and set training patterns might be very distracting.
3. It is often not cheap to participate in extreme sports and since they are more focused on the individual there is often no sponsorship. This might not be the case if the athlete is one of the leading figures in the sport, but more often athletes need to be ready to spend a lot of their own money.

19.4 MOTIVATION BEHIND EXTREME SPORTS

Extreme sports have been perceived to be exciting, and this is partly because they come with a lot of risk and danger. But there is another side to how people view extreme sports. It might not be due to risk and danger that people are interested; extreme sports become an extension of mainstream sports since sportspersons are able to lower the dangers and risks by either their skills or experience, or a combination of both, meaning that it is no longer extreme due to a lowering of the risk involved. A lot of good sportspersons are able to manage the risks and even lower the risks to a minimum, which is a question of consequence and likelihood of the risks. Extreme athletes assert that with great ability and practice, the likelihood of injury will be extremely low, even though the consequence is higher. Elite athletes undertake a number of routines in order to minimize the potential risk: (1) Practice the same step/technique over and over (2) Spend countless hours of working on physical strength and technique (3) Use the latest equipment to supplement their training and (4) Eat the right food. In almost all extreme sports the most important success factor is repetition, such as with the routines just mentioned above.

However, another line of thought exists in extreme sports. Often, it is the case that extreme sportspersons are looking for high rewards rather than being focused on the risk. [3]

It has been often found that the extremely high reward of completing an extreme sport is a great influencer for extreme athletes, which they hold in very high regard compared to the attraction of taking risks.

19.5   POPULARITY OF EXTREME SPORTS IN DIFFERENT COUNTRIES

It is very difficult to create a list of countries where extreme sports are popular as there are many. Below is a list of some of these (not necessarily in any order): [4]

1. United States: Open to all new, exciting and innovative ideas. One of the top destinations for extreme sports enthusiasts and spectators.
2. Brazil: One of the largest countries for extreme sports and true adventurists, as well as Rio de Janeiro carnival.
3. Italy: A number of extreme sports enthusiasts either perform in Italy or consider the country as one of the best places to perform extreme sports. Italy has the deep cultural heritage and influence that is powerful and extremely interesting to many, such as extreme sportspersons.
4. Spain: One of the most popular places in Spain for extreme sports is La Furia Roja – extreme sports enthusiasts also flock in large numbers to other parts of Spain to enjoy different extreme sports.
5. Thailand: Even though Thailand is known for a number of adventure sports, but one of the most common adventure sports is diving and its varieties.
6. Greece: Greece has been the epitome of extreme sports for a number of years. A number of activities take place in Greece but extreme sports are also particularly popular in Crete and Kalymnos. Beaches are popular places for extreme sports as well.
7. New Zealand: New Zealand is often known as the 'world capital of extreme sports'. The mountains are great places for bungee jumping, snow-capped mountains are perfect for extreme altitude sports, while the water surrounding New Zealand allows for extreme water sports.
8. Costa Rica: Costa Rica has a huge stretch of rainforest which is a pure delight for a large number of visitors and extreme sports enthusiasts.

9. Mexico: Mexico has a very upbeat, young and adventurous culture, and a number of tourists come to the country to both enjoy the food and take part in a number of sports. At the same time, there are other problems which have caused socioeconomic instability in the country.

10. Australia: Just the sheer size of this country makes it a great space for adventure sports and extreme sports.

11. Argentina: The two places that are extremely popular in Argentina for extreme sports are La Cumbre and Bariloche. Vast open spaces make the country extremely popular for biking and different forms of gliding.

12. Portugal: One of the most common sports in Portugal (apart from soccer) is surfing.

13. Caribbean Islands: Vast open lands, beaches and ocean make the Caribbean a great place for all three types of extreme sports: water, land and air.

14. Philippines: The presence of a large body of water/ ocean makes the Philippines an ideal place for extreme water sports.

15. France: The culture of France makes it a highly exciting place for extreme sports.

16. Ireland: Ireland is another popular destination for extreme sports. The terrain makes it extremely suitable for different extreme sports.

17. UK: The UK has long been one of the most popular locations for extreme sports. Its popularity has been growing more in recent years and it has become one of the most sought-after places for extreme sports.

18. Netherlands: Clean vehicles and bicycles are extremely popular and have taken over the country. The Netherlands is extremely well connected in terms of bicycle paths, which has generally proved to be very successful in bringing many forms of land-based extreme sports to the country.

19. Singapore: Singapore is often seen as the 'newest hub for extreme sports' and the easy access to this country has proved to be extremely beneficial for extreme sports enthusiasts.

20. Peru: Peru has become very popular for zip-lining and has recently become a popular destination for extreme sports.

21. Canada: Canada has numerous places suitable for extreme sports and is extremely favorable for enthusiasts.

19.6 WHICH COUNTRIES FALL BEHIND IN THE POPULARITY OF EXTREME SPORTS

Research has shown that investment in sports is not always the top priority for a developing nation. Often, the education systems of most developing countries are behind where they should be in the required spending for sports. Extreme sports and the infrastructure development necessary for extreme sports is often not the top priority. This is actually a cycle where underdevelopment in sports leads to fewer athletes willing to participate in sports, which leads to less excitement and popularity in general sports and has a high impact on the popularity of extreme sports.

Another important factor in developing extreme sports is the early start in the career of potential sports enthusiasts. School and university sports hold a prominent place in the community for developed nations, which is often not the case with developing nations.

In general, most of the developing nations, even those trying to develop the infrastructure for extreme sports, still have a long way to go to be considered as a power house for extreme sports.

Multiple studies have been done on the development of extreme sports in different countries and it's been shown that the African region (Algeria, Benin, Bostwana, Burkina Faso, Cameroon, Cape Verde, Chad, Comoros, Congo, Côte d'Ivoire, Dem. Rep. Of Congo, Eritrea, Ethiopia, Gabon, Gambia, Ghana, Guinea, Kenya, Madagascar, Malawi, Mali, Mauritius, Mozambique, Namibia, Niger, São Tomé and Principe, Swaziland and Zambia) have a long way to go, followed by the eastern Mediterranean region (Iran, Iraq, Kuwait, Lebanon, Libya and Tunisia). These regions lack extreme sports infrastructure and the popularity level of extreme sports is less than 5 (out of a scale of 1 to 10 where 10 is the highest).

19.7   COMMERCIALIZATION OF EXTREME SPORTS [5]

Whenever we talk about the commercialization of extreme sports, the first thing that comes to mind is ESPN and the X Games. ESPN clearly understood that extreme sports as a category appeals to men and women between the ages of 12 and 35 and this age group both liked to take part in the games as well as see others participating. 1995 saw the first summer X games, which were hugely successful and made ESPN introduce the Winter X games in 1997. This was a win-win situation for both ESPN and the participants. The participants love to be part of the games and also to watch others participating, while ESPN gained a huge fan following and a lot of good press and advertising while having to part with relatively low costs to award the winners. There have been a lot of different players who have played a significant part in the success of the X games: ESPN, the X games body, corporate money and partnership, site/locations choices and cities to host the games. The X games were created to bring in more participants, viewers (both on-site and television) and profit, and was able to make a lot of money through endorsements and strong sponsorships. Some past gold sponsors for the X games have included companies such as AT&T, Adidas, Mountain Dew, Taco Bell and Snickers. There are also associate sponsors, with the only difference between gold and associate sponsors being that associate sponsors don't provide prize money and only sponsor specific events. Some past associated sponsors have been Visa, Sony and Disney.

19.8   SOME POPULAR SPORTS: SPARTAN
RACES AND TOUGH MUDDER

The Spartan race and Tough Mudder are two races which are both similar and very different in their own ways. Spartan races are races that have obstacles over distances which can range from just 3 miles to a full marathon distance. It has four different types, starting from the smallest, known as the Spartan Sprint, to Super Spartan, to the Spartan Beast and the toughest known as Ultra Beast. The Spartan race was basically a spin-off from the Death race which was a 48-hour race; the Spartan was created as a more manageable race involving a much wider audience. The different types of race include the following:

1. Spartan Sprint: 3 miles of racing and at least 20 obstacles
2. Spartan Super: 8 miles of racing and at least 25 obstacles
3. Spartan Beast: 13 miles of racing and at least 30 obstacles
4. Ultra Beast: 26 miles of racing with at least 60 obstacles

Most obstacles include jumping over fire, crawling under barbed wire, a wall climb and mud crawling, to list a few examples, and if athletes are not able to complete any obstacle then there is a penalty of 30 burpees.

Tough Mudder, on the other hand, is structured slightly differently but the general idea is very similar to the Spartan race. The race is approximately 12 miles long and the aim is to test both the physical and mental strength of the athletes. The way that Tough Mudder is designed is based on four factors that the athletes need to overcome: water, fire, electricity and height. Unlike Spartan Races, which can be done as an individual sport, Tough Mudder requires team work, as team members need to help each other in order to complete the race.

The different types of race are as follows:

1. Regular Tough Mudder: 10–12 miles and 25 obstacles.
2. Tough Mudder Half: Five miles and 12 obstacles.
3. Tough Mudder: Timed race which gives prize money to top three finishers across different venues.
4. Tough Mudder 5k: As understood from the name, the distance is 3.1 miles/5km.
5. Toughest Mudder: Eight hours in length and has six events – eligible athletes get entry to 'Contender Category'.
6. Tough Mudder X: Determines the 'Fittest and Fastest athletes' in the world. Combination of Cross-fit, strength and racing.
7. Mini Mudder: Course developed for children. Age group of 7–12 and includes 1 mile and 10 obstacles.
8. Urban Mudder: Five-mile course which introduced the fun aspects of having beer and a DJ in the race.
9. World's Toughest Mudder: a 24-hour length race which includes top male, top female and top team as prize categories.

19.9 NUTRACEUTICALS, SPORTS NUTRITION AND FOOD SUPPLEMENTS

Nutraceuticals, sports nutrition and food supplements have become extremely popular in recent years in all formats of sports – especially extreme sports. There has been a huge growth in the nutraceutical and food supplement industry and the U.S. food and beverage supplement industry shows an annual revenue of $4 billion and an annual growth of between 3% and 5%. Most of the nutraceutical and food supplement companies target the millennial generation who are the largest customers. The marketing strategies of nutrition and supplement companies are extremely elaborate and thorough. On one hand companies like HelloFresh, Blue Apron, etc., have started providing traditional meal packages to cater to the busy generation (who want to be healthy but want to cook their food in least amount of time) and on the other hand various companies are projecting their plant based organic nutritional shakes which are replacements for entire meals. The following are some of the most important features that the nutraceutical companies use to increase the growth of the product portfolio:

1. All about packaging: It's been determined that more than 65% of new customers are attracted to new packaging to give the product a try. Companies spend a huge amount of time and resources to understand the market and then the graphic designers come up with the designs and packaging to attract the customers.
2. All about labeling: The label is one of the most important features of the product. It's extremely costly if the dietary ingredients and percentage of ingredients are incorrect or if there is a need to change any information after the product is launched. Millennials read labels more than anyone else and the label is one of the most important selling features of the product.
3. FDA approval: It's been determined that FDA approval on any product increases the sell through by more than 20%. This is an important feature to attract millennials.
4. Internet marketing and social media marketing: Social media marketing has a huge role to play in the final sell through of the product since most of the millennials research on the web and try to determine the most suitable product for themselves.

Diverse nutraceuticals, amino acids and diverse research sports-based supplements have been developed and marketed over the last two decades, with more in the pipeline. Safety and toxicity are the prime concern, so we recommend that sports nutritionists, nutritionists and athletic coaches should consult with each other before recommending such supplements to the athletes. Furthermore, hydration is very important, which should be conveyed to athletic teams. Finally, it is the responsibility of the coaches to establish an ideal drug-free environment for athletes.

19.10   FUTURE OF EXTREME SPORTS

The future of extreme sports holds a lot of promise. If we look deeper, there are a number of reasons to be very excited about the future of extreme sports, but also some reasons to be concerned. [6, 7]

Reasons to be excited:

1. People wanting to do something exciting and thrilling.
2. A show off attitude: Taking pictures with a camera (phones and Go Pro), which allows easy uploading of photos and videos on YouTube, Facebook, Snapchat and Instagram.

3. Introduction of technology: Technology has definitely played a huge part in the popularity of extreme sports. Technology has helped on both sides, for better preparation to take part in extreme sports and also helping in making extreme sports memorable. There are multiple examples, such as Go Pro, iPhones and Samsung phones, with advanced picture taking abilities, as well as Strava's unique capability.

4. People love danger, excitement and thrills, a trend that is increasing.

What might harm the popularity?

1. Becoming too commercialized: once a particular location or spot becomes popular, access to those locations becomes extremely costly.
2. Often times, places where extreme sports take place are turned into resorts.
3. Climate change often plays a huge part: some sports will not be present in the future and new sports will emerge.

19.11   FUTURE TRENDS [8]

19.11.1   How Will Extreme Sports Look in the Near Future: (< 3 Years)?

Extreme sports will be in both individual and group form. But in the near future, there could be a greater movement towards group activities. Athletes will do more analysis of their performance, save data and use analytics to come up with future driven actions.

19.11.2   How Will Extreme Sports Look in the Longer Term: (> 3 Years)? [9, 10]

There will be more use of automated experiments to firstly understand the risk and dangers before people participate in extreme sports where these are present. Just like self-driving cars currently in the market, where the goal of the future is to minimize accidents through the use of such vehicles, the use of automated robots aims to first understand the impact of the extreme sport in question and then undertake such activity.

REFERENCES

1. Bold Worldwide, Marketing Techniques. https://www.boldworldwide.com/bold-marke ting-blog/six-effective-sports-marketing-techniques (Date accessed: August 2018)
2. Parkinson G, 3 Sports Marketing Strategies to Engage Fans with Fresh Content. https ://www.scribblelive.com/blog/2015/09/16/3-sports-marketing-strategies-engage-fans-fresh-content/ (Date accessed: August 2018)
3. Donovan J, Extreme Sports Athletes Crave the Reward, Not the Risk. https://adventure. howstuffworks.com/extreme-sports-athletes-crave-reward-not-risk.htm (Date accessed: August 2018)

4. Murray T, The 19 Best Countries in the World for Adventure Seekers. https://www.bus inessinsider.com/the-best-countries-in-the-world-for-adventure-seekers-2017-3#2-italy -political-instability-may-have-cost-italy-in-the-best-overall-countries-ranking-but-it-has-not-affected-its-draw-for-adventure-seekers-italy-also-ranked-top-in-the-cultu ral-influence-and-heritage-categories-according-to-italiait-the-country-offers-endless-opportunities-to-practice-all-types-of-extreme-sports-18 (Date accessed: August 2018)

5. Huh C & Byoung L. The commodification process of Extreme Sports : The diffusion of the X-Games by ESPN, https://www.nrs.fs.fed.us/pubs/gtr/gtr_ne289/gtr_ne289_049. pdf (Date accessed: August 2018)

6. Gunner, The Future of Sports. https://factorymedia.com/misc/the-future-of-sports/ (Date accessed: August 2018)

7. Griffith S, Extreme + Adventure Sports. http://futureof.org/sports-2015/extreme-adven ture-sports/ (Date accessed: August 2018)

8. Benedictus L, Why Are Deadly Extreme Sports More Popular than Ever? https://www. theguardian.com/sport/2016/aug/20/why-are-deadly-extreme-sports-more-popular-than-ever (Date accessed: August 2018)

9. Duke University, Sports and Society Course in Coursera. https://www.coursera.org/lectu re/sports-society/the-strange-case-of-extreme-sports-part-1-uNK7R (Date accessed: August 2018)

10. Etter E, Extreme Sports Are More Popular than Ever, Prompting Questions about Legal Liability. http://www.abajournal.com/magazine/article/extreme_sports_are_more_pop ular_than_ever_prompting_questions/ (Date accessed: August 2018)

Index

α-lipoic acid, 209
β alanine, 87–88
β-carotene (vitamin A), 211
   for high altitude sports, 268
β-hydroxy-β-Methyl Butyrate (HMB), 85, 87,
   159, 160–161, 331
β-sitosterol, 89

AAS, *see* Anabolic-androgenic steroids
Above knee amputation (AKA), 118
Abseiling, 244
Acanthopanax senticosus, 89
Accelerade™, 306
ACSM, *see* American College of Sports
   Medicine
ACTH, *see* Adrenocorticotropic hormone
Adaptogen, 88
Adenosine triphosphate (ATP), 76–77, 78–79,
   93, 151
Adequate water (AI), 298
Adidas, 347
Adrenergic receptors, 129
Adrenocorticotropic hormone (ACTH), 89, 91
Adulterants and third-party supplement testing,
   145–146
Adventure racing, nutritional requirement
   and, 6, 53
Aerials and skateboarding, 242
Aerobic pathway, 35
AI, *see* Adequate water
Airborne/mid-air high altitude sports, 272–273
Airstyle kitesurfing, 285
AKA, *see* Above knee amputation
AL, *see* Alpha-linolenic acid
Alanine, 312
Ali, M., 220
Alpha-linolenic acid (ALA), 148
Amateur boxing, 36
American Bicycle Association, 240
American College of Sports Medicine
   (ACSM), 305
American Heart Association, 22
Amino acid mixtures, 161–162
Amputees, 115, 116, 118–123
Anabolic-androgenic steroids (AAS), 200
Anaerobic glycolysis, 79
Anaerobic metabolic pathway, 35
Anaerobic performance, beta-alanine affecting, 43
Andalusia Tour, 52
Androgenic steroids, 85
Androstenedione, 85

Antarctic Ice Marathon, 51
Anthocyanins, 96, 98, 209, 210
Anthropometric characteristics and gender
   differences, open-water swimming,
   15–16
Antioxidants, 205–206
   energy metabolism and, 208–211
   excitation-contraction coupling fatigue and,
   211–212
   exercise-induced muscle damage and,
   207–208
   exercise-induced oxidative stress behavior
   and, 206–207
   perspective, 212–213
Anxiety, 21, 91
   reduction of, 87
AP-I activation, 207, 208
Aquatics, 281–282
Arevalo, S., 15
Argentina, 346
Arginine, 88
Armstrong, L., 194
Ashwagandha, 90, 200
Astaxanthin, 209, 210
AT&T, 347
ATP, *see* Adenosine triphosphate
Australia, 346

Badwater Ultramarathon, 4, 51
Ball games, in ancient Greece, 223
Ball on the line game, 223
Barley, 228
Base jumping, 240, 263
BCAAs, *see* Branched chain amino acids
Beetroot (*Beta vulgaris*), 94–95, 155–156
Berlin Marathon (2014), 50
Beta-alanine, 42–43, 152–153
Big air FMX, 244
Biocell™, 316
BioDapt, 120
Biodex Multi-Joint System B2000, 315
Bioenergetics (energy flow), 76–77
Bitter orange (*Citrus aurantium*), 96
Blades, 120
Blogs, 343
Blood proteins (creatine kinase and myoglobin),
   327–328
Blood transfusions, 199
Blue Apron, 349
BMX (bicycle motocross), 240, 243
Boarding/heli-skiing, 273

Boating, 282–283
Bodyboarding, 284, 288
Body surfing, 284
Boenish, C., 240
Boron requirement, for high altitude sports, 267
Bouldering, 245, 271
Bovine spongiform encephalopathy (BSE), 312
Boxing, 35–36
    in Greek Olympic sports, 221
    training and nutrition for, 36–38
Branched chain amino acids (BCAAs), 80, 81,
    161–162
Brazil, 345
BSE, *see* Bovine spongiform encephalopathy
Budapest World Championship, 18, 19
Bumps races, 286
Bungee jumping, 240, 263, 272

Caffeine, 41–42, 64, 66, 85–86, 90, 94, 149–150,
    156–157
    benefits of, 268
    hydration and, 305–306
Calcium, 84
    requirement, for high altitude sports, 266
Caloric/energy needs evaluation for athletes, 77
Canada, 346
Canoeing, 282, 290
    ice, 239
Canoeists, *see* Nutrient intake, of athletes
Canyoning, 272
Capsaicin, 98
Carbohydrate, 76–77, 79–80, 134, 149, 161
    for athletes for success in extreme sports,
        251–252, 253, 254–255
    considerations, 57–60
    consumed by ancient Greek athletes, 230, 231
    need, for extreme sports athletes, 251
    physical and athletic performance and, 80, 81
    and proteins based on Rasmussen report,
        81–82
    requirements, 25, 77
        boxing, 38
        swimming, 25
Carbohydrate–protein sports drink, 306–307
Cardiovascular endurance exercise testing, 148
Cardiovascular thermoregulatory mechanisms,
    137
Caribbean Islands, 346
Carnitine, 85, 87
Carnosine, 42, 43, 87, 152
Carpenter, J. B., 240
Catalina Channel swim, 12, 15, 21
Catechins, 94, 209
Catecholamines, 129
Cave diving, 289
    freshwater, 272

Caving, 244
CDC, *see* Centers for Disease Control and
    Prevention
Centers for Disease Control and Prevention
    (CDC), 317
Central clock, 130, 135
Chariot games, in ancient Greece, 225
Chasqui Challenge, 51
Cheese rolling, 273
CHO-PRO trial, 306
Chromium (III) requirement, for high altitude
    sports, 266
Chrono-nutrition, 130, 134
Circadian clocks, 130
Citrulline, 95, 98
CK, *see* Creatine kinase
Cliff diving, 282, 290
Coasteering, 272
Coast to Coast (New Zealand), 6
Coca-Cola®, 306
Coconut water (tender), 98
Cody, S., 240
Cold-water swimmers, 23
Collagen hydrolysate, 315–316
Combat sports
    boxing, 35–36
        training and nutrition for, 36–38
    fighter diet plan, 44–45
    food and nutritional requirements for, 254–255
    food consumption by ancient Greek athletes
        for, 231
    kickboxing, 39–40
    mixed martial arts (MMA), 43–44
    sports supplements
        beta-alanine, 42–43
        caffeine, 41–42
        creatine, 40–41
Combustion, 76
Comrades Marathon, 51
Concentric contractions, 321
ConsumerLab.com, 146
Continuing Survey of Food Intakes by
    Individuals (CSFII), 305
Cordyceps sinensis, 92
Cortisol, 135
Costa Rica, 345
Coumarin, 89
Course racing, 285
CPK, *see* Creatine phosphokinase
Creatine, 40–41, 85, 86, 151–152, 158, 160
Creatine kinase (CK), 207
Creatine phosphate, 78, 79
Creatine phosphokinase (CPK), 86
Criterium du Dauphine Libere, 52
CSFII, *see* Continuing Survey of Food Intakes by
    Individuals

Cyanocobalamin (B12), 84
Cycling, 5
    nutritional requirement and, 50, 52

Dehydration, 44, 62, 301, 302
Dehydroepiandrosterone, 85
Delayed-onset muscle soreness (DOMS),
        324–325, 332
DHA, *see* Docosahexaenoic acid
Dietary reference intakes (DRIs), 83
Dietary Supplement Health and Education Act
        (DSHEA), 145
Dietary supplements, 144
    to aid physical performance, 148–149
        beta-alanine, 152–153
        caffeine, 149–150
        creatine, 151–152
        nitrate (beetroot juice), 155–156
        sodium bicarbonate, 153–155
    for cognitive performance, 156
        caffeine, 156–157
        creatine, 158
        ginseng, 157–158
        L-theanine, 158
        Rhodiola rosea, 157
        theacrine, 158
    for exercise recovery, 159
        amino acid mixtures, 161–162
        beta-hydroxy-beta-methylbutyrate
            (HMB), 160–161
        carbohydrates, 161
        creatine, 160
        protein, 159–160
    for overall health, 146–147
        fish oil (omega-3 fatty acids), 148
        multivitamin/mineral supplements
            (MVMs), 147
        protein supplements, 148
        vitamin D3, 147
    regulation of, 144–145
    safety of, 145–146
Dirt BMX, 243
Discus throw, in Greek Olympic sports, 223
Disney, 347
Docosahexaenoic acid (DHA), 148
Doping, by ancient Greek sportsmen, 226, 228
Downhill mountain biking, 271
Drafting, 20, 26
Drifting, 243
DRIs, *see* Dietary reference intakes
DSHEAS, *see* Dietary Supplement Health and
        Education Act

EAA, *see* Essential amino acids
Eagle, for golfing, 120
EAR, *see* Estimated average requirement

Eating fatigue, 58
Eco-Challenge (United States), 6
EGCG, *see* Epigallocatechin-3-gallate
Eicosapentaenoic acid (EPA), 148, 330
EIMD, *see* Exercise-induced muscle damage
Elastographic techniques, 325
Electrolytes
    consumed by ancient Greek athletes, 230
    for extreme sports athletes, 255
Electron transport chain (ETC), 83
Eleutherococcus senticosus, 89–90
Eleutherosides, 89
Elevated vacuum suspension (EVS), 118–119, 122
Elite cyclists, 195
Elite swimmers, 24, 28, 29
Endurance exercise, 193
Endurance speed, 12–13
Endurance sports, 75–76; *see also* Extreme
                endurance sports; Extreme sports
Endurance swimming, energetics and
            biomechanics of, 12–15
Energy drinks, 248
Energy homeostasis, 77
Energy metabolism and antioxidants, 208–211
Energy requirements, for extreme sports athletes,
        252–253
English Channel swim, 12, 15, 20–21
EPA, *see* Eicosapentaenoic acid
Epigallocatechin-3-gallate (EGCG), 94, 97, 210
Epinephrine, 129, 135–136
EPO, *see* Erythropoietin
EPOC, *see* Excess post-exercise oxygen
                consumption
Equestrian games, in Greek Olympic
                sports, 222
Ergogenic compounds, 85
    β alanine, 87–88
    β-Hydroxy-β-Methyl Butyrate (HMB), 87
    caffeine, 85–86
    carnitine, 87
    creatine, 86
    sodium bicarbonate/citrate, 87
    taurine, 86
Ergogenic functional food/neutraceuticals, 93
    beetroot (*Beta vulgaris*), 94–95
    bitter orange (*Citrus aurantium*), 96
    garlic (*allium sativum*), 93
    ginger (*Zingiber officinale*), 93–94
    green tea (EGCG), 94
    hydroxycitric acid (Garcinia), 97
    quercetin, 97
    resveratrol, 97–98
    tapioca, 98
    tart cherry/sour cherry (*Prunus cerasus*), 96
    watermelon (*Citrullus vulgaris/lanatus*),
        95–96

Ergogenic herbs
  biochemical tuning and, 99
  Cordyceps sinensis, 92
  Eleutherococcus senticosus, 89–90
  Eurycoma longifolia, 89
  Panax ginseng, 88–89
  Paullinia cupana, 90
  Rhodiola rosea, 91
  Schisandra chinensis, 91
  Withania somnifera, 90–91
Erythropoietin (EPO), 199
Escape from Alcatraz Triathlon, 5
ESPN, 347
Essential amino acids (EAA), 81, 162
Estimated average requirement (EAR), 83
Eurycoma longifolia, 89
Even pacing, 18, 20
Event medicine, 7
EVS, *see* Elevated vacuum suspension
Excess post-exercise oxygen consumption
    (EPOC), 131
Excitation-contraction coupling fatigue and
    antioxidants, 211–212
Exercise-induced muscle damage (EIMD),
    321–322
  and antioxidants, 207–208
Exercise-induced oxidative stress behavior and
    antioxidants, 206–207
Expedition-length adventure races, 6, 7
Extreme endurance sports, 3–4; *see also*
    individual sports
  adventure races/multi-sport, 6
  cycling, 5
  health and medical support, 7
  running, 4
  swimming, 5
  training and nutrition, 7
  triathlon, 5
Extreme ironing, 271
Extreme sports; *see also individual sports*
  classification of, 241
    air, 241
    earth/land, 241
    eater, 241
    snow and ice, 241
  commercialization of, 347
  evolution and history of, 239–241
  food habits difference of millennials and, 247
    'fast food eater' tag avoiding, 248
    fast service, 248
    food with ethics, 247
    'healthy' definition, 247
  food and nutritional requirements
    combat sports, 254–255
    racing, 253–254
  food requirements for athletes for success in,
      251–253

future of, 256, 292–293, 349–350
growth of, 246–247
land-based, 246
  demographics of, 250
  popular markets for, 255
  reasons for growth/evolution of, 248–249
  top ten in USA, 250–251
market size for land-based, 246
meaning of, 239
performers of, 250
popular, 241–246
and regular sports compared, 249
  difference in athletes, 249
  requirements, 250
risks of, 256

FA, *see* Fatty acids
Fat considerations, 62, 77
  by ancient Greek athletes, 230
  for extreme sports athletes, 252, 253
Fatigue, 15, 22, 43, 58, 88
  carbohydrate, 61
  muscle, 25, 87
Fat loss, 132
Fat metabolism, 82, 92
Fat requirements for athletes, 82–83, 252
Fats and lipids, 82
Fatty acids (FA), 78, 82
FDA, *see* Food and Drug Administration
Fédération Internationale de Natation (FINA),
    15, 22
Female swimmers, 29
  energy intake requirements of, 24
Fiber, significance of, 252
FINA, *see* Fédération Internationale de Natation
FINA Grand Prix (2014), 54
FINA Marathon Swim World Series, 53
FINA Open Water, 51
FINA Open Water Grand Prix (2014), 29, 53
Fish oil (omega-3 fatty acids), 148
  benefits of, 268
  consumed by ancient Greek athletes, 232
  for extreme water sports athletes, 292
Flatland BMX, 243
Flavoenzymes, 83
Flavonoids, 97, 209
Fleet racing, 283
Flip and skateboarding, 242
Flowboarding, 290
Fluid, hydration, and micronutrient
    considerations, 62–64
Fluid loss, 44, 52
Fluid requirements, for athletes for success in
    extreme sports, 253
Fluid turnover, 303
Flyboarding, 291
FMX (freestyle motocross), 243–244

Foil boarding, 284
Folic acid (B9), 84
Food and Drug Administration (FDA), 145
Food and Nutrition Board, 305
Food and Nutrition Board of the National
    Academies of Sciences, Engineering,
    and Medicine, 297
France, 346
Free climbing, 245
Freeride kitesurfing, 285
Freestyle kitesurfing, 285
Freshwater cave diving, 272
Functional foods, 74–75; *see also* Gelatin
  bioenergetics (energy flow), 76–77
  caloric/energy needs evaluation for
    athletes, 77
  disadvantages of, 269–270
  endurance sports, 75–76
  ergogenic, and neutraceuticals, 93
    beetroot (*Beta vulgaris*), 94–95
    bitter orange (*Citrus aurantium*), 96
    garlic (*allium sativum*), 93
    ginger (*Zingiber officinale*), 93–94
    green tea (EGCG), 94
    hydroxycitric acid (Garcinia), 97
    quercetin, 97
    resveratrol, 97–98
    tapioca, 98
    tart cherry/sour cherry (*Prunus
      cerasus*), 96
    watermelon (*Citrullus vulgaris/
      lanatus*), 95–96
  ergogenic compounds, 85
    β alanine, 87–88
    β-Hydroxy-β-Methyl Butyrate (HMB), 87
    caffeine, 85–86
    carnitine, 87
    creatine, 86
    sodium bicarbonate/citrate, 87
    taurine, 86
  ergogenic drugs and agents, 85
  macronutrients
    carbohydrates, 79–80
    carbohydrates and proteins based on
      Rasmussen report, 81–82
    fat requirements for athletes, 82–83
    fats and lipids, 82
    proteins (amino acids), 80–81
  meaning of, 269
  micronutrients, 83
    vitamins, 83
  minerals (electrolytes), 84
    macrominerals, 84
    microminerals and trace elements, 85
  muscle metabolism, 78–79
  myth about lactic acid and muscle pain, 79
  nutritional aid

ephedrine (alkaloid), 92
  ergogenic herbs, 88–92, 99
  sports nutrition, 75
  total energy expenditure (TEE), 77–78
  total energy intake (TEI), 78
  types of, 269
  vitamins to improve athletic performance,
    83–84

Gait-adaptive knee, 118
Garlic (*allium sativum*), 93
Garcinia, *see* Hydroxycitric acid
GAS, *see* General Adaptation Syndrome
Gastrointestinal problems, 65
Gatorade®, 306
Gelatin, 311–312
  anaphylactic reaction and, 316–317
  application in sports nutrition and athletic
    performance, 317
  clinical trials in bone and joint diseases,
    315–316
  delivery modules and, 317
  economics and worldwide trend, 314
  human consumption, 313
  manufacturing, evolution of, 312–313
  uses in food and pharmaceutical industry,
    314–315
GelFilm™, 314
General Adaptation Syndrome (GAS), 127
GI, *see* Glycemic index
Ginger (*Zingiber officinale*), 93–94
Ginseng, 157–158
Giro d'Italia, 52
Gladiator games, in ancient Greece, 224
Glucosamine
  for ancient Greek athletes, 231
  for extreme sports athletes, 255
Glutamine, 88
  consumed by ancient Greek athletes, 232
  for extreme water sports athletes, 292
  for high altitude sports, 268
Glutathione, 209, 210
Glycemic index (GI), 80
Glycerol, 88
Glycogen, 80
  reserve, 78–79
Gorge walking, 272
Greece, 345
Greek Olympic sports, 220
  athletes and, training, 225
    doping, 226
    event location/map, 227
    gymnasiums and training, 227
    nutrition, 226
    self-control and discipline, 227
    skin care, 227
    sports, medicine, and education, 226

wounds, 226–227
ball games in, 223
categories description of, 221
chariot games in, 225
combat sports and food in, 231
comparison with modern athletes, 228–229
    diet comparison for normal people, 233
    athlete training comparison, 233–234
competitors/athletes in, 225
criteria for sportsperson and, 225
end of, 234
food and nutritional requirements
    in ancient Greece, 229–230
    dessert, 228
    diet, 227
    difference with current athletes, 228–229
    doping, 228
    drink/water, 228
    grain, 228
    meat, 228
gladiator games in, 224
history of, 220–221
modern athlete's food requirements and, 234
pentathlon and food in, 232
racing and food in, 230–231
team sports in, 223
transition to modern Olympic games,
    234–235
types of, 221–223
wild animal hunting in, 224
Green bone, 312
Green tea, 94
Grinds and skateboarding, 242
Growth hormones, 85
Guarana, 90
Guaranine, *see* Caffeine

HA, *see* Hydration Assessment Checklist
Hamilton, T., 194
Hang gliding, 240, 264
Harris and Benedict equation, 77
HCA, *see* Hydroxycitric acid
Head races, 286
Health and medical support, 7
Heart rate (HR), 21
Heat shock, 75
HEL, *see* Nᵉ-(hexanoyl) lysine
HelloFresh, 349
Herbal extracts
    consumed by ancient Greek athletes, 230, 232
    for extreme sports athletes, 253
    for extreme water sports athletes, 292
High-intensity power exercise tests, 148
High-intensity prolonged swimming, 27
High-lining, 263
High-protein diets, significance of, 37
Histidine, 87

HMB, *see* β-Hydroxy-β-Methyl Butyrate
Homeopathy, 268
Hooks, for bicycling, 120
'Horse with rider' game, 223
HPG, *see* Hypothalamic-pituitary-gonadal axis
HR, *see* Heart rate
Hydration, 39, 137
Hydration Assessment (HA) Checklist, 303
Hydrodynamic resistance, 13
Hydroxycitric acid (HCA), 97
Hyperglycaemia, 27
Hyper-hydration strategies, 63
Hyperinsulinaemia, 27
Hyperspectral imaging, 116, 122
Hypobaric hypoxia, 137
Hypohydration, 39, 302
Hyponatremia, 63, 84
Hypothalamic-pituitary-gonadal (HPG) axis,
    196, 197
Hypothermia, 22–23

Ice canoeing, 239
Ice climbing, 262, 271
Ice swimming, 272
Iditarod Invitational in Alaska, 52
Indian ginseng, *see* Ashwagandha
Indirect calorimetry, 131
InformedChoice.org, 146, 163
Injuries, prosthesis-related
    common injuries for all amputation levels,
        121
    residual limb injuries, 121
Inline skating, 241, 244
In-Socket Digital Data Recorder (ISDDR), 117
Institute of Medicine (IOM), 297, 298, 301
Insulin resistance, 82
Insulin sensitivity, impairment of, 208
International BMX Federation, 240
International Olympic Committee (IOC), 130
International Rafting Federation, 283
International Society of Sports Nutrition (ISSN),
    37, 41, 81, 151
    on caffeine effects on exercise
        performance, 41
    Position Stand on Nutrient Timing, 38
    Position Stand on Protein, 37
Intravenous fluids (IVF), 6
    fluid rule, 6
IOC, *see* International Olympic Committee
IOM, *see* Institute of Medicine
Ireland, 346
Iron, 85
Ironman Triathlon, 5, 7, 16, 51, 52
    testosterone impact on, 195
Iron requirement, for high altitude sports, 266
ISDDR, *see* In-Socket Digital Data Recorder
Isoleucine, 80

Isometric contractions, 321
ISSN, *see* International Society of Sports
        Nutrition
Italy, 345
IVF, *see* Intravenous fluids

Javelin throw, in Greek Olympic sports, 223
Jet skiing, 285, 291
Johnson, B., 193
Joint flexibility and muscle stiffness, 325–326
Jones, M., 193
Jordan, M., 220
Jungle Marathon, 51
Jungle Ultra, 4

Kayaking, 283, 290
    and canoeing compared, 282
Kazan World Championship, 18
Kickboxing, 39–40
Kimetto, D., 50
Kiteboarding, 289
Kite skiing, *see* Snow kiting
Kitesurfing, 240, 273, 285, 289
Kneeboarding, 284, 291
Knox NutraJoint™, 315

Lactate threshold (LT), 12
Lactic acid and muscle pain, 79
Lactobacillus-fermented milk, 208
La Furia Roja (Spain), 345
Land-based extreme sports, 246
    demographics of, 250
    popular markets for, 255
    reasons for growth/evolution of, 248–249
    top ten in USA, 250–251
Landis, F., 199
Landkiting, 245
Laser Doppler flowmetry (LDF), 123
Laser speckle imaging, 116, 122
LBM, *see* Lean body mass
LDF, *see* Laser Doppler flowmetry
Leadville Trail 100, 4
Leadville Trail 100 MTB, 5
Lean body mass (LBM), 75, 96
Leucine, 80, 87
Lignans, 89
Lilienthal, O., 240
LimbLogic Communicator™ (In-Socket Digital
    Data Recorder), 117
Lipolysis, 96
London Marathon (203), 50
London Olympics, 120
Longboarding, 242
Long-distance swimming races, 13, 22
Longer races, (OWS) (25 km and more), 28–29
Long jump, in Greek Olympic sports, 222
Lower limb, 118

LT, *see* Lactate threshold
L-theanine, 158
Luteinizing harmone (LH), 196, 198
Lysine, significance of, 252

Macrominerals, 84
Macronutrients
    carbohydrates, 79–80
    carbohydrates and proteins based on
        Rasmussen report, 81–82
    fat requirements for athletes, 82–83
    fats and lipids, 82
    proteins (amino acids), 80–81
Maddox, Richard Leach, 313
Magnesium, 84
    requirement, for high altitude sports, 266
    significance of, 252
Manganese, significance of, 252
Manhattan Island Marathon Swim, 12, 15, 21
MAPK, *see* Mitogen-activated protein kinase
Marathon, 4
Marathon des Sables, 4
Marathon-Swim Lake Zurich, 21
Marketing, of extreme sports, 342–343
    challenges with, 343
Match racing, 283
Maximum oxygen uptake ($VO_{2\,max}$), 12, 13, 61,
    86, 90, 95, 152
MCH, *see* Milk casein hydrolysate
Melatonin, 96
Mellouli, O., 15, 20
Merchandise sales, 343
Mexico, 346
Microminerals and trace elements, 85
Micronutrients, 83
    vitamins, 83
Milk casein hydrolysate (MCH), 208
Milo of Croton, 229
Minerals (electrolytes), 84
    consumed by ancient Greek athletes, 230, 231
    macrominerals, 84
    microminerals and trace elements, 85
Mitogen-activated protein kinase (MAPK),
    207, 212
Mixed martial arts (MMA), 43–44
MMA, *see* Mixed martial arts
Monoskiing, 262
Mono-unsaturated fatty acids (MUFA), 82
Monster™, 157
Motivation, behind extreme sports, 345–346
Motocross, 243
Moto Knee and versa Foot, 120
Mountain and high-altitude sports
    classification of, 261–264
    day to day activities for high intensity athletes
        in, 264–265
    evolution of, 260–261

food nutrients and impacts, 268–269
food, nutrition, and micronutrients for,
        265–267
mental strength importance for, 265
nutraceuticals and functional foods
        importance for, 269–270
physical requirement for, 268
places appropriate for, 270
    airborne/mid-air, 272–273
    mountainous terrain, 271
    water terrain at high altitude, 272
snow and ice and air sports and
    statistics, 273
vitamins and antioxidants requirements for,
        267–268
Mountain biking, 244
Mountainboarding, 242–243
Mountain Dew, 347
Mountaineering, 245
Mountainous terrain and high altitude sports, 271
MUFA, *see* Mono-unsaturated fatty acids
Multivitamin/mineral supplements (MVMs), 147
fish oil (omega-3 fatty acids), 148
protein supplements, 148
vitamin D3, 147
Murphy, Shane, 278
Muscle cramp, 75
Muscle glycogen stores, 25, 26
nutrition during race and, 27–28
    longer races, 28–29
    Olympic races, 28
    short races, 28
pre-race nutrition and, 26–27
Muscle metabolism, 78–79
Muscular endurance tests, 148–149

NAC, *see* N-acetylcysteine
N-acetylcysteine (NAC), 212
NADH, *see* Nicotinamide adenine dinucleotide
National Athletic Trainer's Association, 305
National Bicycle League, 240
National Research Council, 253
Negative pacing, 18
Nerve function, 328–329
The Netherlands, 346
New Zealand, 345
NF-κB, 207, 208, 211, 212
Niacin (B3), 83
Nickel requirement, for high altitude sports, 267
Nicotinamide adenine dinucleotide (NADH), 83
Nitrate, 88, 95
    beetroot juice, 155–156
Norepinephrine, 129, 135–136
Norseman Triathlon (Norway), 5
North Pole Marathon, 51
NSF International, 146, 163
Nutraceuticals, 348–349

Nutrient intake, of athletes, 178, 185
dietary pattern, 184
materials and methods
    dietary assessment, 178–179
    statistical analysis of results, 179
    studied population characteristics, 178
mineral compounds, 186–187
morphological and biochemical blood
        parameters, 180, 183–184, 187–188
results, 180, 183–184
    dietary assessment, 180, 181–182
Nutrition; *see also individual entries*
during competitions, 26
    pre-race nutrition, 26–27
    during race, 27–29
for recovery, 29
roles
    carbohydrate requirements, 25
    energy intake requirements, 24–25
    energy requirement estimation in 10 km
        race, 25–26
Nutritional aid
ephedrine (alkaloid), 92
ergogenic herbs, 88–92, 99
Nutritional requirement, for athletes, 49–50
adventure racing, 53
carbohydrate considerations, 57–60
cycling, 50, 52
energy considerations, 55, 57
fat considerations, 62
fluid, hydration, and micronutrient
        considerations, 62–64
physiological characteristics and, 55, 56
protein considerations, 60–62
running, 50
ski mountaineering, 54–55
supplement considerations, 64
swimming, 53–54
triathlon, 52–53
Nutritional requirements, in extreme sports,
        127–128
chrono-nutrition, 130, 134
general health, 129–130
macronutrients/micronutrients, 128
metabolic state, 128–129
nutritional considerations for extreme
        sports, 134
    cortisol, 135
    environment, 136–137
    epinephrine/norepinephrine, 135–136
    hydration, 137
    travel and food availability, 134–135
sport nutrition, 130
    goals, 132–134
    intensity/duration/volume, 130–131
    macronutrient adjustments, 131–132
N^ε-(hexanoyl) lysine (HEL), 207, 209

Octopamine, 96
Official competitions, performance analysis and
        pacing strategies during, 16–20
Offline marketing, 342–343
Ohio Willow Wood Company, 117, 122
Ollie and skateboarding, 242
Olympic Games, 53
    boxing, 36
    and extreme sports compared, 344
    open-water swimming (OWS), 15, 16, 18, 20
Olympic races (OWS) (10 km), 28
Omega-3 fatty acids, 148
    benefits of, 268
    consumed by ancient Greek athletes, 231
    for extreme sports athletes, 255
Online marketing, 342, 343
Opdycke, R. L., 20
Open-water swimming (OWS), 11–12, 282
    anthropometric characteristics and gender
            differences, 15–16
    endurance swimming energetics and
            biomechanics, 12–15
    nutrition during competitions, 26
        pre-race nutrition, 26–27
        during race, 27–29
    nutrition for recovery, 29
    nutrition roles
        carbohydrate requirements, 25
        energy intake requirements, 24–25
        energy requirement estimation in 10 km
            race, 25–26
    performance analysis and pacing strategies
            during official competitions, 16–20
    psychological aspects, 21–22
    risk factors, 22
    ultra-endurance races, 20
        Catalina Channel Swim, 21
        English Channel Swim, 20–21
        Manhattan Island Swim, 21
        Marathon-Swim Lake Zurich, 21
    water temperature and hypothermia, 22–24
Osmoregulation, 300
Outdoor diving, 282
Owens, J., 220
OWS, *see* Open-water swimming
Oxidative stress, exercise-induced, 206–207, 212

Pacing strategy, 18–20
Packrafting, 286
Paddle boarding/paddle sports, 286, 289
PAL, *see* Physical activity level
Panax ginseng, 88–89
Pankration, in Greek Olympic sports, 223
Parabolic-shaped pacing, 18
Paragliding, 263
Paralympics, 118, 256
Paris-Nice, 52

Park BMX, 243
Parkour, 245
Park riding, 285
Patrouille des Glaciers', 51, 54
Paullinia cupana, 90
PDCAA, *see* Protein Digestibility Corrected
        Amino Acid Score
Pentathlon
    food consumption by ancient Greek athletes
            for, 232
    in Greek Olympic sports, 222
Performance density, 17–18
Peripheral clocks, 130, 135
Peroxisome proliferator-activated
            receptor gamma coactivator-1 alpha
            (PGC-1α), 209
Personal floatation devices (PFD), 6
Peru, 346
Peruvian Maca, 200
PFD, *see* Personal floatation devices
PGC-1α, *see* Peroxisome proliferator-activated
            receptor gamma coactivator-1 alpha
Philippines, 346
Phospho-creatine, 151
Phosphorous, 84
Photoperiods, 130
Physical activity level (PAL), 78
Physical performance, dietary supplements to
            aid, 148–149
    beta-alanine, 152–153
    caffeine, 149–150
    creatine, 151–152
    nitrate (beetroot juice), 155–156
    sodium bicarbonate, 153–155
Pikes Peak Marathon, 51
Pinch Hitter, for baseball, 120
Pink-locking suspension system, 119
Pistorius, O., 120
Polish Food and Nutrition Institute, 178
Polyphenolic compounds, 96
Polyunsaturated fatty acids (PUFA), 82
Pomegranate juice, 98
POMS, *see* Profile of mood states
Pool diving, 282
Popularity, in different countries, 345–346
Pork skins, 312–313
Portugal, 346
Positive pacing, 18, 20
Post-exercise carbohydrate supplementation, 161
Post-exercise intervention (post-intervention), 331
Post-exercise meal, 81–82
Potassium, 84
    requirement, for high altitude sports, 265
Power Play, for hockey, 120
Pre-exercise intervention (prevention), 329–331
Pre-exercise meal, 58, 81
Pre-exercise snack, 81

Primal Quest (United States), 6
Proanthocyanidins, 98
Probiotics
    consumed by ancient Greek athletes, 232
    for extreme water sports athletes, 292
Profile of mood states (POMS), 22
Propelling efficiency, 13–14
Prosthetics, 115–118
    device function, 120–121
    in extreme sports, 120
        blades, 120
        Moto Knee and versa Foot, 120
        upper-limb prosthetics, 120
    related injuries
        common injuries for all amputation
            levels, 121
        residual limb injuries, 121
        residual limb health outcomes measurement,
            121–123
    socket systems, 118–119
    types, design, and materials, 118
Protein, 159–160
    for athletes for success in extreme sports,
        251, 254
    balance, 81
    considerations, 60–62, 77
    consumed by ancient Greek athletes, 231, 232
    for extreme water sports athletes, 291–292
    need, for extreme sports athletes, 251
    powder, 269
Protein Digestibility Corrected Amino Acid
    Score (PDCAA), 37
Proteins (amino acids), 80–81
Protein supplements, 148
PUFA, *see* Polyunsaturated fatty acids
Pyridoxine (B6), 84

QoL, *see* Quality of Life short form
Quality of Life short form (QoL), 316
Quassinoids, 89
Quercetin, 97, 209, 210
Quinoa, 251–252

Race Across America, 5, 51, 52
Racing
    food and nutritional requirements for, 253
    food consumption by ancient Greek athletes
        for, 230–231
Radcliffe, P., 50
Rafting, 283
RAGBRAI, 5
Raid Gauloises (New Zealand), 6
Range of motion (ROM), 323, 325–326, 332
Rating of perceived exertion (RPE), 22
RBC, *see* Red blood cell
RBE, *see* Repeated Bout Effect
RDA, *see* Recommended daily allowance

Reactive oxygen species (ROS), 205, 206, 208,
    210, 211
    -induced defense system, 212
Recommended daily allowance (RDA), 83
Recommended daily intake (RDI), 147
Red blood cell (RBC), 84
Regular diving, 281–282
Rehydration, 84, 98
    techniques, 304–307
'Repeated Bout Effect (RBE)', 330–331
Repeated sprint tests, 149
RER, *see* Respiratory exchange ratio
Residual limb health outcomes measurement,
    121–123
Residual limb injuries, 121
Respiratory exchange ratio (RER), 94, 132
Resting metabolic rate (RMR), 77
Resveratrol, 97–98, 211
Rhodiola rosea, 91, 157
Riboflavin (B2), 83
    significance of, 252
Rio Olympic race, 18, 25
RMR, *see* Resting metabolic rate
Rock climbing, 245
Roman games, 223–225
ROS, Reactive oxygen species (ROS)
Rottnest Channel Swim (Western Australia), 23
Rowing, 286
RPE, *see* Rating of perceived exertion
Rules of travel, 6
Running, 4
    nutritional requirement and, 50
Running/foot race, in Greek Olympic sports, 222
Running-based Anaerobic Sprint Test, 151
Ryanodine receptor, 211–212

Sailing, 283
Sandboarding, 242
Saponins, 89
Sarcoplasmic reticulum (SR), 211
    calcium-dependent ATPase (SERCA), 211
Schisandra *chinensis*, 91
Schultz, M., 120
Scuba diving, 290
Sculling, 286
SDH, *see* Succinate dehydrogenase enzyme
Sea jousting, 286–287
Search engine optimization, 343
Seattle to Portland (STP), 5
SEC, *see* Surface electrical capacitance
Selenium requirement, for high altitude sports, 267
Selye, H., 127
Sesamin, 89
Sheltered position, in swimming, 20
Shivering, 22
Short-distance swimming races, 13
Short races (OWS) (5 km or less), 28

Side by side rowing, 286
Silicone gel probe holder, 123
Singapore, 346
Skateboarding, 240, 242
Skeletal muscle damage and recovery, from
        eccentric contractions, 321–322
    damage
        blood proteins (creatine kinase and
            myoglobin), 327–328
        delayed-onset muscle soreness (DOMS),
            324–325, 332
        joint flexibility and muscle stiffness,
            325–326
        muscle function, 322–324
        nerve function, 328–329
        swelling and edema, 326–327
    post-exercise intervention (post-
        intervention), 331
    pre-exercise intervention (prevention),
        329–331
Skiff racing, 283
Skiing, 239, 262
Skimboarding, 284, 291
Ski mountaineering, nutritional requirement
        and, 54–55
Skin hydration, 116
Skin oxygen saturation, 116
Skin perfusion, 116, 122
Sky diving, 263, 273
SL, see Stroke length
Slacklining, 244
    at high altitude, 271
Snickers, 347
Snowblading, 261
Snowboarding/snurfing, 240, 261
Snow kiting, 262
Snowmobiling, 262, 271
Socket fitting process, 116
Socket systems, 118–119
Sodium bicarbonate, 153–155
Sodium bicarbonate/citrate, 87
Sodium requirement, for high altitude sports, 265
Solo-swims, 5
Sony, 347
Spain, 345
Spartan Race, 252, 279, 347–348
Speed racing, 285
Sport nutrition, 75, 130
    goals, 132–134
    intensity/duration/volume, 130–131
    macronutrient adjustments, 131–132
Sports supplements
    Beta-alanine, 42–43
    caffeine, 41–42
    creatine, 40–41
SR, see Sarcoplasmic reticulum
Stake races, 286

Stand-up surfing, 284
STP, see Seattle to Portland
Street BMX, 243
Strength tests, 148
Stroke length (SL), 14–15
Stroke rate, 15
Succinate dehydrogenase (SDH) enzyme, 93
Surface electrical capacitance (SEC), 116, 122
Surfing, 239, 284, 288
Surf matting, 284
Sweat loss, 84
Sweep rowing, 286
Swelling and edema, 326–327
Swimming, 5
    nutritional requirement and, 53–54
Synchronized diving, 281
Synchronized swimming, 282
Synephrine, 96
Syringaresinol, 89

Tachycardia, 22
Taco Bell, 347
Tapioca, 98
Tart cherry/sour cherry (*Prunus cerasus*), 96
    juice, 269
Taurine, 85, 86
TCA, see Tricarboxylic acid cycle
TCOM, see Temperature, transcutaneous oxygen
        measurement
Team racing, 283
Team sports, in ancient Greece, 223
TEE, see Total energy expenditure
Tegaderm™, 123
TEI, see Total energy intake
Temperature, transcutaneous oxygen
        measurement (TCOM), 123
Terpenoids (quassinoids), 89
Testosterone, 90, 193–194
    androgen response
        to acute extreme endurance exercise and,
            194–196
        to prolonged extreme endurance training,
            197–199
        to ultra-endurance exercise in extreme
            conditions, 196–197
    nutritional strategies, functional foods, and
        dietary supplements for androgen
        augmentation, 200
    as performance enhancing drug (PED) in
        extreme endurance sport, 199
TEWL, see Transepidermal water loss
TG, see Triglyceride
Thailand, 345
Theacrine, 158
Theobromine, 90
Theodosius I, 234, 235
Theophylline, 90

Thermogenesis, 77
Thiamine, 83
Ticket sales/free giveaway/scratch and get code, 343
Time-to-exhaustion tests, 149
Tissue injury, 119
Total energy expenditure (TEE), 77–78
Total energy intake (TEI), 77, 78
Tough Mudder race, 252, 347–348
Tour de France, 52, 55
Training and nutrition, 7
Transcontinental Race in Europe, 5
Transepidermal water loss (TEWL), 116, 122, 123
Trans Pyr, 52
Transtibial amputation, 118
Triathlon, 5
    nutritional requirement and, 52–53
Tribulus terrestris (*TT*), 200
Tricarboxylic acid (TCA) cycle, 78, 83
Triglyceride (TG), 82
'Triple Crown of Open Water Swimming', 12, 16
TT, *see Tribulus terrestris*
Tubing, 287

UGT, *see* Uridine diphospho-glucuronosyl transferases
Ultra-distance cycling, 5, 193
Ultradistance swimming, 5
Ultra-endurance exercise, 195
Ultra-endurance races, 12, 20, 22
    Catalina Channel Swim, 21
    English Channel Swim, 20–21
    Manhattan Island Swim, 21
    Marathon-Swim Lake Zurich, 21
Ultra-endurance triathlons, energy considerations in, 55
Ultra-events, 50
Ultramarathons, 4, 193
    testosterone levels impact on, 194–196
Underwater games, 284–285
United Kingdom, 346
United States, 345
United States Parachuting Company (USPA), 263
Unsaturated fatty acids, 82
Upper-limb prosthetics, 120
Uridine diphospho-glucuronosyl transferases (UGT), 200
USA Swimming, 53
USP, 146
USPA, *see* United States Parachuting Company

$VO_{2\,max}$, *see* Maximal oxygen uptake
Vacuum suspension, *see* Elevated vacuum suspension
Valine, 80

Vanadium requirement, for high altitude sports, 267
Van Rouwendaal, S., 15
Variable pacing, 18
Vegans, 148
Viau system, for swimming, 120
Videos/ads, during advertising breaks, 343
Visa, 347
Vitamin C, 212
    for high altitude sports, 267
Vitamin D3, 147
Vitamin E, 211, 212
    for high altitude sports, 267
Vitamins
    consumed by ancient Greek athletes, 232
    to improve athletic performance, 83–84
Vuelta a Espana cycling, 52, 195

WADA, *see* World Anti-Doping Agency
Wakeboarding, 287, 289
Wakeskate kitesurfing, 285
Wakestyle kitesurfing, 285
Water/hydration, 297–298
    biochemical and physiological functions of, 298–299
    fluid intake and replacement and, 307–308
    measurement and, 303–304
    optimal health and, 300–301
    rehydration techniques and, 304–307
    salient beneficial features of, 299
    status, and athletic performance, 301–302
    thirst and, 299–300
Water aerobics, 287
Water ball, 287
Water basketball, 287
Watermelon (*Citrullus vulgaris/lanatus*), 95–96
Water motor sports, 287
Water polo, 282
Water skiing, 287–288
Water sports, extreme
    based on difficulty, 279
    based on elements, 278
    based on location, 279
    based on risk, 278–279
    definition of, 279
    evolution of, 280–281
    food and nutritional requirements for, 291–292
    future of, 292–293
    meaning of, 278
    types of, 280–291
Water temperature and hypothermia, 22–24
Water terrain at high altitude, 272
Waveriding kitesurfing, 283, 285
Webb, Matthew, 11
Weertman, F., 15
Western diet, 129–130

Western Ontario and McMaster Universities
　　Osteoarthritis Index (WOMAC), 316
Western States Endurance Run (WSER), 4, 196
Wheat, 228
White water rafting, 272, 290–291
Wild animal hunting, in ancient Greece, 224
Wildflower Triathlon (California), 5
Wilimovsky, J., 15
Windsurfing, 240, 285, 289
Wing suiting, 263
Withania somnifera, 90–91
WOMAC, *see* Western Ontario and McMaster
　　Universities Osteoarthritis Index

World Anti-Doping Agency (WADA), 86, 145,
　　200
Wrestling, in Greek Olympic sports, 221–222
WSER, *see* Western States Endurance Run

X Games, 347

Yachting, 283
Young, G., 21

Zinc requirement, for high altitude sports, 266
Zip-lining, at high altitude, 271
Zorbing, 245–246, 271

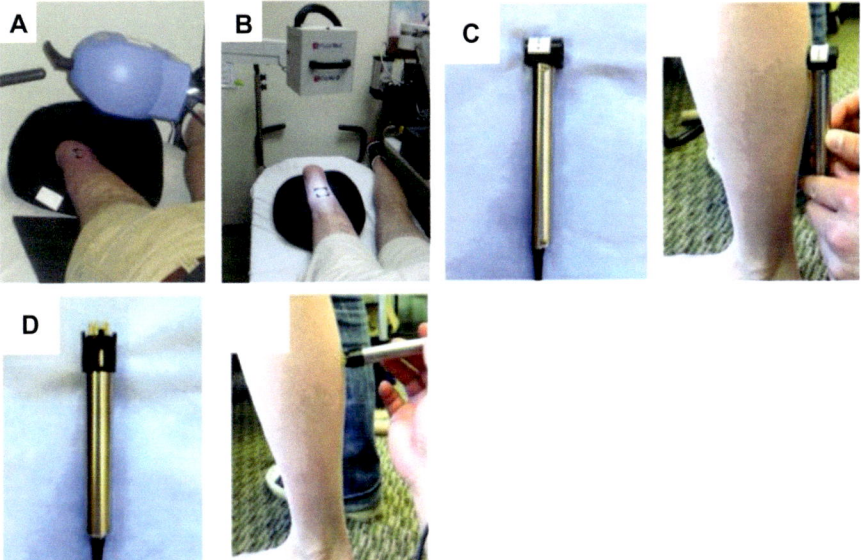

FIGURE 6.1 Non-invasive imaging to monitor residual skin health. **A.** Laser speckle imaging (LSI) for skin perfusion. **B.** Hyperspectral imaging for skin oxygen saturation. **C.** Transepidermal water loss (TEWL) for skin barrier function. **D.** Surface electrical capacitance for skin hydration. (Reprinted with permission from Rink CL, et al. Standardized approach to quantitatively measure residual limb skin health in individuals with lower-limb amputation. (New York, Mary Ann Liebert, 2017), 225–232).

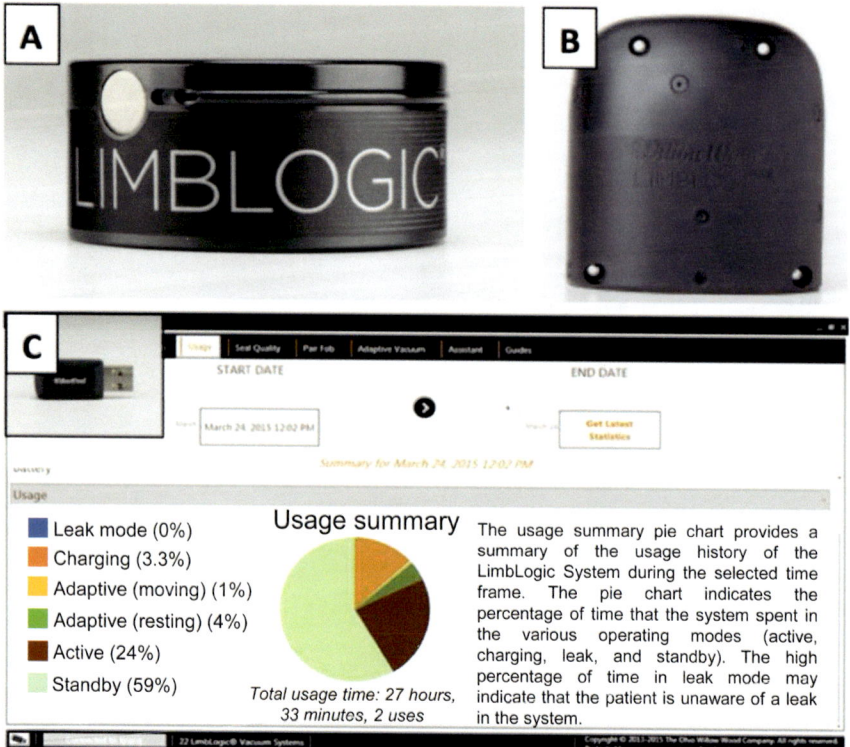

FIGURE 6.2 The ISDDR Platform. ISDDR is a commercially available Willow Wood technology enabling real-time, in-socket recording of patient- centric data. The device consists of two components: **A.** and **B.** a controller, and **C.** a communicator. The controller consists of a **A.** distal or **B.** side-mounted housing that contains a six-axis accelerometer along with a vacuum pressure sensor capable of resolving global changes in the socket pressure waveform that correlate with in-socket motion and prosthesis fit. Using the communicator **C.** quantitative data related to socket motion and prosthesis usage can be transferred to a workstation in order to provide relevant patient centric data to both the user and clinician about prosthesis performance.

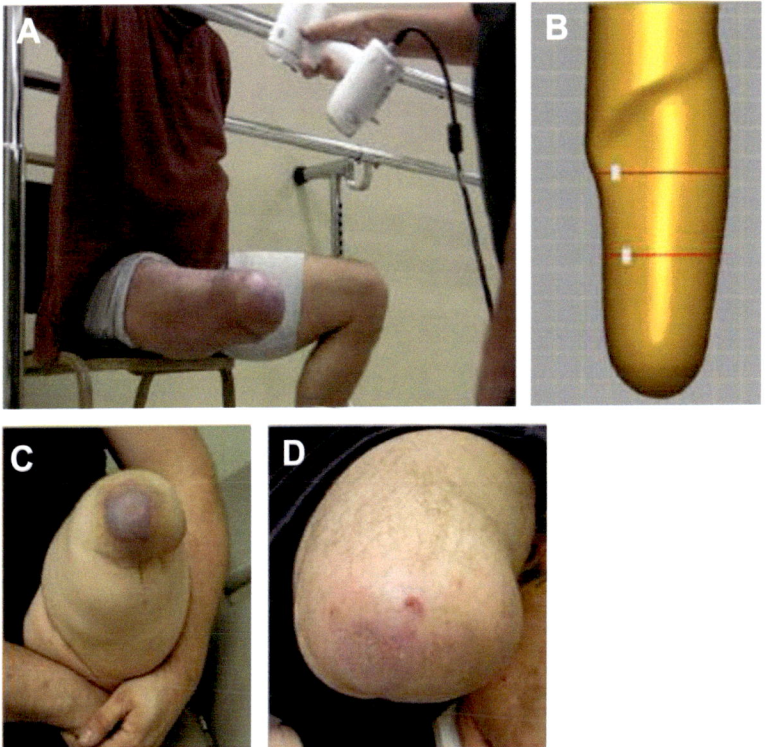

FIGURE 6.3 **A.** Prosthetists use a scanning device to digitize limb shape. **B.** Digital model is modified to create a positive mold for socket fabrication tailored to the residual limb. **C.** Tissue injury as a result of using a pink-locking suspension system. **D.** Injury healed once the amputee was fit and began wearing an elevated vacuum suspension socket (EVS).

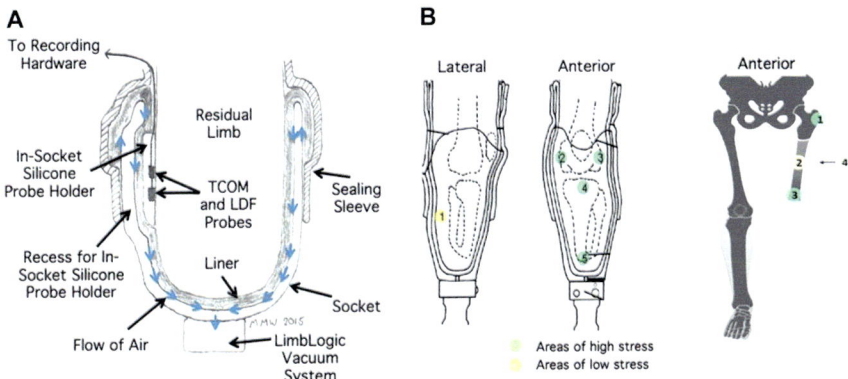

FIGURE 6.4 Elevated vacuum suspension schematic and probe measurement points. **A.** Illustration of test socket with recess for in-socket silicone probe holder. **B.** Residual-limb measurement sites. Green and yellow indicate measurement sites of high and low stress, respectively. LDF = laser Doppler flowmetry, TCOM = transcutaneous oxygen measurement. (Reprinted with permission from *Rink C, et al. Elevated vacuum suspension preserves residual-limb skin health in people with lower-limb amputation: Randomized clinical trial.* (California, PLOS, 2016), 1121–32) *JRRD is now PLOS Veterans Disability & Rehabilitation Research Channel.*

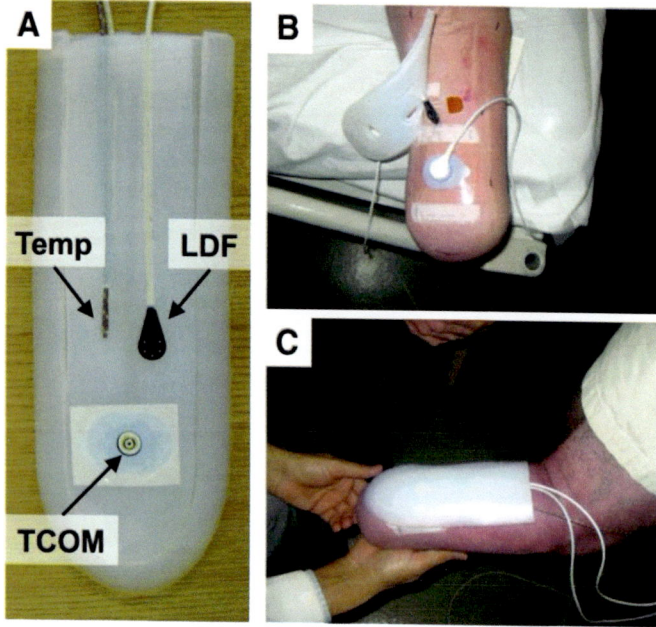

FIGURE 6.5 Silicone gel probe holder for in-liner measurement. **A.** Temperature, transcutaneous oxygen measurement (TCOM) and laser Doppler flowmetry (LDF) probes were embedded in a silicone gel insert to enable real-time measurement of limb temperature, oxygenation, and perfusion respectively. **B.** Placement of probes on residual limb of trans- tibial participant. Oxygen permeable Tegaderm™ was used to adhere the TCOM probe to the limb. **C.** The silicone gel insert enabled reproducible placement and spacing of probes and buffered against the liner from pressing probes tightly against skin. (Reprinted with permission from Rink CL, et al. Standardized approach to quantitatively measure residual limb skin health in individuals with lower limb amputation. (New York, Mary Ann Liebert, 2017), 225–32).

Specific Pre/Mid/Post Nutrition Strategy

Strength	Conditioning	Strength & Cond.
1:1 CHO/Pro	3:1 CHO/Pro	2:1 CHO/Pro
0.25g/lb CHO 0.25 g/lb Pro	0.75g/lb CHO 0.25 g/lb Pro	0.50g/lb CHO 0.25 g/lb Pro
Example: 175 lb 44g CHO 44g Pro	Example: 175 lb 135g CHO 44g Pro	Example: 175 lb 88g CHO 44g Pro